Stillbirth: Prediction, Prevention and Management

Stillbirth: Prediction, Prevention and Management

EDITED BY

Catherine Y. Spong MD

Bethesda, MD, USA

WILEY-BLACKWELL

A John Wiley & Sons, Ltd., Publication

Library of Congress Cataloging-in-Publication Data

Spong, Catherine Y.
Stillbirth : prediction, prevention, and management / edited by Catherine Y. Spong.
     p. ; cm.
   Includes bibliographical references and index.
   ISBN 978-1-4443-3706-8 (hardcover : alk. paper) 1. Stillbirth. I. Title.
   [DNLM: 1. Stillbirth. 2. Pregnancy Complications—etiology. 3. Pregnancy Complications—prevention & control. WQ 225]
     RG631.S66 2011
     618.3′92—dc22

2010047408

A catalogue record for this book is available from the British Library.

This book is published in the following electronic formats: ePDF 9781444398014; Wiley Online Library 9781444398038; ePub 9781444398021

Set in 9/12 Meridien Roman by MPS Limited, a Macmillan Company, Chennai, India

Printed and bound in Malaysia by Vivar Printing Sdn Bhd

1   2011

Contents

List of Contributors

Hannah Blencowe
London School of Hygiene and Tropical Medicine,
London, UK

Janice L.B. Byrne MD
Division of Maternal-Fetal Medicine,
Department of Obstetrics and Gynecology, Division of Medical Genetics, Department of Pediatrics,
University of Utah Health Sciences Center,
Salt Lake City, UT, USA

Joanne Cacciatore PhD, FT, LMSW
Center for Loss and Trauma,
Arizona State University,
Phoenix, AZ, USA

Deborah L. Conway MD
Department of Obstetrics and Gynecology,
Division of Maternal-Fetal Medicine,
University of Texas School of Medicine at San Antonio,
San Antonio, TX, USA

Simon Cousens
London School of Hygiene and Tropical Medicine,
London, UK

Michael L. Draper MD
Division of Maternal-Fetal Medicine,
Department of Obstetrics and Gynecology,
University of Utah Health Sciences Center,
Salt Lake City, UT, USA

Donald J. Dudley MD
Department of Obstetrics and Gynecology,
University of Texas Health Science Center at San Antonio,
TX, USA

Fabio Facchinetti
Mother-Infant Department,
Unit of Obstetrics and Gynecology,
University of Modena and Reggio Emilia,
Modena, Italy

Ruth Fretts MD, MPH
Harvard Vanguard Medical Associates,
Wellesley,
MA, USA

Jason Gardosi MD, FRCOG
West Midlands Perinatal Institute,
Birmingham, UK

Robert L. Goldenberg MD
Department of Obstetrics and Gynecology,
Drexel University College of Medicine,
Philadelphia, PA, USA

Joy E. Lawn
Saving Newborn Lives/Save the Children-US,
Cape Town,
South Africa
Health Systems Research Unit,
Medical Research Council,
South Africa
Institute of Child Health,
London, UK

Elizabeth M. McClure MEd
Department of Statistics and Epidemiology,
RTI International,
Research Triangle Park, NC, USA

Francesca Monari
Mother-Infant Department,
Unit of Obstetrics and Gynecology,
University of Modena and Reggio Emilia,
Modena, Italy

Robert Pattinson
International Stillbirth Association Scientific Board,
Medical Research Council, University of Pretoria,
Pretoria, South Africa

Uma M. Reddy MD, MPH
Eunice Kennedy Shriver National Institute of Child Health and Human Development, National Institutes of Health,
Bethesda, MD, USA

Raymond W. Redline MD
Department of Pathology and Reproductive Biology,
Case Western Reserve University School of Medicine,
Cleveland, OH, USA
Department of Pediatric and Perinatal Pathology,
University Hospitals Case Medical Center,
Cleveland, OH, USA

Carol J. Rowland Hogue PhD, MPH
Women's and Children's Center,
Department of Epidemiology,
Rollins School of Public Health, Emory University,
Atlanta, GA, USA

George Saade MD
Division of Maternal Fetal Medicine,
Department of Obstetrics and Gynecology,
University of Texas Medical Branch,
Galveston, TX, USA

Robert M. Silver MD
Division of Maternal-Fetal Medicine,
Department of Obstetrics and Gynecology,

University of Utah Health Sciences
Center,
Salt Lake City, UT, USA

Cynthia Stanton
Johns Hopkins Bloomberg School of
Public Health,
Baltimore,
MA, USA

Michael Varner MD
Division of Maternal-Fetal Medicine,
Department of Obstetrics and Gynecology,
University of Utah Health Sciences Center,
Salt Lake City, UT, USA

Ronald Wapner MD
Division of Maternal Fetal Medicine,
Department of Obstetrics and Gynecology,

Columbia University,
College of Physicians and Surgeons,
New York, NY, USA

Marian Willinger PhD
Eunice Kennedy Shriver National Institute
of Child Health and Human Development,
National Institutes of Health,
Bethesda, MD, USA

Preface

Stillbirth is a tragic event, affecting not only the mother and father, but also their families, health care team, and community. The loss is felt immediately and persists long term, including during subsequent pregnancies. Stillbirth affects 1 in 200 pregnancies, accounting for more deaths than those due to preterm birth and sudden infant death syndrome (SIDS) combined. Despite this, no single resource for the caregiver has been available. Stillbirth has been neglected far too long. Recently, there has been a welcome surge of interest in investigating stillbirth and its causes, and this momentum has generated sufficient evidence to deserve a comprehensive assessment in a book format. This book has been crafted to fill the void as a single resource for caregivers, addressing the academic issues, psychological effects, and practical clinical management.

I would like to thank the many patients and their families who have shared their experiences with me. Their stories and the interest of other clinicians demonstrated the need for this book. Much gratitude to my colleagues and friends who wrote chapters—their expertise and passion for this topic are unparalleled. I must also thank my family for giving me the time to devote to this work and my parents and sister for their encouragement.

I hope that this contribution will assist multispecialty providers when caring for women with a stillbirth, both immediately and in subsequent pregnancies. I welcome comments on this edition (positive and negative) as I strive to improve it for the future.

Catherine Y. Spong
Bethesda, MD

PART I
Epidemiology and Scope of the Problem

CHAPTER 1

High Income Countries

Ruth Fretts, MD, MPH
Harvard Vanguard Medical Associates, Wellesley, MA, USA

Stillbirth and the definition "problem"

One of the difficulties in the study of stillbirth is that stillbirths are universally undercounted especially at lower ages of gestation. What constitutes a "stillbirth" varies considerably between countries, and while a universal definition has been desired, it is unlikely that a globally accepted definition will be agreed upon. The lower gestational age limit that divides a "miscarriage" from a "stillbirth" depends if a country has resources to collect information and if the intention of the data collection is to count the deaths that could possibly have "survived." In the United Kingdom, reporting of deaths begins at 24 weeks (presumably because the mortality of those born prior to 24 is so high); in most developing countries there is very little data about losses prior to 28 weeks of gestation.

The term fetal death, fetal demise, stillbirth, and stillborn all refer to the delivery of a fetus showing no signs of life. The World Health Organization (WHO) defines stillbirth as a "fetal death late in pregnancy" and allows each country to define the gestational age at which a fetal death is considered a stillbirth for reporting purposes [1]. A moderate proportion of countries have extrapolated from the WHO's definition of what constitutes the "perinatal period" to define stillbirth ($\geqslant 500\,g$, or if the weight is not known, with a gestational age greater than 22 completed weeks (154 days)). But even among developed countries the gestational age at which fetal losses are reported ranges from 16 weeks (The Netherlands) to 28 weeks (Sweden) [2]. Sweden recently revised their reporting laws because of pressures from parental advocacy groups and increasing numbers of live-born infants born prior to 28 weeks, but the stillborn counterparts were not included in national statistics. Other factors that influence the reported stillbirth rate are the accuracy of gestational age dating; whether obstetric providers are accurately educated on the definition of a "liveborn" or "stillborn"; if terminations of pregnancy for lethal or sublethal anomalies are specifically excluded; and if the inevitable previable spontaneous losses that results in a stillborn had labor augmented are included.

Within the United States, terminations of pregnancy for anomalies and augmented previable losses are specifically excluded from the stillbirth statistics but misclassification of these losses is common. Duke et al. compared fetal death reports to the reports generated from the active birth defects surveillance program in the Atlanta area. They found that 13% of fetal deaths should have been excluded from the fetal death statistics because the losses involved induction or augmentation of labor [3]. It is probable that providers recognize the intention of parents (the strong desire to have had a viable healthy pregnancy) and may fill out a fetal death report rather than report the loss as a termination of pregnancy or abortion.

In the United States, because the definition of stillbirth is determined by each state, there are significant variations which can substantially

Stillbirth: Prediction, Prevention and Management, First Edition. Catherine Y. Spong.
© 2011 Blackwell Publishing Ltd. Published 2011 by Blackwell Publishing Ltd.

change the reported stillbirth rate by as much as 50% [4]. National reporting uses 20 weeks of gestation or 350 g if the gestational age is not known. The standardized definition for fetal mortality used by the U.S. National Center for Health Statistics (NCHS) is similar to the WHO definition but adds that a stillbirth must have "the absence of breathing, heart beats, pulsation of the umbilical cord, or definite movements of voluntary muscles" [5]. As advances in obstetrics occur both the neonatal and stillbirth rates decrease but the stillbirths less so, leaving stillbirth the largest contributor to perinatal mortality [6].

Scope of the problem

Compared to other health outcomes and the disease burden, the scope of stillbirth has been overlooked by many, including those who have the opportunity to prioritize spending for research and ultimately to devise and implement prevention strategies. In the United States, the chances that a pregnancy will end as a stillbirth is about 1/200 for white women and 1/87 for black women [7]. Stillbirth occurs more often than deaths due to AIDS and viral hepatitis combined; stillbirth is 10 times more common than sudden infant death syndrome, nearly 5 times more common than infant deaths related to congenital anomalies, and 5 times more often than postnatal deaths due to prematurity [8].

There are many downstream consequences of stillbirth, the most significant and long lasting being experienced by mothers. Women who experience stillbirth are at an increased risk of multiple maladies including depression, anxiety and posttraumatic stress disorder, somatization disorder, and family disorganization [9] (see Chapter 13).

The reason that the scope of the problem has been overlooked is multifactorial. Many people still consider stillbirths as "God's Will" and that death before birth counts less than those after, but for many parents a stillbirth represents loss of chance and a family member. Until recently goals for the reduction of stillbirth were not included

as an important health indicator, yet stillbirths are a measurable "tip of the iceberg." Stillbirth rates reflect a woman's preconceptual health and nutrition status, her access to good care including contraception, first-trimester care, screening for infectious diseases and congenital anomalies, disease identification and management, and adequate care during labor which includes fetal monitoring, timely access to cesarean section and IV antibiotics.

Trends in stillbirth rates

The study of stillbirth trends in historical cohorts and among developing countries identifies factors that affect stillbirth rates and are therefore most amenable to change. Countries where longitudinal data on stillbirths are kept (Denmark, Sweden, Norway, England, and Wales among others), many stillbirth rates remained relatively stable from the 1900s until the early 1940s [10]. After this time period there began a significant decline which continued but then leveled out in the mid-1980s (Figure 1.1) [10]. Interestingly, the increasing focus on the study of stillbirth in the United Kingdom was thought to be a reflection on the decline of the fertility rate; J.A. Ryle, Professor of Social Medicine at Oxford, wrote in 1949 that there was a need to reduce stillbirths as they were a "wastage of human life" and "as a matter of national accountancy we can no longer afford to lose so many potential citizens" [10].

Vallgarda reviewed the characteristics of stillbirths that were 32 weeks of gestation or greater in Denmark from 1938 to 1947 and found that during this time period, stillbirths were reduced from 24.9 to 16.3/1,000 births (a 35% reduction). This correlated with a reduction in the numbers of women having births at home (reduced from 50% to 35% of births). In addition, in 1945, Denmark introduced a law that provided free antepartum care, which was widely used by women (70% of women initially attended prenatal care and by the 1960s this had risen to almost 100%). The types of stillbirths most noted to have decreased were those

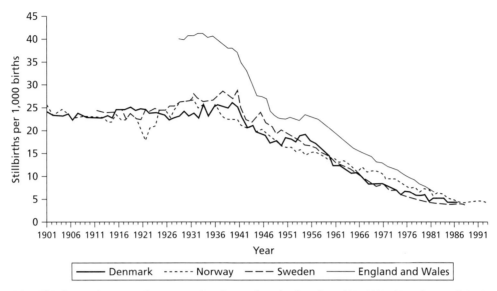

Figure 1.1 Stillbirth rates in Denmark, Norway, Sweden, and England/Wales, 1901–1990. (Data from Ref. [10].)

due to asphyxia in labor, malformations, bleeding, and disease of the mother [10].

Asphyxia in labor

In a Canadian hospital based study that evaluated specific causes of death of babies 20 weeks (or 500 g) or more over more than three decades, there were two causes of fetal death that were reduced by more than 95% (Figure 1.2) [11]. During the 1960s, intrapartum stillbirth was the third most common type of stillbirth (with those that were unexplained and related to growth restriction being more common). With the introduction of intrapartum monitoring and the availability of emergency cesarean section, the proportion of stillbirths that were due to asphyxia in labor dropped from 11% to 2% of total stillbirths with a rate of 0.2/1,000 births [11]. In general, intrapartum asphyxic deaths in term or near-term babies that occur more often than 1/1,000 births suggests a significant potential for improvements in quality of care in the labor and delivery unit [12, 13].

Rh iso-immunization

Stillbirth due to Rh iso-immunization has become a rare event in developed countries. In the same

Canadian dataset that tracked changes in stillbirth over time, the authors noted a 95% reduction of these deaths during the study period of the 1960s to the early 1980s [11]. Initially Rhogam administration was given after the birth of an Rh-positive baby, and this helped reduced Rh iso-immunization considerably, but when the 28-week administration was introduced in the 1970s, the number of stillbirths were reduced even further making this now a very rare cause of stillbirth (less than 1/10,000 births) (Figure 1.2).

Congenital anomalies

The third cause of death that was notably reduced were those related to malformations. The rates of perinatal deaths due to congenital anomalies varies significantly based on maternal nutrition, environmental exposures, resources in the health systems, varied policies on screening for congenital anomalies, and the availability of terminations of pregnancy [12–15]. Within 10 European population-based cohorts for the MOSAIC study, 85% of terminations after 22 weeks of gestation were for congenital anomalies with 50% of these occurring between 22 and 23 weeks of gestation

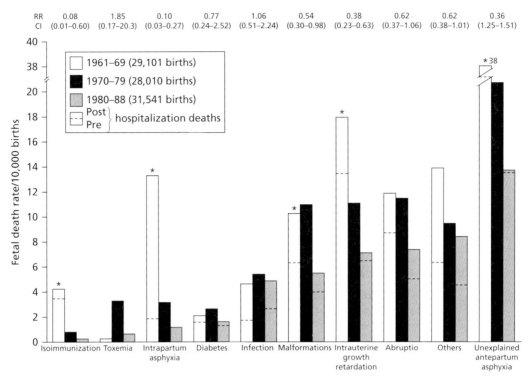

Figure 1.2 Specific causes of stillbirth during three decades in a Canadian hospital, both prior to and after hospitalization per 10,000 births. (Data from Ref. [11].)

and the rest later [15]. Exclusion of terminations of pregnancy reduced the reported stillbirth rate by half. Within the 10 European countries, the percent of stillbirths related to congenital anomalies varied significantly. In Poland where the policy for termination of pregnancies is quite restrictive, the proportion of stillbirths related to congenital anomalies was 34%, in the United Kingdom where the policies for terminations of pregnancy for congenital anomalies is more liberal, these deaths account for only 3.8% of stillbirths [14]. Obviously for parents a termination of pregnancy for congenital anomalies is a traumatic event, the pregnancy outcome however is not typically included in the stillbirth statistics [3, 14, 15].

Over the past 50 years in the United States there was an approximately 70% reduction of late losses (defined as 28 weeks or more), whereas there has been virtually no decrease in early losses (20–28 weeks), since the 1990s the decline has slowed with the number of early fetal deaths exceeding the number of late losses (Figure 1.3) [16]. Unfortunately, within the United States there has not been a large longitudinal study of the specific causes of stillbirth, but there is a large body of evidence which demonstrates that some types of stillbirths have been reduced when prevention strategies have been developed. A prerequisite to designing a prevention strategy however is a thorough stillbirth evaluation which is not routinely performed in the United States. The stillbirth evaluation includes placental and fetal pathology, selected laboratory evaluation, a narrative on what lead up to the diagnosis of stillbirth, including maternal medical and social risk factors, access to care, the quality of care (see Chapter 12–14).

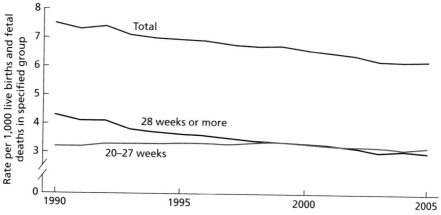

Figure 1.3 Fetal mortality rates by period of gestation: United States, 1990–2005. (Data from Ref. [4].)

Common causes of stillbirth

There has been considerable evolution on how the causes of stillbirth have been classified (see Chapter 3) and whether or not associated conditions are considered causes or risk factors for stillbirth. The severity of pathology whether it is within the placenta or in a disease state such as pregnancy-induced hypertension may be variably interpreted as a cause or as a contributor to the demise. There are notable differences in the types of stillbirth that occur at different gestational ages. Notwithstanding these issues, the most common types of still-birth remain those that are "unexplained." Again the proportion of those that are left unexplained depends on the rigorousness of the stillbirth evaluation. Unexplained losses are those pregnancies that have not been complicated by fetal, maternal, or placental conditions and occur in an appropriately grown baby without evidence of infection or antepartum bleeding [17, 18]. The second and third most common causes of stillbirth are both related to problems related to placental function, with the difference being rated to the acuity of the pathology. Babies that are severely growth restricted (without evidence of chromosomal anomalies or perinatal infection) die presumably due to placental dysfunction [19]. This process is gradual enough that the baby's growth falls off of the expected growth curve and eventually succumbs (see Chapter 7). The third most common cause of fetal death is related

to abruptio placenta. This is a more acute process, with the diagnosis made clinically in the setting where there is antepartum bleeding and premature separation of the placenta that is severe enough to cause a fetal demise.

Causes of stillbirth by gestational age

Spontaneous preterm losses from 20 to 24 weeks of gestation

This is one of the largest categories of loss that occur between 20 and 24 weeks. Reviews of these losses reveal an over-representation of black women, of multiple gestations, and a history of a pregnancy achieved using advanced reproductive technologies (Figure 1.4) [7, 20]. Depending on when a women presents for evaluation, she may be diagnosed with premature rupture of membranes, cervical incompetence, chorioamnionitis, antepartum bleeding with or without premature labor. While a fair number of women will also have a living fetus at the beginning of the birth process, very often the baby is born dead.

Stillbirths less than 28 weeks of gestation

Using the Canadian McGill Obstetrical and Neonatal Database, Fretts et al. evaluated the timing of specific causes of stillbirth. In their study,

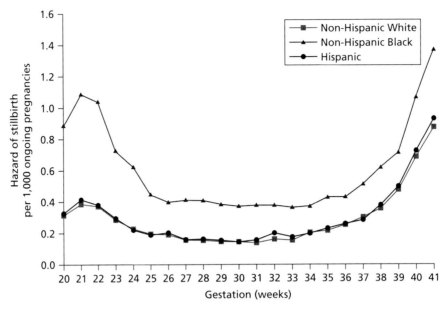

Figure 1.4 Fetal mortality rates by maternal age in singleton pregnancy and multiple pregnancies, 2005. (Data from Ref. [4].)

there was a 97% autopsy rate and a primary cause of death was assigned in the setting of a perinatal review committee [11]. In general, unless there was obvious and significant cord pathology so that a cord accident was the only logical explanation for stillbirth, those births that lose cord loops or knots noted were classified as unexplained.

These so-called "early fetal deaths" have been most difficult to influence with rates much unchanged over the past 30 years. The most common causes of death prior to 28 weeks of gestation include infection (19%), malformations (14%), abruptio placenta (14%), severe growth restriction (7%), and intrapartum asphyxia (7%). While for most of these deaths a cause of death can be assigned, about 20% were unexplained [11].

Stillbirths from 28 to 36 weeks
In the Canadian dataset between 28 and 36 weeks of gestation, unexplained stillbirths remained the most common type of demise (26%), the next most common type of stillbirth were those that occurred in babies with severe growth restriction

(19%), followed by abruptio placenta (18%), infection (8%), malformations (8%), and maternal disease (6%) [11].

Stillbirths at and beyond 37 weeks of gestation
At term, the proportion of unexplained stillbirths increased to 40%, 14% died from severe growth restriction, 13% resulted from abruptio placenta, 8% from maternal disease, 16% were "other causes" including umbilical cord abnormalities, nonimmune hydrops and vasa previa, and twin-to-twin transfusion [11].

Unexplained stillbirths

An "unexplained stillbirth" is the most common type of stillbirth and in some ways are the most troubling. Typically these tend to occur late in pregnancy [17, 18]. Because the unexplained stillbirth is a diagnosis of exclusion, it is subject to the thoroughness of the stillbirth evaluation.

Incomplete examinations will underestimate the role of infection, chromosomal and congenital anomalies. Some classification systems exclude fetal deaths that occurred in the very growth-restricted fetus (less than the 3rd percentile or the 10th percentile) from those that are categorized as "unexplained" while others do not [19].

Where good data exists, late pregnancy (after 36–37 weeks of gestation), advanced maternal age (OR 3.3–5.1), and obesity (OR 2–3) are all risk factors for these unexplained deaths [17, 18]. There are several theories on why these late stillbirth occur but none have been proven and it is likely that the mechanisms of death are heterogenous. The observation that these deaths occur more often in older women late in pregnancy suggests diminished placental function [21, 22] (Figure 1.5). One preventive strategy in this setting is consider these pregnancies "postdates" sooner and follow either with antepartum testing or induction of labor prior to the typical "postdate" period. Theoretically the optimal timing of delivery could be modified according to the patients risk factors for stillbirth; unfortunately there have been no randomized controlled trial evaluating the risks

and benefits of such approach that are powered to address stillbirth reduction. Nicholson et al. [23] did demonstrate that the strategy of the active management of risk while associated with a significantly elevated risk of induction of labor was not associated with an increased risk of cesarean section; they reported a lower risk of fetal adverse outcomes but this study was not powered to look at perinatal mortality.

Other researchers have evaluated the role of the inflammatory response in the unexplained stillbirth. In an ideal setting, if there is fetal hazard such as infection, lymphokines will initiate labor, thus "rescuing" the baby by birth. But the factors in the mother and the baby that are responsible for the initiation of labor are not well known. There are a proportion of late "explained" stillbirths that appear to be related to infection, but for some reason the mother's body did not mount the appropriate response to initiate labor prior to the baby's death [24].

The relationship between elevated blood pressure and stillbirth has been well described, but more recently some researchers have noted that relative hypotension may be a risk for stillbirth [25]. Warland et al. performed a matched case–control study of

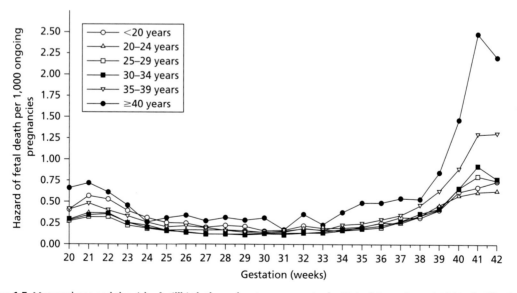

Figure 1.5 Maternal age and the risk of stillbirth throughout pregnancy in the United States hazard (risk) of stillbirth for singleton births without congenital anomalies by gestational age, 2001–2002. (Data from Ref. [22].)

124 women who had a stillbirth with 243 women who had a liveborn. Interestingly in their study, hypertension (systolic blood pressure of greater than or equal to 130 mmHg) was associated with a lower rate of stillbirth (RR 0.4, 95% CI 0.37–0.43), presumably this was due to increased pregnancy monitoring and appropriate induction. But they also found that women whose diastolic blood pressure fell in the borderline range 60–70 mmHg had an elevated risk over their normotensive controls (OR 1.8, 95% CI 1.1–3.0) [25]. While this relationship has not been a consistent finding in studies, it deserves further attention [26].

Placental dysfunction and fetal growth restriction

Approximately half of stillbirths have failed to reach their expected growth potential as measured by birthweight less than the 10th percentile (corrected for gestational age and parental characteristics) [27]. Preterm stillbirths are more likely to be small-for-gestational age and have other placental pathology such as abruptio placenta, although certainly growth restriction also occurs at term [12, 27]. The detection of growth restriction remains a major challenge since most stillbirths that are severely growth restricted were not recognized as growth restricted prior to the diagnosis of the stillbirth [13, 19]. When fetal growth restriction is detected antepartum and preterm, the overall perinatal mortality remains elevated because of the underlying placental pathology, the risk of iatrogenic preterm birth, and its related morbidity and mortality (see Chapter 7).

In the Confidential Enquiry of Stillbirths and Deaths in Infancy 2001, the most common finding in the review of stillbirths was the failure to detect fetal growth restriction; this was seen in 10% of stillbirths in their review. Other deficiencies of care involved the management for fetal growth restriction, the management of hypertension, deficiencies of the interpretation of fetal monitoring (3% for each), and the failure to adequately manage pregnancies complicated by decreased fetal movement [28].

Abruptio placenta

Premature separation of the placenta is the third most common cause of stillbirth. Fatal abruption is more common in the preterm fetus and is strongly associated with placental problems and inflammation [29]. The rates of abruption appear to be increasing in the United States and elsewhere. Maternal drug use is the strongest association among the maternal risk factors, but there are other important risk factors, such as smoking, hypertension, and preeclampsia. Cessation of smoking and drug use are important strategies, and past drug use should be gathered as part of the obstetric history [13]. Also, women who report second- and third-trimester bleeding need to be considered "high risk," and have appropriate fetal monitoring, including periodic assessments of fetal growth.

Infection

The rates of stillbirths due to infection in high resource settings have been relatively unchanged over the past number of decades (Figure 1.2), most of these have occurred in early stillbirths (20–28 weeks) [11]. A substantial proportion of these deaths are related to bacterial ascending infections with *Escherichia coli*, group B streptococci, and *Ureaplasma urealiticum* [30]. When viruses are looked for with polymerase chain reaction (PCR), a moderate number of stillbirths will have placental tissue that is positive for cytomegalovirus (CMV), herpes simplex virus (HSV), or Parvovirus 19. In a study of 96 stillbirths and 35 healthy full-term controls, 33% of stillbirths had positive placental evidence for viruses (16% CMV, 13% Parvovirus 19, 5% HSV), whereas only 6% of healthy controls had placental tissue that was positive. Findings at autopsy such as fetal hydrops and chronic villitis were strongly associated with positive PCR testing [31] (see Chapter 5).

Cord accidents

The study of cord accidents has been difficult because at the birth of a stillborn baby careful systematic evaluation of the cord is not usually carried out. We know that about one-third of live-born babies have one or more cords wrapped around his or her neck. With a live baby this is considered an incidental finding, but it is difficult to determine in the setting of a stillbirth if cord pathology is the *cause* of the death or an incidental finding. Because whether a stillbirth has been related to a cord accident is subjective, there has been considerable variation on the proportion of stillbirths that are attributed to stillbirth, but on average, 20% of stillbirths are attributed to cord accidents by physicians (see Chapter 10). Until we know more, it is important that when a still-born baby is delivered with the presence of a cord-related issue (cord loops, knots, torsion, knotting, or entanglement) a thorough evaluation of baby, mother, placenta, and cord be conducted in order to determine if there were other factors or conditions that could have contributed to the stillbirth. Some have recommended evaluation of the cord location by ultrasound after the diagnosis of still-birth is made so the number or cord loops can be assessed. Photographs taken just after are also useful because they can be viewed during a perinatal review and placed in context with other pathological findings. These would be important steps in the study of cord accidents and make this diagnosis more systematic and less subjective.

Multiple gestations

Over the past two decades, U.S. rates of twin pregnancies have more than doubled and higher-order multiples have increased 6- to 12-fold [20, 33]. The increasing number of multiples is due to increased use of assisted reproductive technologies and an increasing proportion of older mothers (Figure 1.6). The stillbirth rate among multiples is fourfold higher than singletons (19.6/100 vs. 4.7/1,000) [32]. The higher rates are due to both complications specific to multiple pregnancies (such as twin-to-twin transfusion syndrome) and increased risks of complications common to single-tons and multiples, in particular fetal abnormalities and growth restriction. Triplet or higher numbers of gestations are at high risk for multiple complications, including preterm birth and the death of one or more of the babies. Among twin gestations, it is recommended that fetal growth be monitored periodically, and even in uneventful twin pregnancies, delivery is recommended by 39 weeks because of late unanticipated stillbirths [33]. Higher order multiples are associated with even higher rates of perinatal death. One important strategy to reduce stillbirth may be to reduce the number of embryos transferred during an induced reproductive cycle to reduce the number of multiple gestations [20].

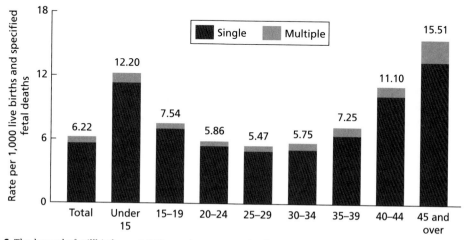

Figure 1.6 The hazard of stillbirth per 1,000 ongoing pregnancies for non-Hispanic white, non-Hispanic black, and Hispanic women. (Data from Ref. [7].)

Maternal risk factors for stillbirth

Risk factors for stillbirth are the same in both developed and developing countries, but the prevalence of these risk factors varies significantly. Unrecognized and uncontrolled hypertension or diabetes, lack of prenatal care, the lack of access to timely cesarean delivery are risk factors everywhere, but this occurs much less often in developed countries. In developed countries, hypertension and diabetes are the most common medical conditions in pregnancy [34] (see Chapter 8). Common social risk factors are obesity, smoking, low maternal education, and first birth (Table 1.1). Extremes in maternal age are risk factors for stillbirth (Figure 1.5). In developed countries, older women over the age are more likely to be starting a family.

Maternal age and parity

In most countries there is a U-shaped relationship between maternal age and stillbirth (Figure 1.5) [4]. Older maternal age is an independent risk factor for stillbirth even after controlling for factors that occur more often in older women, such as obesity,

Table 1.1 Common risk factors for stillbirth in the United States.

Risk factor	Prevalence (%)	Odds ratio
Obesity		
BMI 25–29.9	21–24	1.4–2.7
BMI >30	20–34	2.1–2.8
Nulliparity compared to second pregnancy	40	1.2–1.6
Fourth child or greater compared to second	11	2.2–2.3
Maternal age		
35–39	15–18	1.8–2.2
40+	2	1.8–3.3
Multiple gestation		
Twins	2.70	1.0–2.2
Triplets or greater	0.14	2.8–3.7
Advanced reproductive technologies (all)	1–3	1.2–3.0
Smoking	10–20	1.7–3.0
Alcohol use (any)	6–10	1.2–1.7
Illicit drug use	2–4	1.2–3.0
Low education/socioeconomics status	30	2.0–7.0
Antenatal visits <4*	6	2.7
Black (reference white)	15	20–2.2
Hypertension	6–10	1.5–4.0
Diabetes	2–5	1.5–3.0
Large for gestational age >97% without diabetes	12	2.4
Fetal growth restriction		
<3%	3.00	4.8
3–10%	7.50	2.8
Previous growth-restricted infant	6.70	2.0–4.6
Previous preterm birth with growth restriction	2	4.0–8.0
Decreased fetal movement	4–8	4.0–12.0
Previous stillbirth	0.50	2.0–10.0
Previous cesarean section	22–25	1.0–1.5
Postterm pregnancy (>42 weeks) compared to 38–40 weeks	6	2.0–4.0

Data from Ref. [35].
*Stillbirth 37 weeks or greater.

gestational diabetes, hypertension, and multiple gestations [21]. Advanced maternal age also interacts negatively with first birth, smoking and black rate to further increase the risk of stillbirth. Similar to maternal age, maternal parity (first birth and high parity) are risk factors for stillbirth. Women in the United States having their fourth child (or greater) experience 2.3 times the risk of stillbirth when compared to a woman having her second child [36].

Previous obstetric history

A prior adverse obstetric outcome, such as a preterm birth (spontaneous or induced for medical reasons) or delivery of a growth-restricted infant have common etiological factors to those pregnancies that end in stillbirth. In terms of placental pathology, stillbirth is on the spectrum of disease; a history of a baby being born both very preterm and growth restricted confers a higher risk of subsequent stillbirth than a history of a term stillbirth that was well grown [37] (Table 1.1).

The role of a previous cesarean delivery on the future risk of stillbirth is unclear at present with different risk estimates seen in different populations [38, 39]. It is not certain if the scarring from cesarean delivery reduces placental reserve increasing the risk of a subsequent stillbirth or if having a primary cesarean is a marker of underlying pathology.

Obesity

Obesity is a modifiable risk factor for stillbirth. In developed countries, modern society is "obesogenic"; this is related to a more sedentary lifestyle and the easy access to calorie-rich foods. In the United States, the National Health and Nutrition Examination Survey (NHANES) estimates of obesity (BMI of ≥30) rose from 14% in adults 20 years of age or older in the early 1960s to 34% in 2005. Extreme obesity (BMI of 40.0 or greater) rose from 1% to 5.7% in the same time period [40]. Prepregnancy obesity is associated with a 3.5- to 4.6-fold increased risk for stillbirth after 37 weeks of gestation [41, 42]. The reason for this increased risk is not known, but placental

dysfunction, sleep apnea, metabolic abnormalities, and inability to easily monitor fetal growth or fetal movement are proposed mechanisms [32].

Preconception care

Access to contraception, screening for sexually transmitted diseases, optimizing maternal weight and health, prenatal folic acid supplementation, optimal spacing of pregnancies, all have measurable effects on pregnancy outcome, and stillbirth. It would be an oversight not to recognize the above opportunities for improved health and are likely to have a substantial effect on stillbirth rates.

Alcohol, drug use, smoking and stillbirth

The use of alcohol, illicit drug use, and smoking all have known adverse pregnancy effects; these effects are worse with multiple substance use. Taking the opportunity to counsel and support women to reduce these risky behaviors can improve pregnancy outcomes, although resuming substance use after pregnancy is common. Underreporting of substance abuse is common. Smoking is a common and modifiable risk factor for stillbirth. While prospective studies of smoking cessation interventions are generally underpowered to detect a reduction in stillbirth, consistent epidemiological data supports the conclusion that smoking is associated with preterm birth, fetal growth restriction, and stillbirth, and smoking cessation remains a simple and straightforward stillbirth prevention strategy [43].

Racial factors and stillbirth

There are many social determinants that affect the health of women and her baby, so it can be difficult to tease out what might be primarily biological risk factors within a racial group, from the racial disparities in economic status, health, literacy, and immigration status. A study of more than five million American births demonstrated that black women had more than twice the rate of stillbirth (11.6/1,000) when compared to white (4.9/1,000) or Hispanic women (5.5/1,000) [7]. While education conferred a 30% reduction in stillbirth risk for white women who had more than 12 years of education, there was only a 9% reduction seen for black women and a 4% reduction for Hispanic women (which was not statistically significant) [7]. Black women who experienced a stillbirth were also more likely to have experienced medical, obstetrical, or labor complications than white and Hispanic women (30.1%, 19.5%, and 19.3%, respectively). While black women had higher rates of stillbirth throughout pregnancy than white and Hispanic women (Figure 1.4), this was greatest at 20–23 weeks of gestation (relative risk of hazard) for black compared to white women (RR 2.7 95% CI 2.6–2.9), but an increase was also seen late in pregnancy (>40 weeks, RR 2.2, 95% CI 2.1–2.3) [7].

Evaluating the reasons for these differences both in early and late stillbirths would provide important insight into the chain of events, and mechanisms of loss. One suspects that there may be biological reasons for early losses specifically for black women Since these women are more likely to have uterine fibroids than white women and fibroids are associated with pregnancy complications do influence the risk of stillbirth. In the United States, black women are less likely to undergo an induction of labor after 40 weeks than white women [7].

Decreased fetal movements

Approximately 4–10% of women will report decreased fetal movements sometime during their pregnancy [44, 45]. While most pregnancies will have a normal outcome, recent studies estimate that approximately one quarter of pregnancies will have a less than optimal outcome (growth restriction 14–23% and stillbirth 1.5–4.3%) [45]. Women who presented more than once with this complaint, who had had a history of obstetric problems and who had a fundal height smaller than expected had the worst outcome with a relative risk of 22 for experiencing a poor obstetric outcome [45].

Certainly the management of this complaint is an area of significant opportunity for stillbirth reduction. In a study where information was given to patients at their 18-week appointment and providers were given clinical guidelines for the management of decreased fetal movement (including a timely evaluation of fetal wellbeing with both a nonstress test and an assessment of fetal growth with ultrasound), a 33% reduction of stillbirths was found in 14 delivery units in Norway [44]. During this study period, the number of women who waited 48h or more prior to contacting her provider was reduced from 54% to 49%, and the number of women who received an ultrasound during the course of her evaluation rose from 86% to 94% [44]. While it is not known which aspect of this intervention had the greatest benefit for stillbirth reduction, it is obvious studying stillbirth and the management of high-risk conditions is likely to have a significant benefit on stillbirth rates.

Suboptimal care

In developed countries, the failure to detect severe fetal growth restriction is the most common "missed" opportunity in audits of perinatal mortality after 28 weeks of gestation (estimates range from 6.2% to 14% in the European working group). Maternal smoking (and perinatal mortality related to growth restriction and placental pathology) was noted in 6–21% of cases [13]. The management of hypertension, deficiencies of the interpretation of fetal monitoring during labor and delivery, and the failure to adequately manage pregnancies complicated by decreased fetal movement were also areas where there was reasonable evidence that had the factor been appropriately managed, that a fatal outcome could have been avoided [28, 46].

Strategies for prevention

Until recently, stillbirths have been understudied, but if the outcome of a stillbirth is viewed as the "tip of the iceberg" many improvements in obstetric care can be generated (Table 1.2, Figure 1.7). Strategies for stillbirth prevention begin with a

Table 1.2 Strategies for stillbirth prevention in high income countries.

Improve the systematic review and evaluation of stillbirths similar to other sentinel events

Develop a "stillbirth package" which includes the optimal stillbirth evaluation and support materials for the parents

Improve access and quality of obstetric care for minorities, recent immigrants, poor- and less-educated women

Offer screening for congenital/karyotypic anomalies with the availability of termination of pregnancy

Promote healthy habits with smoking cessation and optimizing weight before pregnancy

Reduction of multiple gestations by reducing the number of embryos transferred in the reproductive technologies

Improve strategies for the detection and management of fetal growth restriction

Optimize the management of decreased fetal movement in the preterm and term pregnancies

Improve management of high-risk conditions with the use of a high-risk roster, develop outreach for noncompliant patients

Adopt evidence-based algorithms monitoring high-risk pregnancies

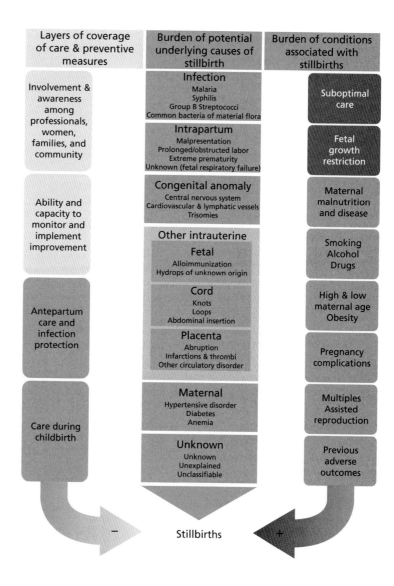

Figure 1.7 Stillbirth determinants. A framework of the setting and conditions that constitute the data sources needed for the understanding of stillbirth mortality. The classification of significant proportions of underlying causes of death globally is reproduced from CODAC. (Reproduced from Ref. [47], with permission from Biomed Central.)

systematic evaluation of each case, which includes the review of medical, obstetric, and social risk factors. A systematic evaluation often leads to the identification of areas of "opportunity." Late prenatal care may result in poor obstetric dating, and a missed opportunity for prenatal diagnosis and an improvement in healthy habits. If there are too many early losses related to higher-order multiple gestations, then feedback to the infertility providers may reduce the number of embryos that are transferred.

There are often opportunities to improved documentation so that the patient and her provider can develop a strategy for antepartum monitoring if a future pregnancy is planned. A more thorough stillbirth evaluation will help assess the risk of recurrence (see Chapter 12). Obstetric providers and labor room nurses need to be educated on the cultural barriers to obtaining autopsy; many parental concerns can be addressed by accommodating and respecting the patient's beliefs while also maximizing the opportunities to find a cause or contributor to the stillbirth.

Improved roster systems for high-risk patients will improve outreach for noncompliant or disorganized patients, thus improving the detection of worsening fetal or maternal status. Improved evidence-based algorithms for high-risk conditions will facilitate care (i.e., delivering twin gestations prior to the estimated due date) [33]. Until recently the management of decreased fetal movement involved only the assessment of imminent fetal jeopardy (with a nonstress test) but missed the opportunity to review other potential risk factors and the opportunity to assess fetal growth. Development of a "stillbirth package" which includes information and support for both the provider and the patient will help facilitate care during this stressful time.

References

1. World Health Organization. Definitions and indicators in Family Planning Maternal & Child Health and Reproductive Health. Geneva: WHO Press; 2001.
2. Gordijn SJ, Korteweg FJ, Erwich JJHM, et al. A multilayered approach to the analysis of perinatal mortality using different classification systems. Eur J Obstet Gynecol Reprod Biol 2009;144:99–104.
3. Duke W, Williams L, Correa A. Using active birth defect surveillance programs to supplement data on fetal death reports: improving surveillance data on stillbirths. Birth Defects Res 2008;82:799–804.
4. MacDorman MF, Kirmeyer S. The challenge of fetal mortality. NCHS data brief, no 16. Hyattsville, MD: National Center for Health Statistics; 2009.
5. National Center for Health Statistics. State Definitions and reporting for live births, fetal deaths, and induced terminations of pregnancy. Revision. Hyattsville, MD: NCHS; 1997.
6. World Health Organization. Neonatal and perinatal mortality. Country, regional and global estimates. Geneva: WHO Press; 2006.
7. Willinger M, Chia-Wen K, Reddy UM. Racial disparities in stillbirth across gestation in the United States. Am J Obstet Gynecol 2009;201:469e.1–8.
8. Kung HS, Hoyert DL, Xu J, Murphy SL. Deaths: final data for 2005. National Vital Statistics Report 56, Number 10; 2008.
9. Cacciatore J, Schnebly S, Froen JF. The effects of social support on maternal anxiety and depression after stillbirth. Health Social Care Community 2009;17:167–76.
10. Vallgarda S. Why did the stillbirth rate decline in Denmark after 1940? Popul Stud. Accessed 12 May 2010, 1–14, iFirst Styovlr, link to article 10.1080/00324721003746484.
11. Fretts RC, Boyd M, Usher RH, Usher HA. The changing pattern of fetal death 1961–1988. Obstet Gynecol 1992;79:35–9.
12. Bell R, Glinianaia SV, Rankin J, et al. Changing patterns of perinatal death, 1982–2000: a retrospective cohort study. Arch Dis Child Fetal Neonatal Ed 2004;89:F531–6.
13. Richardus JH, Graafmans WC, Verloove-Vanhorick P, Mackenback JP, the EuroNatal International Audit Panel, the Euronatal Working Group. Differences in perinatal mortality and suboptimal care between 10 European regions: results of an international audit. BJOG 2003;110:97–105.
14. Papiernik E, Zeitlin J, Delmas D, et al. Termination of pregnancy among very preterm births and its impact on the very preterm mortality: results from 10 European population-based cohorts in the MOSAIC study. BJOG 2008;115:361–8.

15. Boyd PA, DeVigan C, Khoshnood B, et al. Survey of prenatal screening policies in Europe for structural malformations and chromosome anomalies, and their impact on detection and termination rates for neural tube defects and Down's syndrome. BJOG 2008;115:689–96.

16. MacDorman MF, Munson ML, Kirmeyer S. Fetal and perinatal mortality United States 2004. National Vital Statistics Reports 56; 2007.

17. Huang DY, Usher RH, Kramer MS, et al. Determinants of unexplained antepartum fetal deaths. Obstet Gynecol 2000;95:215–21.

18. Froen JF, Arnestad M, Frey K, et al. Risk factors for sudden intrauterine unexplained death: epidemiological characteristics if singleton cases in Oslo Norway, 1986–1995. Am J Obstet Gynecol 2001;184:694–702.

19. Froen JF, Gardosi JO, Thurmann A, et al. Restricted fetal growth in sudden intrauterine unexplained death. Acta Obstet Gynecol Scand 2004;83:801–7.

20. Salihu HS, Aliyu MH, Rouse DJ, et al. Potentially preventable excess mortality among higher-order multiples. Obstet Gynecol 2003;102:679–84.

21. Fretts RC, Schmittdiel J, Mclean FH, et al. Increased maternal age and the risk of fetal death. N Engl J Med 1995;333:953–7.

22. Reddy UM, Chia-Wen KO, Willinger M. Maternal age and risk of stillbirth throughout pregnancy in the United States. Am J Obstet Gynecol 2006;195:764–70.

23. Nicholson JM, Stenson MH, Kellar LS, et al. Active management of risk in nulliparous pregnancy at term, association between a higher preventive labor induction rate and improved birth outcomes. Am J Obstet Gynecol 2009;200:254.e1–13.

24. Lahra MM, Gordon A, Jeffery HE. Chorioamnionitis and fetal response in stillbirth. Am J Obstet Gynecol 2007;196:229.e1–e4.

25. Warland J, McCutcheon H, Baghurst P. Maternal blood pressure in pregnancy and stillbirth: a case control study of third trimester stillbirth. Am J Perinatol 2008;25:311–17.

26. Chen A, Basso O. Does low maternal blood pressure during pregnancy increase the risk of perinatal death? Epidemiology 2007;18:619–22.

27. Gardosi JO. Prematurity and fetal growth restriction. Early Hum Dev 2005;81:43–49.

28. Confidential enquiry into stillbirths and deaths in infancy 2001 in Northern Ireland. Maternal and Child Health Research Consortium, Eight Annual Report, London; 2001.

29. Oyelese Y, Ananth CV. Placental abruption. Am J Obstet Gynecol 2006;108:1005–16.

30. Goldenberg RL, Thompson C. The infectious origins of stillbirth. Am J Obstet Gynecol 2003;189: 861–73.

31. Syridou G, Spanakis N, Konstantinidou A, et al. Detection of cytomegalovirus, parvovirus B19 and herpes simplex viruses in cases of intrauterine fetal death: association with pathological findings. J Med Virol 2008;80:1776–92.

32. Smith GCS, Fretts RC. Stillbirth. Lancet 2007;370: 1715–25.

33. Robinson J, Healy B, Beatty T, Cohen A. The optimal gestational age for twin delivery. Am J Obstet Gynecol 2005;193:S183.

34. Simpson LL. Maternal medical disease: risk of antepartum fetal death. Semin Perinatol 2002;26:42–50.

35. Fretts RC. Stillbirth epidemiology, risk factors and opportunities for stillbirth prevention. Clinical Obstet Gynecol 2010;3:588–596.

36. Aliyu MH, Salihu HM, Keith LG, et al. Extreme parity and the risk of stillbirth. Obstet Gynecol 2005;106:446–53.

37. Surkan PJ, Stephansson O, Dickman PW, Cnattingius S. Previous preterm and small-for-gestational-age births and the subsequent risk of stillbirth. N Engl J Med 2004;350:777–85.

38. Smith CS, Pell JP, Dobbie R. Cesarean section and the risk of unexplained stillbirth in a subsequent pregnancy. Lancet 2003;362:1779–84.

39. Bahtiyar MO, Julien S, Robinson JN, et al. Prior cesarean delivery is not associated with an increased risk of stillbirth in a subsequent pregnancy: analysis of U.S. perinatal mortality data, 1995–1997. Am J Obstet Gynecol 2006;195:1373–8.

40. Flegal KM, Carroll ND, Ogden CL, Curtin LR. Prevalence and trends in obesity among US adults, 1999–2008. JAMA 2010;303:235–41.

41. Chu SY, Kim SY, Lau J, et al. Maternal obesity and the risk of stillbirth: a metaanalysis. Am J Obstet Gynecol 2007;197:223–8.

42. Nohr EA, Bech BH, Davies MJ, et al. Prepregnancy obesity and fetal death: a study within the Danish national Birth Cohort. Obstet Gynecol 2005; 106:250–9.

43. Salihu HM, Wilson RE. Epidemiology of prenatal smoking and perinatal outcomes. Early Hum Dev 2007;83;713–29.

44. Holm Tveit JV, Saastad E, Stray-Peterson B, et al. Reduction of late stillbirth with the introduction

of fetal movement information and guidelines—a clinical quality improvement. BMC Pregnancy Childbirth 2009;32:2–11.

45. O'Sullivan O, Stephen G, Martindale E, Heazell AEP. Prediction poor perinatal outcome in women who present with decreased fetal movements. J Obstet Gynecol 2009;29:705–10.

46. Saastad E, Vangen S, Froen JF. Suboptimal care in stillbirths—a retrospective audit study. Acta Obstet Gynecol 2007;86:444–50.

47. Froen JF, Gordjin SA, Abel-Allem, et al. Making stillbirth count, making numbers talk-issues in data collection for stillbirths. BMC Pregnancy Childbirth 2009;9:58, doi:10.1186/1471-2393-9-58.

CHAPTER 2

Low Income Countries*

Joy E. Lawn, MBBS, MRCP (Paeds), MPH PhD[1,2,3], Hannah Blencowe, MBChB, MRCPCH, MSc[4], Robert Pattinson, FCOG SA[5], Cynthia Stanton, MPH PhD[6], and Simon Cousens, Dip Math Stat[4]

[1]Saving Newborn Lives/Save the Children, Cape Town, South Africa
[2]Health Systems Research Unit, Medical Research Council, South Africa
[3]Institute of Child Health, London, UK
[4]London School of Hygiene and Tropical Medicine, London, UK
[5]International Stillbirth Association Scientific Board, Medical Research Council, University of Pretoria, Pretoria, South Africa
[6]John Hopkins Bloomberg School of Public Health, Baltimore, MD, USA

Stillbirth visibility in global data and policy

The estimated number of third-trimester stillbirths is similar to the 3 million annual early neonatal deaths in the first week of life and larger than the annual number of deaths due to HIV/AIDS (Figure 2.1). This paradox of low policy imperative despite the high burden, and despite close links to other issues with policy momentum, raises an unaddressed question. Do the data gaps, lack of consensus for program priorities, or lack of champions explain the attention gap, or are there other specific factors that limit attention to stillbirths? Shiffman's article on the political imperative for safe motherhood raised the question "Why do some global health initiatives receive priority from international and national political leaders whereas others receive little attention?" [1]. Table 2.1 adapts Shiffman's framework to examine some of the factors shaping low visibility and political priority for stillbirths.

Despite 30 years of attention to child survival interventions [3], over 20 years of attention to safe motherhood [4], and increasing recent attention to newborn survival [5], global attention has remained on survival after live birth and stillbirths remain a largely ignored loss of life, not counting on policy, program, and investment agendas both internationally and often also at national level [6]. In many societies and on the global and national policy agendas, stillbirths are virtually invisible yet are very real to those families who experience a death instead of the expected live baby. Neonatal deaths have risen on the global policy agenda, largely because of the Millennium Development Goals (MDGs) and recognition of the increasing proportion of deaths for children under 5 years that happen in the first month—now at 41% [7], up from 38% in 2000 [8]. If a baby dies just after birth, they count, but a baby who dies in the last trimester or even during labor they do not count. Neither the MDGs nor the Global Burden of Disease exercise mention stillbirths. Stillbirth data are not routinely compiled by the United Nations. Even when stillbirths are measured in surveys, stillbirths are frequently combined with early neonatal deaths and reported as perinatal mortality, a combination which reduces visibility and may mask reporting differences, systematic

---

*This chapter draws on a paper for *The Lancet* Stillbirth series [2] and we are grateful to *The Lancet* and *Elsevier* for permission to use this material.

Stillbirth: Prediction, Prevention and Management, First Edition. Catherine Y. Spong.
© 2011 Blackwell Publishing Ltd. Published 2011 by Blackwell Publishing Ltd.

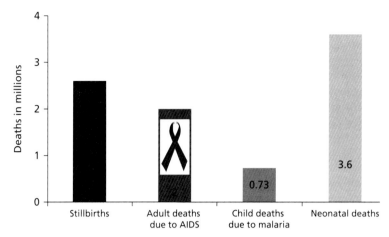

Figure 2.1 The global number of stillbirths compared to other linked global mortality burdens in the year 2008. (Adapted from Ref. [9] [updated with 2008 data].)

misclassification, variation in trends and differing solutions [10]. Stillbirths are not just a low-income country problem. Rates in the United Kingdom and the United States have decreased little in recent years and stillbirths now account for the majority of perinatal deaths [11].

In this chapter we present epidemiological data to prioritize actions to reduce stillbirths, especially in low- and middle-income countries where most of these deaths occur. We discuss the limitations of the data and identify key research questions with respect to improving estimates of stillbirth rates (SBR). Determining *what* to do in which context, and *how* to do it requires data-based priority setting, in both high- and low-income countries. Yet the data is most limited where the burden is highest, the so-called inverse information law.

Counting stillbirths

Definitions and international comparability

Inconsistent application of terminology has contributed to confusion regarding stillbirths [6]. The terminology has changed over time and despite clear global guidelines, there is marked variation between countries, and ironically the variability is greatest between high-income countries [12].

The International Classification of Diseases, 10th revision (ICD 10) [13] refers to fetal deaths and does not mention stillbirths. Fetal death is defined *death prior to the complete expulsion or extraction from its mother of a product of conception . . . the fetus does not breathe or show any other evidence of life, such as beating of the heart, pulsation of the umbilical cord, or definite movement of voluntary muscles.* In ICD measurement focus is on fetal deaths in the last two trimesters of pregnancy and defined by: birthweight ≥500 g, or if birthweight is unknown, gestational age ≥22 completed weeks of gestation, or if both previous criteria are unknown, crown-heel length ≥25 cm (Figure 2.2). If gestational age (22 weeks) is used rather than birthweight (500 g), the stillbirth rate is higher—for example, by about 15% in Norway [14]. In low-income settings, 60 million births at home are usually unweighed even if liveborn. Even in hospitals, a stillborn is often unweighed, and rarely measured. Hence in many low-income settings gestational age is the most commonly used criterion, often based on last menstrual period or estimation based on uterine size.

To assure international comparability, WHO recommends reporting of late fetal deaths (≥1,000 g, ≥28 completed weeks of gestation). However, it is also recommended that countries record outcomes at thresholds lower than 28 weeks as this increases completeness of reporting for ≥28-week threshold.

Table 2.1 Stillbirths counting as a policy and program priority.

Determinants	Description	Factors favoring prioritization of stillbirths	Factors diminishing prioritization of stillbirths
Issues	Framing the problem	National stillbirth rate estimates and numbers Large numbers of deaths—at least 2.65 million Closely linked to maternal and newborn deaths, and maternal complications such as fistula Public attention for parental grief following stillbirths, and data about prolonged grief reactions	Poor visibility of the estimates, and no direct mention of stillbirths in MDGs or Global Burden of Disease to give political framework to drive attention Social importance attached to stillbirths—do the numbers count? Social taboos for grieving stillbirths, and indeed also for neonatal deaths
Ideas	Prioritizing and communicating solutions	Close linkages with maternal health and especially intrapartum care Stillbirth prevention includes antenatal and intrapartum care, and will lead to further prevention of neonatal and maternal deaths	Poorly framed solutions even for the 1.2 million intrapartum stillbirths, affected by conflicts within maternal health community regarding maternal health policy and implementation
Power of the actors	The strength of individuals and organizations concerned with the issue	Active family bereavement groups Some more attention from professional organizations, e.g., obstetricians and midwives More coalescence of United Nations and partner messages with respect to maternal newborn and child health, and some stronger agency and advocacy voices	Parent lobby groups have limited power, especially outside industrialized countries Stillbirths have no professional body that "owns" them—e.g., obstetricians and midwives often perceive their allegiance to be more to the mother, pediatricians to the live-born child Focus is on mothers, and children, some attention to newborns with few mentions of stillbirths, and no clear voice from agencies or professional organizations or individuals
Political context	Political and investment opportunities, or political conflicts	Increasing investment in maternal care services	Stillbirths possibly considered as competition to maternal health priorities, instead of a massive linked burden that also affects the woman due to grieving and stigma Political and ideological conflicts of interest when gestational ages of stillbirth overlap with legal terminations of pregnancy

Adapted from Ref. [1].

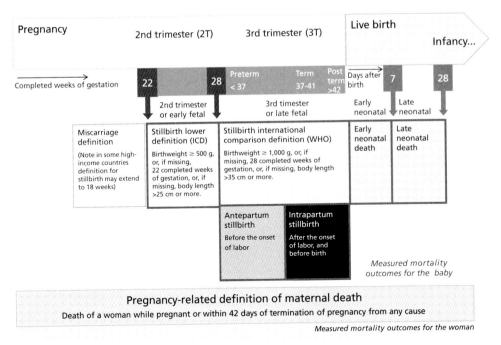

Figure 2.2 Defining stillbirths and related pregnancy outcomes for international comparison. Definitions from International Classification of Diseases, 10th revision (ICD-10). (Based on Ref. [2], used with permission.)

This ≥28 week gestation (third trimester) still-birth threshold has international relevance for public health policy and programs. In low- and middle-income countries where 98% of neonatal deaths occur, neonatal intensive care is not widely available [8] and few babies born alive before 28 weeks gestation survive [15]. After 32 weeks gestation the majority of newborns can survive with basic care, especially given increasing success with kangaroo mother care [16]. In high-income countries with intensive care, neonatal viability has increased dramatically. Although few babies born alive at 22 weeks may survive, by 25 weeks the majority of liveborn babies in high-income countries survive [17]. The Nuffield Council on Bioethics recommends that below 22 weeks of gestation resuscitation should not be attempted, even if a baby is born with signs of life [18]. This shift in neonatal survival has driven down the gestational age cutoff for registering stillbirths in most high- and some middle-income countries.

Thresholds vary from 18 to 28 weeks even in Europe [19], and such inconsistency has a large effect on the number of stillbirths reported, for example, moving from 28- to 22-week threshold can lead to a 40% increase in the number of still-births [20].

In this chapter we use the term stillbirth to include all fetal deaths ≥500g or over 22 weeks gestation. However, where data are reported or discussed, we use the stillbirth definition recommended for international comparison, that is, ≥1,000g birth-weight or 28 or more weeks gestation.

Where do the numbers come from?

Prior to 2006, no global estimates of stillbirths had been published. In 1983 WHO published a global estimate of 8 million perinatal deaths [21] and in 1996 WHO released perinatal mortality estimates with a rate of 58 per 1,000 in developing countries and a stillbirth rate of 32 per 1,000, suggesting a global number of 4.3 million stillbirths [22].

Although a literature review of stillbirth rates was published [23], up to that point, no organization had ever presented estimates of country-specific rates and numbers of stillbirths and this has been a major impediment to visibility and action.

In 2006, two sets of estimates of third-trimester stillbirth rates for the year 2000 were published. One set was developed through a collaborative effort between the Saving Newborn Lives/Save the Children and the Initiative for Maternal Mortality Programme Assessment at the University of Aberdeen, Scotland (immpact) [24]. The second set was developed by the Making Pregnancy Safer Department of WHO [25]. Remarkably, these two stillbirth estimates gave almost the same global totals, 3.3 million [25] and 3.2 (uncertainty range [UR]: 2.5–4.1 million [24]). However, there were major differences for some individual countries [24–26].

Recent estimates for 2008 have been undertaken by a collaboration of researchers from several teams including the Child Health Epidemiology Reference Group, Saving Newborn Lives, the Global Alliance for Prevention of Prematurity and Stillbirth (GAPPS), and WHO. Improved estimates were generated through identifying more data, including more recent data from low-income settings, and refining the modeling methods to comply as closely as possible with published

recommendations regarding systematic and transparent global estimates. The model was then applied to estimate trends. The details of the inputs and methods are published elsewhere [26].

Current global status for stillbirths

Where do stillbirths occur?

Regional and national variation

In the year 2008, a global total of 2.65 (UR: 2.08–3.79) million stillbirths were estimated to occur [26]. Almost all (98%) of these third-trimester stillbirths occurred in low- and middle-income countries, and over three-quarters are in South Asia and sub-Saharan Africa, with regional rates of 26.7 and 29.0 per 1,000 total births, representing 1.1 and 0.9 million third-trimester stillbirths, respectively (Table 2.2, Figure 2.3). In high-income countries the stillbirth rate is under 5 per 1,000 (3.1: UR: 3.0–3.3) [26].

Variation in stillbirth rates between countries is considerable. Finland has the lowest reported rate at 2.0 per 1,000 births, and the highest rates are estimated for Pakistan (46.1 per 1000) and Nigeria (41.9 per 1000)—a greater than 20 fold difference in risk. Even within the same region there is great variation in stillbirth rates. For example, among

Table 2.2 Estimated stillbirth rates and percent intrapartum stillbirth by world region for the year 2008.

Region	Estimated stillbirth rate per 1,000 total births	Number of stillbirths	Uncertainty range		Estimated % intrapartum stillbirths
			Low	High	
High income countries	3.1	36,300	35,500	38,200	13.7%
East Asia	9.0	171,400	116,200	278,600	20.0%
Latin America/Caribbean	9.4	101,800	83,300	125,400	23.1%
Eurasia	9.0	33,500	31,300	42,700	20.0%
Southeast Asia and Oceania	14.2	164,300	130,400	235,700	30.9%
N Africa and W Asia (Middle East)	12.9	112,300	88,900	165,100	16.4%
Sub-Saharan Africa	29.0	943,900	701,800	1,388,800	46.5%
South Asia	26.7	1,083,300	835,900	1,671,000	56.6%
Worldwide	19.1	2,646,800	2,077,010	3,790,420	1,190,700 45.0%

Based on Ref. [2], used with permission.

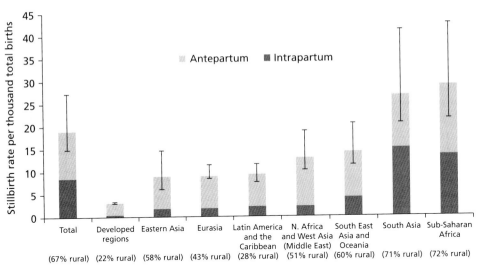

Figure 2.3 Country variation in third-trimester stillbirth rates for the year 2008. (Based on Ref. [2], used with permission.)

sub-Saharan African countries, Mauritius has a reported third-trimester stillbirth rate of 8.9 per 1,000 total births compared with estimated rates of over 30 per 1,000 total births in Cote D'Ivoire, DR Congo, Djibouti, Senegal and Nigeria. (Figure 2.4) [26]. It must be emphasized, however, that national estimates have wide uncertainty, especially those with limited national input data. For example, the estimate for Afghanistan is 29.4 per 1,000 total births, giving 38,000 stillbirths with a range from 24,000 to 72,000.

Stillbirths are heavily concentrated in a few countries. Ten populous countries (India, Pakistan, Nigeria, Bangladesh, China, Ethiopia, DR Congo, Indonesia, Afghanistan, and Tanzania) account for two-thirds of all stillbirths (1.8 million, 66%)—as well as 62% of global maternal [27] and 67% of global neonatal deaths [28] (Table 2.3). The top five countries account for over half of all stillbirths and maternal and neonatal deaths and are critical for progress toward global goals. It is notable that during the last decade China has dropped from second to fourth highest burden of stillbirths due to both a rapid reduction in stillbirth rate and a low total fertility rate. Nigeria has moved up to the second

highest as both the national stillbirth rate and total fertility rate remain very high. Therefore, both family planning and care at birth are important in reducing deaths for mothers, newborns, and stillbirths and these strategies give triple value in lives saved.

Within country variation

Within countries there are also marked differences. India alone contributes an estimated 613,500 third-trimester stillbirths each year with a rate of 22 (UR: 17–36), but variation between states is large with third-trimester stillbirth rates of under 20 per 1,000 births reported from Kerala and rates of 66 per 1,000 or more reported in central India. Differentials in Nigeria may be even more marked—the rates in rural Northern communities are considerably higher than for urban teaching hospitals in Southern Nigeria. In China, the stillbirth rate for rural, ethnic minority groups may be threefold higher than for urban residents [2].

In high-income countries and Latin America most stillbirths are urban, reflecting the urbanized population. In South Asia and sub-Saharan Africa the predominantly rural populations means that

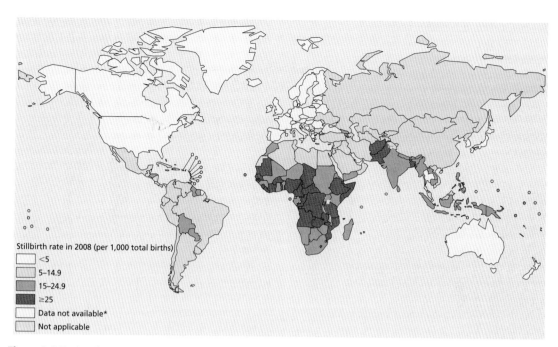

Figure 2.4 Regional variation in stillbirth rates and the proportion of stillbirths that are intrapartum. (Based on Ref. [2], used with permission.)

Table 2.3 Top 10 countries for stillbirths, maternal deaths, and neonatal deaths in 2008.

Country	Rank for number of stillbirths			Rank for number of maternal deaths			Rank for number of neonatal deaths		
India	1			1			1		
Nigeria	2			2			2		
Pakistan	3	1.8 million stillbirths		7	221,000 maternal deaths		3	2.4 million neonatal deaths	
China	4			12			4		
Bangladesh	5			8			7		
Dem Rep Congo	6			3			5		
Ethiopia	7	66% of global total		5	62% of global total		6	67% of global total	
Indonesia	8			9			8		
Afghanistan	9			4			9		
Tanzania	10			6			14		

Data sources: Stillbirths from Ref. [26], neonatal from Ref. [28], and maternal from Ref. [27].
Based on Ref. [2], used with permission.

over two-thirds of all stillbirths in these regions are rural (771,000 in South Asia, 681,000 stillbirths in sub-Saharan Africa).

Urban–rural differentials in stillbirth rates are consistent with urban–rural differentials in skilled attendance at birth, which is at least 50% lower for rural women in Africa and South Asia [29]. The urban–rural gap for cesarean section is even greater. South Asia has an urban cesarean section rate of 14%, with 5% for rural women. Africa has very low cesarean section rates at 5% for urban and only 1% for rural [30]. Indeed, Burkina Faso, Chad, Ethiopia, and Niger all have rural cesarean section rates of almost zero [29].

Association of stillbirth with maternal and newborn mortality and health systems context

When the countries are categorized by stillbirth rate (<5, 5–14.9, 15–24.9, and >25 per 1,000), there are clear correlations with maternal and neonatal mortality and health system indicators (Table 2.4) [26]. Stillbirth rates are under 5 per 1,000 in 45 high-income countries, accounting for 2% of global stillbirths [2]. In these countries the median number of nurses/midwives per 1,000 population is 7.7, virtually all births are with a skilled attendant and neonatal and maternal deaths are also very rare events. In contrast, 28 low-income countries with stillbirth rates greater than 25 per 1,000 account for 43% of global stillbirths. In these countries the median number of nurses/midwives per 1,000 population is 0.5, compared with a minimum of 2.0 recommended by WHO, and half of births occur at home without skilled care [2]. These are also the countries with the health systems and the weakest data to set priorities, improve outcomes, and track progress.

Timing of stillbirth

The simplest grouping of stillbirths is by time of death—antepartum (before the onset of labor) or intrapartum (during labor and birth). The hours during labor and the actual time of birth are a period of high risk, with an estimated 1.19 million (UR: 0.82–1.97 million) intrapartum stillbirths, representing 45% of the world's third-trimester stillbirths annually [2] and slightly higher than the last global estimate for 2000 of 1.02 (UR: 0.66–1.48) million [31]. The inputs, methods, and limitations of these estimates are detailed elsewhere and use median regional intrapartum stillbirth percentage based on 94 datasets. A sensitivity analysis limited to 53 datasets with a stricter definition ($\geq$1,000 g or $\geq$28 weeks) made little difference to most regional estimates, but included no data points for North Africa and West Asia. The data available do not support more complex models accounting for more than just region. More data are urgently required to track this important outcome which is a sensitive measure of care at birth.

There is large variation between regions for intrapartum stillbirths. In rich countries, intrapartum stillbirth rates are typically less than 0.5 per 1,000 births or around 14% of late stillbirths, compared with rates of 12 per 1,000 births or higher (over 50% of stillbirths) in many countries in South Asia and sub-Saharan Africa (Table 2.2, Figure 2.3) [2]. Most of the babies dying during labor are term babies who should survive if born alive and their deaths are often associated with suboptimal care [31].

Birth and the first few hours and days following birth are also the times of highest risk of death for the mother and newborn baby. The period around birth and the early postnatal period is the key time for programmatic action to reduce third-trimester stillbirths, maternal [32], and neonatal deaths [8], as well maternal morbidity (such as obstetric fistula), neonatal morbidity, and lifelong disability subsequent to neonatal complications.

Variation in causes of stillbirth

To reduce deaths, basic information on causation is critical [6]. National neonatal cause-of-death estimates have been published, are regularly updated by the United Nations [28] and disseminated through Countdown to 2015 national data profiles (http://www.countdown2015mnch.org/). This process has played a role in focusing on the three major causes of neonatal death (infections, intrapartum-related, and preterm birth complications) [33]. However, national stillbirth cause estimates do not exist. Two

Table 2.4 Countries grouped by stillbirth rate level and showing variation of GNI, skilled attendance, human resource density, etc. by stillbirth rate level.

	Stillbirth rate (per 1,000 total births)	Stillbirth rate levels			
		<5	5–14.9	15–24.9	>25
Stillbirth status	Numbers of stillbirths occurring in countries with this stillbirth rate	45,000	470,000	1,010,000	1,120,000
				80% of global stillbirths	
	(numbers of countries)	(48)	(74)	(43)	(28)
	Intrapartum stillbirth rate (weighted per 1,000 total births)	0.5	2.4	11.0	17.6
	(% of stillbirths that are intrapartum)	(16.4)	(23.4)	(50.4)	(50.3)
Economic status	Median gross national income per capita	$29,540 High income	$3,710 Middle income	$910 Low and middle income	$450 Low income
Maternal and newborn health status	Median maternal mortality ratio per 100,000 live births	7.7	38.1	257.3	567.3
	Median neonatal mortality rate per 1,000 live births	2.7	10.1	25.5	38.9
	Median percent of births with a skilled birth attendant	100%	98%	65%	50%
	Median percent of births by caesarean section	20.0%	15.3%	4.8%	3.2%
	Median nurse/midwife density per 1,000 population	7.6	3.3	1.0	0.5

Based on Ref. [2], used with permission.

fundamental challenges must be addressed. Firstly, consensus of which causal categories to use and how to link these with maternal conditions, and secondly, lack of comparable population-based data consistent with these categories.

Stillbirth classification systems have proliferated with over 35 published in the last 50 years, more than half in the last 15 years [14]. Approaches vary with some focusing on direct fetal causes (Wigglesworth based), others on maternal causes (Aberdeen based) or placental pathology, or a combination. Most recent classification systems have been devised for high-income countries, are complex, and require fetal surveillance, advanced diagnostics, and postmortem services. Some allow more than one cause per death which is useful for

programs but not compatible with ICD rules [34]. The International Stillbirth Alliance (ISA) has examined the utility of several classification systems to identify the most prevalent causes in high-income settings [35]. Wigglesworth performed worst and yet is the most widely used in low- and middle-income countries [35]. Even in Malaysia and South Africa, newer classifications were hampered by reliance on maternal history, a total lack of postmortem data and limited other investigations such as karyotyping, placental histology, thrombophilia screening, etc. [35]. Another problem even in high-income countries is detection of fetal growth restriction due to placental failure as a frequent antecedent of stillbirth [11]. With a complex system including fetal growth restriction combined with rigorous investigation the unidentified cause group can be reduced to under 30% [35] or even under 20% [36].

The lack of comparability between multiple classification systems is the most significant barrier to any meta-analysis and estimates for stillbirth causation. Hence agreement is required to map increasingly complex cause-of-death classifications used in high-income settings onto simple programmatic categories that are feasible and relevant in low-income settings.

The simplest approach is based on time of death (antepartum and intrapartum). These times can be identified in low-income settings, including home births, and are programmatically relevant. Antepartum stillbirths require improved care during pregnancy while intrapartum stillbirths require better obstetric care. At the next level of complexity, each time period would include a restricted menu of clinically identifiable direct causes which can be differentiated in a hospital or with a fairly advanced verbal autopsy tool (e.g., major congenital abnormalities, chorioamnionitis, etc.). Finally, in settings with high capacity more detailed direct causes of death can be distinguished with laboratory investigation and detailed examination of the placenta, using existing complex classification systems and ICD codes.

Despite limited data, a recent comparison of datasets published in *The Lancet* highlights apparent variations by stillbirth rate (Table 2.5) [2]. The proportion of intrapartum stillbirths increases as the stillbirth rate increases from around 15% in low SBR settings (<5) to over 50% in high SBR settings and in some datasets is up to two-thirds of stillbirths. However, some of the observed variations in distributions within may be real and some are more likely to be artifact related to measurement gaps. For example, the proportion of stillbirths attributed to infection is apparently higher in rich- and middle-income settings than in low-income countries which may reflect detection bias and lack of laboratory investigation. Syphilis is unlikely to be identified in the absence of serological testing. There are no obvious differences in proportion of stillbirths attributed to congenital abnormalities, which may reflect both a real

reduction in High Income Countries (HIC) due to termination and better care, or could be due to missed cases in low-income settings where only very obvious external abnormalities are noted [37].

Among antepartum stillbirths "unidentified condition" is the largest category and increases with increasing SBR. Analyses of classification systems have shown that the "identified" proportion of stillbirths varies according to the classification system used [35], and with the level of laboratory investigation and perinatal autopsy [38]. Fetal growth restriction is more commonly detected in high-income countries as ultrasound is more sensitive than a tape measure. Of these antepartum stillbirths with an unidentified cause, around one-third in South Africa and Bangladesh had a maternal event such as antepartum hemorrhage, easily identifiable through history, also showing the value of collecting data on maternal condition [2].

The importance of maternal conditions for stillbirths and neonatal deaths

Pregnancy outcomes for mothers and babies are closely linked, yet remarkably few datasets present information on all the relevant outcomes. ICD recommends that each stillbirth and neonatal death should be given a code for a direct cause and a separate code for maternal cause, allowing better assessment of attributable risk and programmatic implications. For example, fetal growth restriction is common and may be linked with maternal hypertension, yet the information is lost if only fetal growth restriction is coded. In high-income settings coding and analyzing all the associated conditions is possible. In low-income settings, it is feasible to record at least one stillbirth/neonatal cause and one associated maternal condition, as recommended by ICD, yet this is poorly implemented. The list of maternal conditions potentially related to stillbirth is long. Some, such as hypertension and diabetes, are important in all countries. Others are context specific; for example, high syphilis prevalence, malaria or HIV [39] or maternal undernutrition in low-income countries, and obesity or smoking in middle- and high-income countries [11]. Maternal infections in pregnancy

Table 2.5 Variation in the distribution of stillbirth causation and associated conditions according to increasing levels of stillbirth rate from <5 to >25 per 1,000 total births.

Countries	SBR < 5 6 HIC datasets*	SBR 15–24 South Africa national	SBR > 25 Bangladesh rural hospital
Stillbirth rate of input data	2–4	19	39
Year of input data	2008–2009	2008–2009	2007–2009
Antepartum (total)	316 (91% of all stillbirths)	11,085 (61%)	138 (34%)
a. Antepartum stillbirths			
Stillbirth category (%)			
Congenital	11	2	1
Infection	6	6	5
Fetal growth restrict/placental insuff	32	3	28
Other fetal specific	8	1	13
No stillbirth condition identified (maternal event identified)	43	88 (18)	54 (17)
Associated maternal condition (%)			
Abnormal labor or uterine rupture	–	0	9
Maternal hypertension	11	20	9
Maternal infection (e.g., syphilis)	0	4	1
Chorioamnionitis	5	2	3
Maternal diabetes	8	2	0
APH (abruptio placenta/previa)	15	6	9
Maternal preexisting (e.g., cardiac)	0	2	2
Spontaneous preterm labor	–	–	1
Other maternal specific	9	1	1
No maternal condition identified	62	62	65

(Continued)

Table 2.5 (Continued).

	SBR < 5 6 HIC datasets*	SBR 15–24 South Africa national	SBR > 25 Bangladesh rural hospital
Countries			
Stillbirth rate of input data	2–4	19	39
Year of input data	2008–2009	2008–2009	2007–2009
Intrapartum (total)	*30 (9% of all stillbirths)*	*7,083 (39%)*	*264 (66%)*
b. Intrapartum stillbirths			
Stillbirth category (%)			
Congenital	10	4	4
Infection	17	5	2
Fetal growth restrict/placental insuff	26	1	6
Other fetal specific	4	1	17
No stillbirth condition identified	43	88 (59)	71 (58)
(maternal event identified)			
Associated maternal condition (%)			
Abnormal labor or uterine rupture	10	29	44
Maternal hypertension	0	19	14
Maternal infection (e.g., syphilis)	0	3	0
Chorioamnionitis	17	2	2
Maternal diabetes	0	1	0
APH (abruptio placenta/previa)	10	17	15
Maternal preexisting (e.g., cardiac)	0	1	2
Spontaneous preterm labor	7	5	0
Other maternal specific	0	1	4
No maternal condition identified	56	22	19

The table does not present all conditions, since only one fetal and/or one maternal condition were registered as per ICD recommendations. If more conditions are identified using a complex system and more investigations are available then fewer than 20% of stillbirths have an unidentified condition.
*SBR < 5 includes data from Australia (Queensland Maternal Perinatal Quality Council), Canada (Alberta Perinatal Health Program), the Netherlands (Foundation Perinatal Audit), Norway (Norwegian Birth Registry), UK (CEMACE), USA (CDC).
Based on Ref. [2], used with permission.

are important [40] although stillbirth outcomes are understudied. More distal risk factors such as female literacy and socioeconomic status are also important and are discussed in other papers in this series [11, 41, 42]. Given the high proportion of stillbirths of unknown cause, cross tabulation with maternal condition is valuable, especially for antepartum stillbirths. For example, 20% of antepartum stillbirths, almost one-third of those with "unidentified cause," had mothers with hypertension, and an additional 1% had diabetes or other medical conditions. Given a prevalence of 5% for diabetes in pregnancy, it appears that diabetes may be being missed. More than half of the intrapartum stillbirths without an identified cause were associated with abnormal labor or maternal hypertension. Only 3% of early neonatal deaths were due to an unknown cause [2].

National perinatal audit data are relatively rare in middle-income countries, but can provide useful information to guide programs. The South African perinatal audit database covers over half of South Africa's births [43], and in 2008–2009 included 19,976 stillbirths (39% intrapartum) and 8,562 early neonatal deaths [44]. An important programmatic message from this audit is that 80% of early neonatal deaths, 75% of intrapartum stillbirths, and around half of antepartum stillbirths were associated with an identified maternal condition, and the most common conditions are those that also kill women. For example, hypertensive disease of pregnancy was associated with around 20% of intrapartum and 10% of antepartum stillbirths as well as 6% of neonatal deaths. Maternal conditions most often associated with perinatal death in South Africa are, in order, (1) obstructed labor, (2) hypertensive disease of pregnancy, (3) preterm labor, (4) antepartum hemorrhage, and (5) maternal infections and chorioamnionitis [2]. This information can be used to direct national and regional maternal, stillbirth, and newborn programs.

Stillbirth rate trends

Recent estimates of stillbirth trends from 1995 to 2008 suggest that the average global stillbirth rate has reduced by 1.1% annually, which is lower than the reduction for under-five mortality (2.3% per year) [7], and similar or less than that for maternal mortality reduction at 1.3% (1990–2008 [45]) or 2.1% (1990–2008, U.N. estimates [27]). The slowest decline in stillbirths is seen in sub-Saharan Africa with limited change in South Asia [2]. This mirrors slow progress in neonatal mortality rate reduction for these regions especially Africa, unsurprisingly as neonatal mortality rate was a predictor in the stillbirth rates model. In contrast, Eastern Asia has witnessed a 50% reduction in stillbirth rate driven by a large reduction in China. Latin America, Eurasia, and East Asia have made progress in reducing stillbirths as well as under-five and neonatal mortality. [2].

Assuming that trends from 1995 to 2008 remain constant, the global stillbirth rate in 2020 is projected to be around 16.7 per 1,000 with the slowest progress in sub-Saharan Africa. South Asia and sub-Saharan Africa would still have very high stillbirth rates (over 24 per 1,000) with 18 countries in these regions still in the highest stillbirth rate band (>25 per 1,000) and a widening gap between these regions and Latin America. If no new efforts are made to reduce stillbirths or to reduce unwanted pregnancies particularly for the poorest, rural families, then we estimate that in 2020 over 2 million stillbirths will still occur every year with potentially 90% in sub-Saharan Africa and South Asia [2].

Long-term trends in selected high-income countries, from 1750 to 2000, show that most of these countries had a stillbirth rate of around 30 per 1,000 in 1900 [12], which is similar to current stillbirth rates in many low-income countries (Figure 2.5). High-income countries experienced dramatic, two-third reductions in stillbirth rates between 1950 and 1975 related to infection prevention and treatment and improved obstetric care [12]. This was before the advent of more complex fetal surveillance and diagnostics and also coincided with reductions in maternal and neonatal mortality. Seventy years later, the lack of such progress to reduce all three of these pregnancy outcomes in low-income countries is not a knowledge gap but an action gap.

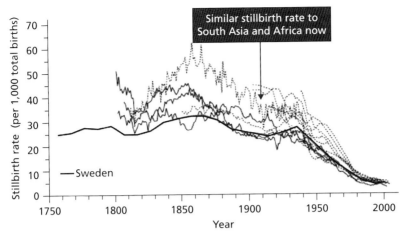

Figure 2.5 Long-term trends for stillbirth rates in 11 selected high-income countries (1750 to 2000). (Data from Ref. [12], used with author permission.)

Making stillbirth data count

Improving the estimation of stillbirth rates

In the absence of national vital registration data, exercises to estimate global third-trimester stillbirth rates are important for global policy and program prioritization. However, these do not address the urgent need for high quality, recent data at the country level. While there is no doubt that stillbirths are a large problem, much of our information depends on estimates and focuses on third-trimester stillbirths. Current estimates are likely to be an underestimate, particularly in the highest mortality settings where the data are sparse and many births occur outside facilities—60 million every year.

The quantity and quality of pregnancy outcome data including stillbirth data must be improved (Table 2.6) [26, 46]. Improving civil registration systems, adding specific perinatal death certificates, and advancing the ICD codes for stillbirth during ICD 11 planning are all critical especially for middle-income countries [47]. Since 98% of global third-trimester stillbirths occur in countries without reliable vital registration, reliance on other data sources is inevitable in the immediate future [26]. Hence the largest and most rapid increase in data available for low-income countries

now would be through inclusion of reliable stillbirth capture in existing household surveys [48]. These surveys especially Demographic Health Surveys (DHS) and UNICEF's Multiple Indicator Cluster Surveys (MICS) provide over 75% of global data for neonatal and child deaths. DHS relies on retrospective pregnancy histories over the last 5 years and are currently unreliable for stillbirth data, although some surveys do capture stillbirths more accurately [46]. Important evaluations include assessing the validity, reliability, and interview duration for a pregnancy history compared to live birth history, and assessing the validity and reliability of a truncated (e.g., last 5 years) history versus a complete pregnancy history. The expanded number of demographic surveillance sites currently in operation in various low-income countries, particularly the INDEPTH sites, offer opportunities to examine these issues comparing retrospective reporting of pregnancy outcomes against prospective, "gold standard" data, and also to assess time taken and cost [2, 46].

Causal data for stillbirths

National estimates of causes of stillbirths are urgently needed to guide programmatic priorities, as have been used for neonatal cause-of-death data [49]. In addition, improved understanding of maternal conditions associated with stillbirth and

Table 2.6 Improving national stillbirth data—what can be done now?.

		Stillbirth rate levels		80% of global stillbirths	
	Stillbirth rate (per 1,000 total births)	<5	5–14.9	15–24.9	>25
Counting stillbirth	Comparable definition	All countries to report ≥1,000 g or ≥28 weeks gestation definition for international comparison and intrapartum stillbirth rate for same stillbirth definition			
	Collecting stillbirth number and denominator (total births)	Vital registration (VR) using specific stillbirth/ neonatal death certificates with birthweight and gestational age		Ensure that large-scale retrospective household surveys include more reliable measure of stillbirth (e.g., pregnancy history as opposed to live birth history). Consider including stillbirth data in MICS surveys	
		Health facility surveillance with detailed dataset		Consider developing or modifying nationally representative sentinel surveillance sites for pregnancy, child and other health outcomes (prospective)	
		Cross-link VR and health facility databases to maximize capture		Improve vital registration systems and include stillbirths. Use specific stillbirth/neonatal death certificates for stillbirths/ neonatal deaths	
	Counting priority	22 weeks for high- and middle-income countries (lower limit improves capture of ≥1,000 g or ≥28 weeks)		Prioritize collection of representative data for ≥1,000 g or ≥28 week stillbirths and intrapartum stillbirths	
		Local definition (e.g., 18 or 20 weeks) can be used locally		Track urban/rural and other key disparities	
		Analyze to track disparities			
Counting for programmatic action	Comparable system mapping for antepartum and intrapartum stillbirths	Consensus on a limited number of programmatically relevant, comparable causal categories that can be distinguished through verbal autopsy, but can be further specified by clinical data in mid mortality settings and link to complex classification systems and ICD codes. Include both direct fetal/neonatal causal group and maternal condition so can cross tabulate			
	Collecting data on cause and maternal condition	Data collected through VR and facility surveillance		Develop or modify and scale up facility audit systems linking maternal, stillbirth, and neonatal data	Data collected through special verbal autopsy studies (e.g., after household surveys, or in sentinel surveillance sites)
		ICD 11 to improve codes for use for stillbirth and neonatal death			

(Continued)

Table 2.6 (Continued).

Stillbirth rate (per 1,000 total births)	Stillbirth rate levels			
			80% of global stillbirths	
	<5	5–14.9	15–24.9	>25
	Agreement on standard protocol for pathological investigation of stillbirth for high-income setting and adaptation for middle income Detailed causes, major focus on early stillbirth and growth restriction		Improve VR coverage and quality for cause attribution Increase laboratory and other capacities for investigation	Agree on standard verbal autopsy tool, case definitions, and hierarchical attribution, linked to neonatal deaths and maternal conditions/deaths Focus on simple programmatically relevant categories
Assessing and addressing avoidable factors		National audit systems, consider confidential enquiry Link to a committee accountable for follow-up actions	Develop or scale up facility audit systems linking maternal, stillbirth, and neonatal data and with accountability mechanisms for action	Start facility audit in large centers Consider special social autopsy studies examining delays at home, on the way and in facilities
Coverage data		Detailed assessment of coverage and quality of care, with analysis to target and reduce disparities	Improve data to track coverage of antenatal and intrapartum quality of care	Consider focus on few indicators initially focused on intrapartum care access and basic antenatal care (e.g., syphilis prevalence, identification, and treatment)

VR, vital registration; DHS, Demographic Health Surveys; MICS, Multiple Indicator Cluster Surveys.
Based on Ref. [2], used with permission.

neonatal death would provide a better foundation for prioritizing interventions to benefit all three outcomes (mother, fetus, and neonate).

Two steps are critical (Table 2.6). Firstly, we need consensus regarding a core list of programmatically relevant causes of stillbirth to cross tabulate with maternal conditions, and that can be distinguished through clinical observations, and through verbal autopsy [46]. Secondly, the quantity and quality of input data especially from low- and middle-income settings must be improved in order to generate enough data to develop national estimates. Current ICD 10 codes do not capture important categories for stillbirths and the revision of ICD now underway provides an important opportunity to improve these codes. In addition, those vital registration data that are collected by countries are not routinely sent to the United Nations or compiled, unlike data for neonatal and child deaths.

In low-income, high-mortality settings, verbal autopsy tools have been used to help distinguish fresh stillbirths from macerated ones as a recognized proxy for intrapartum stillbirth. Some studies have found this to correlate well with hospital data [37], but other studies suggest that verbal autopsy may systematically overestimate the intrapartum proportion [50]. Categories with enormous public health relevance, such as intrapartum events, may be identified through maternal history in verbal autopsy, but other significant causes, for example syphilis, cannot. Advances in verbal autopsy tools and hierarchies for neonatal cause-of-death classifications over the last 5 years have resulted in increased data and improved comparability of data for national estimates [28] and the same advances are required for stillbirth data.

Using data for action in reducing stillbirths

More reliable data are essential to enhance the effectiveness of health systems to monitor both implementation and impact. Ignoring stillbirths is also a missed opportunity to measure maternal and newborn program impact. Many of the 350,000 or so maternal deaths each year are associated with a lack of appropriate intrapartum care. Intrapartum

stillbirth rates have been proposed as a measure of quality of intrapartum care [51], and will remain a useful tool in settings where maternal deaths are relatively rare. A failure to record stillbirths may also obscure interpretation of changes in early neonatal mortality; given that a significant proportion of neonatal deaths may be misclassified as stillbirths [52]. When obstetric and immediate newborn care including resuscitation improve neonatal deaths are less likely to be misclassified as stillbirths [53]. Information for population-level planning requires a reliable denominator which is a challenge in the lowest-income countries where the majority of births are at home [48]. Novel approaches are needed to track pregnancies and outcomes accurately—for example, in sentinel surveillance sites as now used in India [54].

Given the huge differences in stillbirth rates by urban/rural residence, ethnicity, and socioeconomic metrics, data for action need to be as local and specific as possible for program design and tracking [2]. Even in high-income settings, there are major inequalities in stillbirth rates. For example, in the United Kingdom black women are twice as likely to have an intrapartum stillbirth as white women [11]. Stillbirth rates have been proposed as a sensitive marker of inequity and are closely linked to social deprivation and poor maternal health, as well as to service availability and quality [56].

Mortality audit is a potentially powerful process to monitor health care within health systems [57]. Some maternal audits currently include stillbirths and others could be adapted to incorporate stillbirth and neonatal data. There are multiple examples from high-income countries, for example, the United Kingdom's national enquires [58]. There are fewer examples from low- or middle-income countries, particularly of national-scale mortality audit. In South Africa as well as the Confidential Enquiry into maternal deaths, there is a voluntary, facility-based audit of stillbirths and neonatal death [44]. The last step in the audit process (accountability and action) is the most critical and is often lacking especially at national scale [43].

Another important data gap involves indicators for coverage of stillbirth interventions that should be provided during antenatal or intrapartum care.

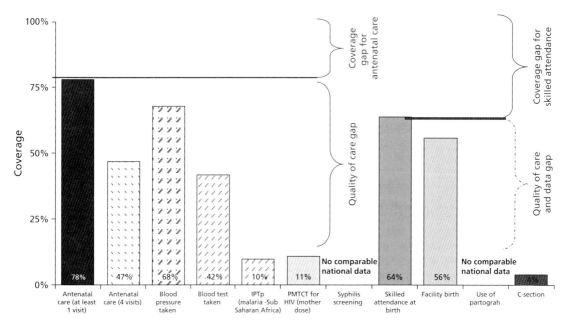

Figure 2.6 Coverage and quality gaps for antenatal care and skilled attendance in developing countries around the year 2008. (Adapted from Ref. [55] data on antenatal care and facility births from UN databases for 2008. Data on blood pressure test (50 countries), blood test (41 countries), and cesarean section (44 countries) based on DHS statcompiler http://www.statcompiler.com/.)

Many of the interventions that would markedly reduce stillbirths [41] are not routinely measured at population level in low- and middle-income countries (Figure 2.6). For women receiving care there are often missed opportunities between the contact point (e.g., antenatal care or facility birth) and the provision of high-impact, evidence-based interventions to prevent them experiencing a stillbirth. These include syphilis screening and treatment, or, for intrapartum care, monitoring of the fetal heart and timely instrumental or cesarean delivery, if indicated [21]. A few large-scale assessments of provider skills have been conducted, and data suggest that service provision may be less effective than expected due to deficiencies in quality of care. For example, an assessment of 1,358 skilled birth attendants in Nicaragua showed that the median competency score was only 52% for five key skills [59]. While these special studies, audits, and routine clinical data are useful for monitoring and addressing quality of care deficiencies, they are often restricted to specific program sites,

leaving program planners blind to the quality of care received by the majority of women and babies. Increasing data on coverage and quality for individual components within pregnancy and childbirth care is a crucial next step for effective population-level tracking of programs [60]. DHS includes a detailed module of antenatal care quality, and given the current overload in DHS survey questions, adding more would be challenging, but a process to review which are highest impact and reprioritize the questionnaire is becoming increasing urgent given global dependence on DHS for mortality and coverage data.

Research priorities for stillbirth epidemiology in low- and middle-income countries

A recent Pubmed review revealed that only 3% of publications on stillbirth relate to low-income countries [14], although these countries account for almost 90% of the burden. This 3/90 gap is more marked than the 10/90 gap that has been well described for global health research [61]. In addition there are missed opportunities to include stillbirth outcomes in other related studies. A recent analysis of Cochrane reviews showed that apart from trials on cervical cerclage, only a minority of pregnancy and intrapartum maternal intervention trails reported stillbirth or neonatal outcomes [9].

The Lancet Stillbirth Series reported an exercise to define and rank research questions regarding improved epidemiological measurement and understanding in low- and middle-income countries using a priority setting methodology developed by the Child Health and Nutrition Research Initiative (CHNRI) [62]. The CHNRI method has been used for a wide range of topics that include childhood pneumonia, diarrhea, neonatal infections, zinc supplementation, mental health, disability, primary health care, and also country-level priority setting in South Africa.

A total of 47 research questions were identified based on recent reviews [46, 63]. These questions were then refined and scored by 20 experts [62] for each of five domains: answerability, effectiveness, deliverability, disease burden reduction, and effect on equity [2]. The top-ranked questions for advancing epidemiological understanding of stillbirth were dominated by questions regarding stillbirths and infection, including the relationship between stillbirths and HIV, malaria, and syphilis [2]. This is logical since although interventions to address infection in pregnancy are feasible, there are limited high-quality data related to stillbirth as an outcome of maternal infections. For example, no high-quality studies of malaria in pregnancy were identified that reported stillbirths. Even syphilis, a disease that inspired the development of pathology, has low-quality data for prevalence in pregnancy and few studies with adjusted risk of stillbirth. Other high-ranked epidemiological gaps pertain to maternal anemia in pregnancy and to prediction of obstetric risk factors. Obstetric risk dominated the Development and Delivery research agendas for low- and middle-income countries [42], but was not so highly ranked in

the epidemiology lists suggesting that this was seen as an implementation research gap rather than an epidemiological understanding gap. Other themes in the top 10 ranked epidemiology options included understanding the interaction of infection and hypoxic injury.

The research options regarding epidemiological measurement advances tended to be ranked lower as the effect on disease burden reduction is scored lower. The top-ranked option for improving epidemiological measurement was a stillbirth causation mapping system. Ranked 2–5 were improved methods for counting stillbirths in surveys, demographic surveillance, and consistency in verbal autopsy, also linking in maternal conditions. More details of this exercise are published elsewhere [64].

Conclusion

Stillbirths remain invisible on programmatic and policy priorities and yet are highly relevant to current investments for maternal and neonatal health, especially for care at the time of birth when a combined 2 million deaths occur. Not counting stillbirths, and especially the 1.2 million occurring during labor, may result in missed program impact and misinterpretation [51]. There are now more than enough data to substantiate the need for attention and action to reduce this large burden of 2.65 million stillbirths in the last 12 weeks of pregnancy [26], linked to around 3 million early neonatal deaths during the first week of life and 350,000 maternal deaths (Box 2.1) [8].

However, although there is ample evidence here to show that action is required now, current stillbirth data are far from adequate to track trends or program effectiveness. A new focus is needed on *all* deaths around the time of birth (not just deaths among liveborn children). Having one unified set of global stillbirth estimates is an important short-term step, but better counting of stillbirths is the real priority [34]. In the medium- to longer-term improvements in vital registration, more specific ICD codes and routine reporting and collation of stillbirth data are crucial, and require leadership within the United Nations. Immediate advances in global data availability and quality could be achieved through surveys but has not been given attention in recent revisions of the main global survey tools. Estimates for stillbirth causation are hampered by noncomparable classification systems, yet are necessary to guide programmatic priorities across contexts with varying data complexity including using verbal autopsy. Facility-based data especially collected through national audit systems is another important source of data,

especially for improving quality of care but need to include stillbirths, be used at scale and result in change. Stillbirth research investment even in rich countries is limited compared to burden, and almost entirely lacking in low-income countries, even within studies examining maternal or neonatal outcomes [14, 65].

Millions of families experience stillbirth and yet remain uncounted, unsupported, and the solutions understudied. The case could not be clearer—both for better counting and also for action to make stillbirths count in programmatic action.

Box 2.1 Data-based priorities for the reduction of stillbirths

Where? At least 2.65 million stillbirths are estimated to occur each year, 98% in low- and middle-income countries, and 55% in rural families in sub-Saharan Africa and South Asia where skilled attendance and especially cesarean sections are much lower than for urban births. The stillbirth rate varies from 2.0 per 1,000 total births in Finland to more than 40 in Nigeria and Pakistan.

When? Globally around 1.2 million stillbirths are estimated to occur during labor (intrapartum) with higher rates in low-income countries where almost a half of stillbirths are term intrapartum babies, viable with better care during birth. Antepartum stillbirths (1.45 million) require improved care during pregnancy, targeting maternal infections, hypertension, and poor fetal growth.

Why? National and global estimates for stillbirth causation and linked maternal conditions are impeded by >35 classifications systems. Despite limitations in the available data, the "big five" to target for global stillbirth reduction are clear: (1) childbirth complications, (2) maternal infections, (3) maternal conditions especially hypertension, (4) fetal growth restriction, and (5) congenital abnormalities.

Improving the data? The majority of the world's stillbirths occur in countries without adequate vital registration. Urgent focus is needed to increase the quality of pregnancy outcome data collected through alternative data sources especially household surveys—to count stillbirths, estimate causes (using a simple, programmatic classification that can be used with verbal autopsy), and also improve coverage and tracking data for key maternal, neonatal, and stillbirth interventions.

Progress? The average annual rate of reduction has been slower for stillbirths (estimated 1.1% between 1995 and 2008) than maternal and child mortality reduction. Without an acceleration of current progress, by 2020 over 90% of all stillbirths will be in South Asia and sub-Saharan Africa.

Adapted from Ref. [2].

Acknowledgments

We are grateful to The Lancet for allowing use of material from The Lancet stillbirth series and we thank our other coauthors on *The Lancet* Stillbirth Series epidemiology paper (Louise Day, Jason Gardosi, and Rajesh Kumar), and *The Lancet* Stillbirth Series steering team (Zulfiqar Bhutta, Frederik Froen, Vicki Flenady, Robert Goldenberg, Monir Islam, and Joy Lawn) for contributions during the development of the series. Appreciation to Mikkel Oestergaard and Florence Rusciano at WHO for assistance with Figure 2.3. Joy Lawn is funded by the Bill & Melinda Gates Foundation via Saving Newborn Lives/Save the Children-US. Cynthia Stanton was partially funded by the Global Alliance for the Prevention of Prematurity and Stillbirths (www.gappsseattle.org). Some of the work was funded through a grant from the Bill & Melinda Gates Foundation to the International Stillbirth Alliance secretariat for this series. The views expressed herein are solely those of the authors.

References

1. Shiffman J. Generating political priority for safe motherhood. Afr J Reprod Health 2004;8(3):6–10.
2. Lawn JE, Blencowe H, Pattinson R, et al, for *The Lancet's* Stillbirths Series steering committee. Stillbirths: Where? When? Why? How to make the data count? *Lancet* 2011; published online April 14. DOI:10.1016/S0140-6736(10)62187-3.

3. Rohde J, Cousens S, Chopra M, et al. 30 years after Alma-Ata: has primary health care worked in countries? Lancet 2008;372(9642):950–61.

4. Ronsmans C, Graham WJ. Maternal mortality: who, when, where, and why. Lancet 2006;368(9542):1189–200.

5. Shiffman J. Issue attention in global health: the case of newborn survival. Lancet 2010;375(9730):2045–9.

6. Frøen JF, Cacciatore J, McClure EM, et al. Stillbirths: Why they matter. Lancet - in press.

7. Rajaratnam JK, Marcus JR, Flaxman AD, et al. Neonatal, postneonatal, childhood, and under-5 mortality for 187 countries, 1970–2010: a systematic analysis of progress towards Millennium Development Goal 4. Lancet 2010;375(9730):1988–2008.

8. Lawn JE, Cousens S, Zupan J. 4 million neonatal deaths: when? where? why? Lancet 2005;365(9462):891–900.

9. Lawn JE, Yakoob MY, Haws RA, et al. 3.2 million stillbirths: epidemiology and overview of the evidence review. BMC Pregnancy Childbirth 2009;9(Suppl. 1):S2.

10. Kramer MS, Liu S, Luo Z, et al. Analysis of perinatal mortality and its components: time for a change? Am J Epidemiol 2002;156(6):493–7.

11. Flenady V, Middleton P, Smith G. Reducing avoidable stillbirths in high income countries. Lancet - in press.

12. Woods R. Long-term trends in fetal mortality: implications for developing countries. Bull World Health Organ 2008;86(6):460–6.

13. WHO. International statistical classification of diseases and realted health problems: tenth revision, Volume 2: Instruction manual 1, 2. Geneva: WHO; 1993.

14. Froen JF, Gordijn SJ, Abdel-Aleem H, et al. Making stillbirths count, making numbers talk—issues in data collection for stillbirths. BMC Pregnancy Childbirth 2009;9:58.

15. Yasmin S, Osrin D, Paul E, Costello A. Neonatal mortality of low-birth-weight infants in Bangladesh. Bull World Health Organ 2001;79(7):608–14.

16. Lawn JE, Mwansa-Kambafwile J, Horta BL, et al. 'Kangaroo mother care' to prevent neonatal deaths due to preterm birth complications. Int J Epidemiol 2010;39(Suppl. 1):i144–54.

17. Costeloe K. EPICure: facts and figures: why preterm labour should be treated. BJOG 2006;113(Suppl. 3):10–12.

18. Critical care decisions in fetal and neonatal medicine: ethical issues. Nuffield Council on Bioethics; 2006. http://www.nuffieldbioethics.org/neonatal-medicine.

19. Gissler M, Mohangoo AD, Blondel B, et al. Perinatal health monitoring in Europe: results from the EURO-PERISTAT project. Inform Health Soc Care 2010;35(2):64–79.

20. Goldenberg RL, McClure EM. Reducing intrapartum stillbirths and intrapartum-related neonatal deaths. Int J Gynaecol Obstet 2009;107(Suppl. 1):S1–3.

21. Edouard L. The epidemiology of perinatal mortality. World Health Stat Q 1985;38(3):289–301.

22. WHO. Perinatal mortality: a listing of available information. Report No.: WHO/FRH/MSM/96.7. Geneva, Switzerland: WHO; 1996.

23. Say L, Donner A, Gulmezoglu AM, et al. The prevalence of stillbirths: a systematic review. Reprod Health 2006;3:1.

24. Stanton C, Lawn JE, Rahman H, et al. Stillbirth rates: delivering estimates in 190 countries. Lancet 2006;367(9521):1487–94.

25. WHO. Perinatal and neonatal mortality for the year 2000: country, regional and global estimates. Geneva: WHO; 2006.

26. Cousens S, Blencowe H, Stanton C, Chou D, Ahmed S, Steinhardt L, et al. National, regional and global estimates of stillbirth rates in 2009 with trends since 1995. Lancet (in press).

27. World Health Organization, UNICEF UNFPA and the World Bank. Trends in maternal mortality: 1990 to 2008; 2010. http://www.who.int/reproductive-health/publications/monitoring/9789241500265/en/index.html.

28. Black RE, Cousens S, Johnson HL, et al. Global, regional, and national causes of child mortality in 2008: a systematic analysis. Lancet 2010;375(9730):1969–87.

29. Countdown. Countdown to 2015 decade report (2000–2010): taking stock of maternal, newborn and child survival. Geneva: WHO; 2010.

30. Lawn JE, Lee AC, Kinney M, et al. Two million intrapartum-related stillbirths and neonatal deaths: where, why, and what can be done? Int J Gynaecol Obstet 2009;107(Suppl. 1):S5–18, 19.

31. Lawn J, Shibuya K, Stein C. No cry at birth: global estimates of intrapartum stillbirths and intrapartum-related neonatal deaths. Bull World Health Organ 2005;83(6):409–17.

32. Li XF, Fortney JA, Kotelchuck M, Glover LH. The postpartum period: the key to maternal mortality. Int J Gynaecol Obstet 1996;54(1):1–10.

33. Lawn J, Kerber K, Enweronu-Laryea C, Cousens S. 3.6 Million Neonatal Deaths – What is progressing and what is not? Seminars in Perinatology. 2010;34(6):371–86.

34. Gardosi J, Kady SM, McGeown P, et al. Classification of stillbirth by relevant condition at death (ReCoDe): population based cohort study. BMJ 2005;331(7525):1113–17.

35. Flenady V, Froen JF, Pinar H, et al. An evaluation of classification systems for stillbirth. BMC Pregnancy Childbirth 2009;9:24.

36. Vergani P, Cozzolino S, Pozzi E, et al. Identifying the causes of stillbirth: a comparison of four classification systems. Am J Obstet Gynecol 2008;199(3):319e1–4.

37. Edmond KM, Quigley MA, Zandoh C, et al. Diagnostic accuracy of verbal autopsies in ascertaining the causes of stillbirths and neonatal deaths in rural Ghana. Paediatr Perinat Epidemiol 2008;22(5):417–29.

38. Petersson K, Bremme K, Bottinga R, et al. Diagnostic evaluation of intrauterine fetal deaths in Stockholm 1998–99. Acta Obstet Gynecol Scand 2002;81(4):284–92.

39. Ticconi C, Mapfumo M, Dorrucci M, et al. Effect of maternal HIV and malaria infection on pregnancy and perinatal outcome in Zimbabwe. J Acquir Immune Defic Syndr 2003;34(3):289–94.

40. Goldenberg RL, McClure EM, Saleem S, Reddy UM. Infection-related stillbirths. Lancet 2010;375(9724):1482–90.

41. Bhutta Z. What will it take to reduce the burden of stillbirths in developing countries? Lancet (in press).

42. Pattinson R, Kerber K, Buchmann E, et al. Stillbirths: how can health systems deliver for mothers and babies? Lancet - in press.

43. Pattinson R, Kerber K, Waiswa P, et al. Perinatal mortality audit: counting, accountability, and overcoming challenges in scaling up in low- and middle-income countries. Int J Gynaecol Obstet 2009;107(Suppl. 1):S113–21, S121–2.

44. Saving Babies 2008–2009: seventh perinatal care survey of South Africa (in press).

45. Hogan MC, Foreman KJ, Naghavi M, et al. Maternal mortality for 181 countries, 1980–2008: a systematic analysis of progress towards Millennium Development Goal 5. Lancet 2010;375(9726):1609–23.

46. Lawn JE, Gravett MG, Nunes TM, et al. Global report on preterm birth and stillbirth (1 of 7): definitions, description of the burden and opportunities to improve data. BMC Pregnancy Childbirth 2010;10(Suppl. 1):S1.

47. AbouZahr C, Cleland J, Coullare F, et al. The way forward. Lancet 2007;370(9601):1791–9.

48. Hill K, Lopez AD, Shibuya K, Jha P. Interim measures for meeting needs for health sector data: births, deaths, and causes of death. Lancet. 2007 Oct 26;370(9600):1726–35.

49. Lawn JE, Wilczynska-Ketende K, Cousens SN. Estimating the causes of 4 million neonatal deaths in the year 2000. Int J Epidemiol 2006;35(3):706–18.

50. Aggarwal, A., V. Jain, et al. (2010). "Validity of verbal autopsy for ascertaining the causes of stillbirth." Bull World Health Organ http://www.who.int/bulletin/online_first/10-076828.pdf.

51. Fauveau V. New indicator of quality of emergency obstetric and newborn care. Lancet 2007;370(9595):1310.

52. Spector JM, Daga S. Preventing those so-called stillbirths. Bull World Health Organ 2008;86(4):315–16.

53. Barson AJ, Tasker M, Lieberman BA, Hillier VF. Impact of improved perinatal care on the causes of death. Arch Dis Child 1984;59(3):199–207.

54. Jha P, Gajalakshmi V, Gupta PC, et al. Prospective study of one million deaths in India: rationale, design, and validation results. PLoS Med 2006;3(2):e18.

55. Lawn JE, Kerker KJ. Opportunities for Africa's newborns. Cape Town: Save the Children and PMNCH; 2006. http://www.healthynewbornnetwork.org/ resource/opportunities-africas-newborns.

56. Parsons L, Duley L, Alberman E. Socio-economic and ethnic factors in stillbirth and neonatal mortality in the NE Thames Regional Health Authority (NETRHA) 1983. Br J Obstet Gynaecol 1990;97(3):237–44.

57. Shankar A, Bartlett L, Fauveau V, et al. Delivery of MDG 5 by active management with data. Lancet 2008;371(9620):1223–4.

58. Centre for Maternal and Child Enquiries (CMACE). Perinatal mortality 2008. London: CMACE; 2010. http://www.cmace.org.uk/getattachment/4a8ae5ec-3e24-469c-8aba-260c3db4a729/Perinatal-Mortality-2008.aspx.

59. Harvey SA, Blandon YC, McCaw-Binns A, et al. Are skilled birth attendants really skilled? A measurement method, some disturbing results and a potential way forward. Bull World Health Organ 2007;85(10):783–90.

60. Bryce J, Daelmans B, Dwivedi A, et al. Countdown to 2015 for maternal, newborn, and child survival: the 2008 report on tracking coverage of interventions. Lancet 2008;371(9620):1247–58.

61. Doyal L. Gender and the 10/90 gap in health research. Bull World Health Organ 2004;82(3):162.

62. Rudan I, Gibson J, Kapiriri L, et al. Setting priorities in global child health research investments: assessment of principles and practice. Croat Med J 2007; 48(5):595–604.

63. Global Alliance to Prevent Prematurity and Stillbirth. Global report on preterm birth & stillbirth: the foundation for innovative solutions and improved outcomes. BMC Pregnancy Childbirth 2010;10:S1.

64. Stillbirth research consortium. A global research agenda to reduce stillbirth. 2010.

65. Goldenberg RL, McClure EM, Bhutta ZA, et al. Stillbirths: the vision for 2020. Lancet - in press.

CHAPTER 3

Classification of Stillbirths

Uma M. Reddy, MD, MPH and Marian Willinger, PhD
Eunice Kennedy Shriver National Institute of Child Health and Human Development,
National Institutes of Health, Bethesda, MD, USA

Although there will always be a degree of uncertainty about whether a particular stillbirth was actually caused by a certain condition, the assignment of a cause of death is important to develop interventions for stillbirth prevention and to monitor their impact. There are currently at least 35 classification systems of stillbirth, many of which have been developed for different reasons. They have differing categories for classifying cause, numerous definitions for relevant conditions, and varying levels of complexity. As a result, no single system is uniformly accepted. Furthermore, the challenge for all classification systems is to not only list risk factors for stillbirth, but also to estimate the degree of certainty that the stillbirth can be ascribed to these factors.

Experts agree that the optimal classification system would identify the pathophysiological entity initiating the chain of events that irreversibly lead to death [1]. Such classification is complex due to the multiple pathophysiological processes encountered in the mother, fetus and placenta, and their interaction. Since the integrity of the classification is based on available pathologic, clinical, and diagnostic data, it is clear that a complete stillbirth evaluation should be performed. Due to lack of sufficient knowledge about disease states and normal fetal physiology, there will be a degree of uncertainty regarding whether a specific condition was actually the cause of the stillbirth.

There are many potential contributing factors as well as multiple disciplines involved in determining the cause of death which add to the complexity. Criteria that can be used to categorize a particular condition as a cause of stillbirth should consider the following principles [1]:

1. There is epidemiologic data demonstrating an excess of stillbirth associated with the condition.

2. There is biologic plausibility that the condition causes stillbirth.

3. The condition is either rarely seen in association with live births or when seen in live births, results in a significant increase in neonatal death.

4. A dose–response relationship exists so that the greater the "dose" of the condition, the greater the likelihood of fetal death.

5. The condition is associated with evidence of fetal compromise.

6. The stillbirth would likely not have occurred if that condition had not been present, that is, lethality.

For optimal utility, classification systems should use uniform definitions, clear guidelines, and a well-defined structure to allow for an unambiguous assignment of a cause of death if appropriate. Ideally, there should be good interrater agreement and classification assignments should be reproducible. In addition, the ability to amend a system to allow for future research developments without altering the basic structure is useful. The remainder of this chapter will discuss some of the stillbirth classification systems used worldwide, focusing on their purpose, principles used to classify stillbirths, and differences between the systems.

Revised Aberdeen classification system

The Aberdeen classification system was developed to analyze the obstetrical factors that lie behind perinatal deaths in Scotland [2]. After 30 years of use in Scotland and England, it was recognized that regional differences in the way the cases were being classified impacted the ability to make valid temporal or regional comparisons. In 1986, Cole and colleagues [3] published updated guidelines that are referred to as the revised Aberdeen classification and are still being used worldwide.

The purpose of this system is to aid in the prevention of perinatal deaths by identifying the factor that probably initiated the events leading to death. The list of causes is hierarchical in that the presence of first cause on the list (Table 3.1, Aberdeen) takes precedence over the next one. The category of causes in order are: (1) lethal or severe congenital defect/malformation; (2) isoimmunization; (3) preeclampsia; (4) antepartum hemorrhage after 20 weeks, excluding hemorrhage due to preeclampsia; (5) mechanical to include uterine rupture, birth trauma, or intrapartum asphyxia; (6) maternal disorder to include trauma, preexisting disease, maternal infection; (7) miscellaneous fetal and neonatal conditions; (8) unexplained according to obstetric history subclassified into 2,500 g or more and <2,500 g; (9) unclassifiable because little is known about the pregnancy or delivery.

If using this order does not identify the initiating factor in the clinician's judgment, then the hierarchy should not be applied. In cases that are difficult to classify the rule applied is that the average experienced clinician agrees that the death would be prevented if the cause under consideration was eliminated.

Wigglesworth classification

There was a need to have a fetal and neonatal classification to be used in tandem with the Aberdeen obstetric classification. Wigglesworth [4] developed a classification scheme that would have as the aim the reduction of perinatal deaths by selecting elements that had the possibility of being influenced by clinical management. The scheme relied on gestational age and time of death. The first step was to group the deaths by birthweight categories. The second part of the classification is to group by causes or modes of death that are "as far as possible mutually exclusive, easy to recognize, and carry implications for perinatal care." Similar to the Aberdeen classification, the scheme is hierarchical.

After implementation of the scheme, Wigglesworth and colleagues [5, 6] revised the classification system to incorporate the autopsy or imaging findings when available but does not rely on them. The modifications, including a decision tree, were made based on the use of clinical information, macroscopic examination at autopsy, and histological, microbiological, and chromosome analysis, and an assessment of interobserver reliability. The cause of death categories are: (1) congenital anomaly; (2) unexplained death prior to the onset of labor; (3) death from intrapartum events that covers any baby that would have survived if not for a catastrophe in labor to include deaths from anoxia, asphyxia, or trauma; (4) immaturity (live births only); (5) specific conditions, other than above to include deaths due to infection or isoimmunization.

Centre for Maternal and Child Enquiries

The United Kingdom's Centre for Maternal and Child Enquiries (CMACE), formerly the Confidential Enquiry into Maternal and Child Health (CEMACH), has been using "extended Wigglesworth" along with the Aberdeen to classify perinatal deaths [7]. Category 5 above becomes categories 5–8 as follows: (5) infection, maternal, fetal, or infant; (6) other specific causes, fetal, or infant; (7) accident or nonintrapartum trauma; (8) sudden infant death, cause unknown (Table 3.2, extended Wigglesworth).

CEMACH and its predecessor, the Confidential Enquiry into Stillbirths and Deaths in Infancy

Table 3.1 Classifying perinatal death: fetal and neonatal factors.

Classification of Butler Bonham (1963)	Current classification	Suggested subclassification*	Category
Congenital malformation	Congenital anomaly	Chromosomal defect	1
		Inborn error of metabolism	2
		Neural tube defect	3
		Congenital heart disease	4
		Renal abnormality	5
		Other malformation	6
Isoimmunization	Isoimmunization	–	7
Antepartum death with autopsy evidence of anoxia	Antepartum asphyxia	–	8
Antepartum death without autopsy evidence of anoxia			
Intrapartum death with autopsy evidence of anoxia	Intrapartum asphyxia	–	9
Intrapartum death with autopsy evidence of anoxia and trauma			
Intrapartum death without autopsy evidence of anoxia or trauma			
Cerebral birth trauma	Birth trauma	–	10
Neonatal death (no autopsy abnormality)	Pulmonary immaturity	–	11
Hyaline membrane	Hyaline membrane disease (HMD)	HMD	12
		HMD with IVH	13
		HMD with infection	14
Intraventricular hemorrhage (IVH)	Intracranial hemorrhage	Intraventricular hemorrhage	15
		Other intracranial bleeding	16
Pulmonary infection	Infection	Necrotizing enterocolitis	17
		Antepartum infection	18
		Intrapartum infection	19
Extrapulmonary infection		Postpartum infection	20
Massive pulmonary hemorrhage Miscellaneous	Miscellaneous	–	21
No necropsy	–	–	–
–	Unclassified or unknown	Cot death	22
		Unattended delivery	23
		Undocumented or unclassified	24

Reproduced from Ref. [3], with permission from Wiley-Blackwell.
*Further detailed subclassification is rendered much easier if each congenital anomaly and each factor contributing to the death is separately coded using the ICD system.

(CESDI), found that a 76.1% of the stillbirths were unexplained with the extended Wigglesworth classification and 74.4% of these unexplained stillbirths remained unexplained after applying the Aberdeen classification for associated obstetric factors [7].

Their classification system was revised to reduce the proportion of deaths to an unexplained or nonspecific cause, while addressing the goal of identifying the condition initiating the series of events that lead to the death, and the resources

Table 3.2 Causes of stillbirths using the Wigglesworth and obstetric classifications; England, Wales, Northern Ireland, Channel Islands, and the Isle of Man: 2007.

Wigglesworth classification	Obstetric classification	Proportions* of stillbirths within each Wigglesworth category
Congenital defect/malformation (lethal or severe)	Congenital anomaly	98.5
	Preeclampsia	0.4
	Maternal disorder	0.8
	Miscellaneous	0.4
Unexplained antepartum fetal death	Congenital anomaly	0.1
	Preeclampsia	4.9
	Antepartum hemorrhage	10.7
	Mechanical	1.5
	Maternal disorder	8.1
	Miscellaneous	0.2
	Unexplained	74.4
Death from intrapartum "asphyxia," "anoxia," or "trauma"	Preeclampsia	2.4
	Antepartum hemorrhage	22.0
	Mechanical	13.7
	Maternal disorder	7.8
	Miscellaneous	0.5
	Unexplained	53.7
Infection	Antepartum hemorrhage	0.9
	Maternal disorder	93.8
	Miscellaneous	0.9
	Unexplained	4.4
Other specific causes	Congenital anomaly	1.3
	Isoimmunization	2.5
	Preeclampsia	1.9
	Antepartum hemorrhage	12.6
	Mechanical	2.5
	Maternal disorder	8.2
	Miscellaneous	66.0
	Unexplained	5.0
Accident or nonintrapartum causes	Antepartum hemorrhage	40.0
	Maternal disorder	40.0
	Unexplained	20.0
Unclassifiable	Antepartum hemorrhage	20.0
	Maternal disorder	10.0
	Unexplained	70.0

Ref. [7].
*Percentages are calculated removing not known.

available [8]. A new Perinatal Death Notification form was also developed to incorporate the new system. The major changes are adding two categories that would have previously been labeled unexplained: specific placental conditions and intrauterine growth restriction (IUGR). It is recognized that postmortem and placental pathology have become more important with the addition of these categories. IUGR is used where a fetus has been clinically recognized as having poor

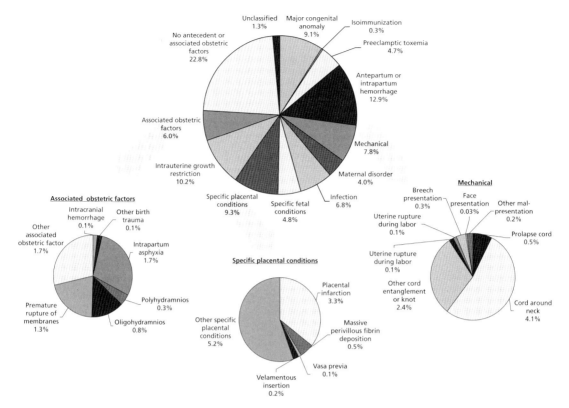

Figure 3.1 Primary cause/associated factor for stillbirths using the CMACE maternal and fetal classification; England, Wales, Northern Ireland, and the Crown Dependencies: 2008 (excluding terminations of pregnancy).

intrauterine growth, for example, a fetus on the 97th percentile dropping to 50th. In their 2008 report, the percentage of unexplained stillbirths using this system was 23%. The major causes/associated factors are antepartum or intrapartum hemorrhage (12.9%), IUGR (10.2%), specific placental conditions (9.3%), and major congenital anomalies (9.1%) (Figure 3.1, CMACE 2010).

Perinatal Society of Australia and New Zealand Perinatal Death Classification

At the 2000 Perinatal Society of Australia and New Zealand (PSANZ) annual conference, a process was initiated to develop a classification scheme that was acceptable on a national level in Australia, where states used different systems, and in New Zealand [9]. The Australian and New Zealand Antecedent Classification of Perinatal Mortality (ANZACPM) was renamed Perinatal Society of Australia and New Zealand Perinatal Death Classification (PSANZ-PDC) in 2003. A neonatal death classification system (PSANZ-NDC) was also developed at that time.

PSANZ-PDC is similar to Aberdeen in that it is based on antecedent obstetric factors and seeks to identify the factor that initiated the sequence of events leading to the death. It is based on clinical and autopsy findings, including placental pathology. It is mainly hierarchical in descending order with some qualifications that are delineated in the guidelines. Each main group contains subcategories. The main groups are: (1) congenital abnormality (structural, functional, or chromosomal) that is considered to have made a major contribution; (2) perinatal infection; (3) hypertension when it is considered the initiating event, including abruption attributed to the hypertensive disorder; (4) antepartum hemorrhage; (5) maternal conditions other than hypertensive disorders or renal disease presenting as hypertension; (6) specific perinatal conditions; (7) hypoxic peripartum death including deaths from acute or chronic hypoxia of normally formed babies; (8) fetal growth restriction less than 10th percentile using Australian birthweight percentiles by gestational age; (9) spontaneous preterm (membranes ruptured before 24 weeks showing evidence of infection would be in category 2 above); (10) unexplained antepartum death; (11) no obstetric antecedent. The PSANZ web site provides guidelines for the use of the classification system (http://www.psanzpnmsig.org/).

TULIP

Named for a well-known Dutch association, the pathophysiologically based TULIP classification system aims to define the underlying cause and mechanism of perinatal mortality based on clinical and pathological findings for the purpose of counseling and prevention [10]. The system was designed to include late fetal losses, stillbirths, early neonatal deaths, late neonatal deaths, and perinatally related infant deaths.

A classification consisting of groups of cause and mechanism of death was devised by a panel through the causal analysis of the events related to 109 perinatally related deaths in a tertiary referral teaching hospital during a 1-year period. Cause of death was defined as the initial, demonstrable pathophysiological entity initiating the chain of events that irreversibly led to death. The classification consists of six main causes with subclassifications: (1) congenital anomaly (chromosomal, syndrome, and single- or multiple-organ system), (2) placenta (placental bed, placental pathology, umbilical cord complication, and not otherwise specified [NOS]), (3) prematurity (preterm prelabor rupture of membranes, preterm labor, cervical

dysfunction, iatrogenic, and NOS), (4) infection (transplacental, ascending, neonatal, and NOS), (5) other (fetal hydrops of unknown origin, maternal disease, trauma, and out of the ordinary), and (6) unknown. Based on 411 perinatally related deaths using the TULIP system, the cause of death was as follows: congenital anomalies (35%), placenta (27%), prematurity (23%), infection (1%), other (3%), and unknown (11%) (Table 3.3). Out of the unknown cases 64% were missing important information.

The mechanism of death was defined as organ failure that is not compatible with life, initiated by the cause of death that has directly led to death. Based on the same 411 cases, the mechanism of death was divided into the following six categories: cardio/circulatory insufficiency (11%), multi-organ failure (7%), respiratory insufficiency (32%), cerebral insufficiency (2%), placental insufficiency (30%), and unknown (19%).

ReCoDe

The ReCoDe classification system (relevant condition at death) was developed to define relevant clinical categories for stillbirth on a dataset of stillbirths in the West Midlands. A total of 2625 stillbirths from 1997 to 2003 were classified [11]. This system (Box 3.1) seeks to identify the relevant condition at the time of death in utero. The system aims to establish what went wrong and not necessarily why (as the classification does not have to rely on finding an underlying cause, more than one category can be coded if the information is available). The hierarchy starts from conditions affecting the fetus and moves outward in simple anatomical groups, which are subdivided into pathophysiological conditions; the primary condition should be the first category on the list that is applicable to stillbirth case.

Fetal growth restriction is included as the last category in group A: a fetus below the 10th customized percentile would be assigned this classification only if no other specific fetal conditions were present. Customized percentiles were calculated using the gestation-related optimal weight software GROW,

Table 3.3 TULIP system.

Cause of death	n (% of total)	Subclassification	
1. Congenital anomaly	142 (35)	1. Chromosomal defect	1. Numerical
			2. Structural
			3. Microdeletion/uniparental disomy
		2. Syndrome	1. Monogenic
			2. Other
		3. Central nervous system	
		4. Heart and circulatory system	
		5. Respiratory system	
		6. Digestive system	
		7. Urogenital system	
		8. Musculoskeletal system	
		9. Endocrine/metabolic system	
		10. Neoplasm	
		11. Other	1. Single organ
			2. Multiple organ
2. Placenta	111 (27)	1. Placental bed pathology	
		2. Placental pathology	1. Development
			2. Parenchyma
			3. Localization
		3. Umbilical cord complication	
		4. NOS	
3. Prematurity/immaturity	95 (23)	1. Preterm Prelabor Rupture of Membranes (PPROM)	
		2. Preterm labor	
		3. Cervical dysfunction	
		4. Iatrogenous	
		5. NOS	
4. Infection	6 (1)	1. Transplacental	
		2. Ascending	
		3. Neonatal	
		4. NOS	
5. Other	13 (3)	1. Fetal hydrops of unknown origin	
		2. Maternal disease	
		3. Trauma	1. Maternal
			2. Fetal
		4. Out of the ordinary	
6. Unknown	44 (11)	1. Despite thorough investigation	
		2. Important information missing	
Total	411		

version 4.6 (www.gestation.net), which calculates the fetal growth potential by adjusting for fetal gender and constitutional characteristics known at the beginning of pregnancy such as maternal height and weight, parity, and ethnic origin. The actual birthweight is then compared with the optimal weight predicted for the corresponding gestation, and a "customized percentile" is calculated. This method aims to improve the distinction between constitutional and pathological smallness for gestational age. Customized smallness for gestational age is then defined as fetal growth restriction.

Box 3.1 ReCoDe classification system

Classification system according to relevant condition at death (ReCoDe)

Group A: Fetus
1. Lethal congenital anomaly
2. Infection
   2.1 Chronic
   2.2 Acute
3. Nonimmune hydrops
4. Isoimmunization
5. Fetomaternal hemorrhage
6. Twin–twin transfusion
7. Fetal growth restriction*

Group B: Umbilical cord
1. Prolapse
2. Constricting loop or knot†
3. Velamentous insertion
4. Other

Group C: Placenta
1. Abruptio
2. Previa
3. Vasa previa
4. Other "placental insufficiency"‡
5. Other

Group D: Amniotic fluid
1. Chorioamnionitis
2. Oligohydramnios†
3. Polyhydramnios†
4. Other

Group E: Uterus
1. Rupture
2. Uterine anomalies
3. Other

Group F: Mother
1. Diabetes
2. Thyroid diseases
3. Essential hypertension
4. Hypertensive diseases in pregnancy
5. Lupus or antiphospholipid syndrome
6. Cholestasis
7. Drug misuse
8. Other

Group G: Intrapartum
1. Asphyxia
2. Birth trauma

Group H: Trauma
1. External
2. Iatrogenic

Group I: Unclassified
1. No relevant condition identified
2. No information available

*<10th customized weight for gestational age centile.
†If severe enough to be considered relevant.
‡Histological diagnosis.

The distribution of ReCoDe categories in the 2,625 stillbirths is seen in Figure 3.2. By the ReCoDe classification, the most common condition was fetal growth restriction (43.0%). 43.7% of all stillbirths were counted in more than one category of relevant conditions. 15.2% of stillbirths remained unclassified with "no relevant condition identified."

The Stockholm classification of stillbirth

The Stockholm classification system of stillbirth identifies the underlying cause of death, that is, the factor that initiated the chain of events leading to death [12]. This system consists of 17 diagnostic categories of underlying conditions related to stillbirth (primary diagnoses) and associated factors which may have contributed to the death (associated diagnoses). The diagnoses are subdivided into definite, probable, and possible causes of death. The grading system is based on the fact that in many cases conditions are identified that can be related to stillbirth, but the findings individually have a relatively weak association or are too few to result in a definite cause of death. In this classification, to overcome this problem, levels of certainty/probability are ascribed to each diagnosis to reflect the status of available evidence and clinical experience. The assessment of cause of death is based on an extensive clinical and laboratory investigation protocol and assumes a high frequency of postmortems and placental examinations.

An evaluation of 382 cases of stillbirth from 22 completed weeks in Stockholm, Sweden, during 2002–2005 using this classification system resulted in 382 primary diagnoses and 132 associated diagnoses. The leading cause of death was IUGR/

A primary ReCoDe classification

Fetus	Lethal congenital anomaly	A1	391	14.9
	Infection	A2	79	3.0
	Nonimmune hydrops	A3	36	1.4
	Isoimmunization	A4	11	0.4
	Fetomaternal hemorrhage	A5	5	0.2
	Twin-twin transfusion	A6	38	1.4
	Fetal growth restriction	A7	1129	43.0
Cord	Prolapse	B1	12	0.5
	Constricting loop or knot	B2	75	2.9
	Velamentous insertion	B3	0	0.0
	Umbilical cord—other	B4	0	0.0
Placenta	Placental abruptio	C1	181	6.9
	Placental previa	C2	6	0.2
	Vasa previa	C3	2	0.1
	Placental insufficiency	C4	18	0.7
	Placental—other	C5	25	1.0
Amniotic fluid	Chorioamnionitis	D1	10	0.4
	Oligohydramnios	D2	7	0.3
	Polyhydramnios	D3	3	0.1
Uterus	Rupture	E1	3	0.1
	Anomalies	E2	0	0.0
	Uterus—other	E3	0	0.0
Mother	Diabetes	F1	35	1.3
	Thyroid diseases	F2	1	0.0
	Essential hypertension	F3	2	0.1
	Hypertensive diseases in pregnancy	F4	21	0.8
	Lupus or antiphospholipid syndrome	F5	1	0.0
	Cholestasis	F6	1	0.0
	Drug misuse	F7	1	0.0
	Other maternal condition	F8	24	0.9
Intrapartum	Intrapartum asphyxia	G1	88	3.4
	Birth trauma	G2	0	0.0
Trauma	External trauma	H1	0	0.0
	Iatrogenic trauma	H2	1	0.0
Unclassified	No relevant condition identified	I1	398	0.0
	No information available	I2	21	0.8
Total			2625	100.0

Figure 3.2 Distribution of ReCoDe categories in the 2,625 stillbirths.

placental insufficiency (23%), followed by infection (19%), malformations/chromosomal abnormalities (12%), and the unexplained group (12%). The unexplained group together with the unknown group comprised 18%. The frequencies for all the groups are presented in Figure 3.3.

Causes of death and associated conditions

The purpose of the causes of death and associated conditions (CODAC) system is the "systematic arrangement of deaths in categories based on

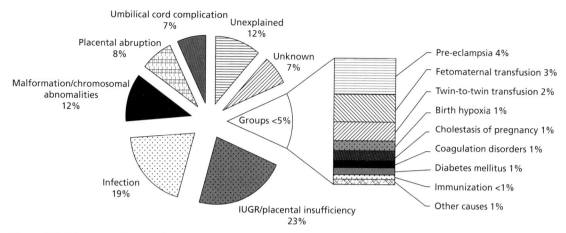

Figure 3.3 Primary conditions related to stillbirth 2002–2005.

the information that is known about them, to aid in the process of information management" [13]. This information can be used for a variety of purposes including health care policy development surveillance, research, and clinical management.

CODAC strives to be useful in a global setting where many stillbirths and newborn deaths are not registered, and was designed to be useful when a range of information is available. It is designed to manage information on terminations, stillbirths, and neonatal deaths, and relate to concepts of underlying causes in the International Classification of Disease (ICD) system.

The objective of CODAC is to capture information on the sequence and relative significance of the events in order to understand why the death occurred. CODAC was developed to code the cause of death (the digits in the first position) and two associated conditions (the digits in the second and third position). The categories for the primary causes of death are not hierarchical: (1) infectious causes; (2) conditions, events, or diseases specific to neonatal life; (3) mechanics and events of parturition or its complications; (4) deaths occurring after the onset of labor; (5) congenital anomalies, chromosomal anomalies, and structural malformations; (6) fetal conditions, diseases and events; (7) cord conditions, diseases and events; (8) maternal conditions, diseases and events; (9) unknown, unexplained, and unclassifiable; (10) terminations

of pregnancy. The associated conditions in either the second or third position are divided into perinatal and maternal. In the full version, there are 94 subcategories, which are further specified in 577 categories. For low-resource countries, a simplified version of 95 categories is available.

The decision on cause of death is based on subjective expert opinion and should "only be coded if the single or combined conditions lead to death in a significant (>0.05) proportion of cases." However, in cases of biological plausibility a lower threshold can be met or if there are complex clinical conditions these criteria do not have to be met.

INCODE (Initial Causes of Fetal Death)

This system was developed to assign the cause of death for stillbirths enrolled in the Stillbirth Collaborative Research Network (SCRN) (Figure 3.4) [14]. A complete evaluation, including postmortem examination, placental pathology, medical record abstraction, and maternal interview, was available on 512 stillbirths among 500 women. SCRN investigators developed a new methodology to assign the defined causes of death of stillbirths using clinical, postmortem, and placental pathology data. It incorporated known causes of death and assigned them as probable or possible based

SCRN	Version 04/ December 21,2009	Form 91A

Review Case ID	Member	Review Number	Form Completion Date
_ _ _ _ _ _ _ _ _ _	_ _	_ _ _	_ _ - _ _ - _ _ _ _
			mm dd yyyy

	01= Present	02= Possible	03= Possible
Instructions: Code findings according to the • designation wher 01=present; 02=possible cause of death; and 03=probable cause of death. Use the highest code for a finding with the criteria met. For example, if there is systemic lupus erythematosus disease activity (flare) during pregnancy and abruption placentae, the SLE should be coded as 1c3 (probable cause).			
5. Placental and/or Fetal Infection (Excluding Fetal Membranes)			
a. **Fetal infection involving vital organs: brain, heart lung & liver** (*Positive bacterial or viral culture, or viral-specific PCR – examples: listeriosis, group B stre ptococcus, Escherichia coli, other viruses, protozoa*) **Specify organism, if known**			
1) Culture or PCR proven infection in vital organs with no documented histologic signs of infection	•		
2) Culture or PCR proven infection in vital organs with signa of infection in the placenta but not organs		•	
3) Histologic evidence of infection in vital organs without culture or PCR proven infection in vital organs		•	
4) Histologic evidence of infection in vital organs with culture or PCR proven infection in vital organs			•
5) Pathognomonic pathologic findings in fetus with or without culture or PCR proven infection			•
b. **Fetal infection that causes congenital anomaly or other fetal condition** (*Fetal infection with a teratogenic organism – examples: parvovirus, varicella, CMV, toxoplasmosis*) **Specify organism, if known** _____			
1) Organism known to cause fetal anomaly/condition, anomaly/condition is present, timing of infection not consistent with specific anomaly/condition	•		
2) Organism known to cause fetal anomaly/condition, anomaly/condition is present, timing of infection is unknown		•	
3) Organism known to cause fetal anomaly/condition, anomaly/condition is present, timing of infection consistent with expected anomaly (including neuronal injury or calcifications)			•
4) Pathognomonic pathologic findings in fetus or placenta with or without culture or PCR proven infection			•
c. **Placental infection - organism likely to lead to decreased placental function** (*Maternal infection with organism known to decrease placental function - examples: malaria, syphilis*) **Specify organism, if known** _____			
1) Culture or PCR proven infection without placental histologic changes characteristic of infection or in the absence of placental histology	•		
2) Culture or PCR proven infection and placental histologic changes characteristic of infection such as villitis and placentitis (minimal placental involvement)		•	
3) Culture or PCR proven infection and placental histologic changes characteristic of infection such as villitis and placentitis (extensive placental involvement)			•
4) Pathognomonic pathologic findings in placenta with or without culture or PCR proven infection			•
d. **Infection-related fetal death by other or unknown mechanisms** (*placental or fetal infection, possible mechanism different from other categories*) **Specify organism, if known** _____			
1) Presence of maternal or fetal infection, no clear pathophysiologic sequence leading to fetal death	•		
2) Presence of maternal or fetal infection, plausible pathophysiologic sequence leading to fetal death		•	
3) Presence of maternal or fetal infection, likely pathophysiologic sequence leading to fetal death			•
4) Pathognomonic pathologic findings in fetus or placenta with or without culture or PCR proven infection			•

Figure 3.4 SCRN cause of death review form. (Reprinted with permission from ref. [13].)

on strict diagnostic criteria, derived from published references and pathophysiologic sequences that lead to stillbirth.

Six broad categories of causes of death are accounted for, including maternal medical conditions; obstetric complications; maternal or fetal hematologic conditions; fetal genetic, structural, and karyotypic abnormalities; placental infection, fetal infection, or both; and placental pathologic findings. Small for gestational age (SGA) was not treated as a cause of death but rather as evidence that a particular maternal or placental condition adversely influenced fetal well-being. Although SGA is commonly associated with stillbirth, it was considered as a consequence of other intrinsic conditions that are possible or probable causes of fetal death and not considered to be a proximate cause of death.

The gestational age at death is critical to determining growth restriction and assigning a cause. Gestational age at delivery is based on last menstrual period and ultrasound criteria and the gestational age of the stillbirth at death is adjusted for the difference between the time when the fetus was last alive and time of diagnosis of death, using pathologic criteria to most accurately determine the time of death. This is an improvement over arbitrarily using the time of delivery to reflect the time of death, as a significant proportion of fetuses (usually preterm) die days or weeks before the actual delivery. If unknown, the time of fetal death was based on postmortem examination.

INCODE deals with the difficulty of assigning a cause of stillbirth by ascribing degrees of certainty. A probable cause of stillbirth is designated when the identified condition is, with high likelihood, the cause of the fetal death. A possible cause of stillbirth is designated when the identified condition cannot, with high likelihood, be considered the cause of death, but there is reasonable certainty that this condition may be involved in a pathophysiologic sequence that led to the stillbirth. Not all conditions of interest can be further classified as a probable or possible cause of death based on the best available evidence or even expert opinion. In this circumstance, the condition is considered present. For the most part, "present" conditions are considered potential risk factors for, rather than causes of, stillbirth. Figure 3.4 provides an example of how probable, possible, and present is designated for infection.

One novel aspect of SCRN is that 1,932 women with live births were enrolled to serve as a contemporaneous control group. These women underwent the same study protocol (except the postmortem examination) as women who had stillbirth. INCODE is designed to be modified based on the knowledge obtained from the case-control data. One of the major goals will be to compare the initial clinical cause of death data with the final cause of death once all data from the study

are available. In addition, there is flexibility to consider potential newly discovered causes or risk factors for stillbirth.

Comparison of classification systems

A retrospective cohort study of 154 stillbirths diagnosed at the San Gerardo Hospital, Italy, from 1995 to 2007 compared ReCoDe, Wigglesworth, and Tulip, as well de Galen-Roosen (not described in this chapter) [15]. Autopsy and placental examination was performed in 98.7% of the stillbirths. The proportion of cases classified as unexplained were 45% for Wigglesworth, 14% for ReCoDe, and 16% for Tulip. The proportion of cause due to congenital anomalies in Wigglesworth and Tulip were similar at 35.7 and 33.8, respectively. The reduction of rates of unexplained in the recent systems has been due to the inclusion of fetal growth restriction and pathology of the placenta. The authors also indicated that the autopsy and placental pathology are of utmost importance for evaluating the stillbirth.

PSANZ-PDC and ReCoDe were compared using the National Women's Health's, New Zealand, stillbirth database for 2004–2007 [16]. There were 306 stillbirths, including 114 terminations of pregnancy, of which 85 were due to congenital anomalies. The autopsy rate was 60.8%. The proportion of unexplained stillbirths was significantly different for the two systems: 8.5% for ReCoDe and 14.1% for PSANZ-PDC. Growth restriction of <10th percentile using customized growth curves was attributed as a primary cause of death for 23% using ReCoDe and 8% using PSANZ-PDC. The predominant cause of death was congenital anomalies in similar proportions (36%) for both systems.

Conclusion

There is still varying and considerable uncertainty in establishing the cause of death for a significant proportion of stillbirths because of our incomplete understanding of the underlying pathophysiology.

New classification systems are developed and old ones revised as more knowledge is gained. However, no matter which classification is used, in virtually all cases there will be a degree of uncertainty regarding whether a specific condition was indeed "the cause of death." To deal with this uncertainty, existing classification systems have elected to note which potentially relevant conditions were present in cases of stillbirth, created a hierarchy of causes, or coded each condition as a certain, probable, or possible cause. When employing a classification system, the degree of uncertainty should be taken into account.

In order to design interventions that will reduce the incidence of stillbirth, it is imperative that studies elucidate the etiology of stillbirth by thorough investigation of how a disease process affects the mother, fetus, and placenta. The value of classification systems is to use this information to establish a likely causal picture of the loss.

References

1. Reddy UM, Goldenberg R, Silver R, et al. Stillbirth classification—developing an international consensus for research: executive summary of a National Institute of Child Health and Human Development workshop. Obstet Gynecol 2009;114(4):901–14.

2. Baird D, Walker J, Thomson AM. The causes and prevention of stillbirths and first week deaths. J Obstet Gynaecol Br Emp 1954;61:433–48.

3. Cole SK, Hey EN, Thomson AM. Classifying perinatal death: an obstetric approach. Br J Obstet Gynaecol 1986;93:1204–12.

4. Wigglesworth JS. Monitoring perinatal mortality. A pathophysiological approach. Lancet 1980;2:684–6.

5. Hey EN, Lloyd DJ, Wigglesworth JS. Classifying perinatal death: fetal and neonatal factors. Br J Obstet Gynaecol 1986;93:1213–23.

6. Keeling JW, MacGillivray I, Golding J, et al. Classification of perinatal death. Arch Dis Child 1989;64:1345–51.

7. Confidential Enquiry into Maternal and Child Health (CEMACH). Perinatal mortality 2007. London, UK: CEMACH; 2009.

8. Centre for Maternal and Child Enquiry (CMACE). Perinatal Murtality 2008. London: CMACE; 2010.

9. Chan A, King JF, Flenady V, et al. Classification of perinatal deaths: development of the Australian and New Zealand classifications. J Paediatr Child Health 2004;40:340–47.

10. Korteweg FJ, Gordijn SJ, Timmer A, et al. The Tulip classification of perinatal mortality: introduction and multidisciplinary inter-rater agreement. BJOG 2006; 113(4):393–401.

11. Gardosi J, Kady SM, McGeown P, et al. Classification of stillbirth by relevant condition at death (ReCoDe): population based cohort study. BMJ 2005;331(7525): 1113–17.

12. Varli IH, Petersson K, Bottinga R, et al. The Stockholm classification of stillbirth. Acta Obstet Gynecol Scand 2008;87(11):1202–12.

13. Froen JF, Pinar H, Flenady V, et al. Causes of death and associated conditions (Codac)—a utilitarian approach to the classification of perinatal deaths. BMC Pregnancy Childbirth 2009;9:22–3.

14. Dudley DJ, Goldenberg R, Conway D, et al.; for the Stillbirth Research Collaborative Network. A new system for determining the causes of stillbirth. Obstet Gynecol 2010;116(2 Pt 1):254–60.

15. Vergani P, Cozzolino S, Pozzi E, et al. Identifying the causes of stillbirth: a comparison of four classification systems. Am J Obstet Gynecol 2008;199:319e.1–4.

16. Lu JR, McCowan L. A comparison of the Perinatal Society of Australia and New Zealand-Perinatal Death Classification system and relevant condition at death stillbirth classification systems. Aust N Z J Obstet Gynaecol 2009;49:467–71.

PART II
Etiology/Causes

CHAPTER 4
Demographics and Exposures

Carol J. Rowland Hogue, PhD, MPH
Women's and Children's Center, Department of Epidemiology, Rollins School of Public Health, Emory University, Atlanta, GA, USA

This chapter focuses on current and historical trends in stillbirth rates in the developed world that may shed light on known or suspected causes of stillbirth in the United States. For example, characteristics of women who are at greater risk for disease (e.g., having greater inflammatory response to an infectious agent) may point in the direction of needed research into the causal pathway for the disease (e.g., stress-associated inflammatory processes). Other observable behavioral characteristics (e.g., smoking), if associated with stillbirth, may suggest areas for primary prevention through preventing or reducing the behavior. In the developing world where the vast majority of stillbirths occur, grinding poverty, lack of access to qualified emergency obstetrics care, inadequate training of birth attendants, and poor access to screening and treatment of syphilis and other preventable infectious diseases are prime targets for reducing global stillbirth risk [1, 2]. Yet even in developed countries where women and infants receive the best possible perinatal health services, improvement in stillbirth rates can be achieved through applying knowledge gained from observational studies of risk factors. Prime targets for reducing stillbirth risk in the developed world are behaviors—individual, medical care-related, and sociocultural.

In her review of the etiology and prevention of stillbirth [3], Fretts identified 15 risk factors: 7 maternal medical conditions (hypertension, diabetes, systemic lupus erythematosus, renal disease, thyroid disease, thrombophilias, and cholestasis of pregnancy); 3 pregnancy-related (previous delivery of a growth-restricted or stillborn infant or multiple gestation of the current pregnancy); and 5 maternal sociodemographic or behavioral characteristics (African-American race, low educational attainment, advanced age, smoking, and obesity). In this chapter we limit the discussion of potential risk factors to those that have a behavioral, sociocultural, medical intervention component, or a logical combination of two or three of those elements (Table 4.1). These factors include the 5 reviewed by Fretts, plus an additional 16 that have been associated in one or more epidemiologic studies, as either potential risk factors or preventive interventions. These are listed in Table 4.1 in order of discussion in this chapter. Before proceeding to describe stillbirth patterns for these demographics and behavior-related exposures, let us consider some methodological issues that pertain to most published work in this area.

Changing demographics and exposures

Demographic characteristics are not static, for example, in age at first childbearing, and time trends may provide clues to stillbirth etiology. This is because different combinations of other exposures may operate for each of the demographic or exposure categories described in this chapter. During the last few decades, teenage childbearing has decreased throughout the developed world [4–6] and is now concentrated in poor communities where young women view their future options as highly limited. Thus, if there is an elevated stillbirth risk among

Stillbirth: Prediction, Prevention and Management, First Edition. Catherine Y. Spong.
© 2011 Blackwell Publishing Ltd. Published 2011 by Blackwell Publishing Ltd.

Table 4.1 Demographics and common exposures reviewed, with level of evidence of effect on stillbirth, presumed source of the exposure, and type of health care intervention that may mitigate the effect.

Common exposure (in order discussed)	Risk factor	Level of evidence	Behavioral	Sociocultural	Health care intervention
Maternal age	35+; young (<2 years from menarche)	+++/+	Y	Y	Monitor for high-risk
Paternal age	45+	+	Y	Y	Monitor for high-risk
Race	African-American	+++	–	Y	Monitor for high-risk
Ethnicity	Hispanic	++	–	Y	Monitor for high-risk
Parity	Nulliparity; grand multiparity	+++/+++	Y	Y	Monitor for high-risk
Prior poor pregnancy outcome	Stillbirth	+++	–	–	Monitor for high-risk
Interpregnancy interval (IPI)	<18 months	++	Y	–	Counsel to ↑ IPI
Socioeconomic/social position	Poor, less educated	+++	Y	Y	Provide support?
Occupation	Selected, low-pay	+	–	Y?	–
Marital status	Unmarried, father not present	+	Y	Y	Provide support?
Acute stressful events	Multiple events	+	Y	Y	Provide support?
Chronic, life-course stress (PTSD)	Early life, daily hassles	+	Y	Y	Provide support?
Caffeine	Heavy during pregnancy	+	Y	Y	Counsel?
Smoking	Smoking during pregnancy	++	Y	Y	Counsel and patch?
Alcohol	Binge drinking during pregnancy	+	Y	Y	Counsel?
Illicit drugs	Multiple	+	Y	Y	–
Prepregnancy obesity	BMI > 30	+++	Y	Y	Preconception ↓ wt
Iron deficiency	Preconception supplement protective?	+	–	Y?	Preconception?
Maternal mental disorders	Several	+	–	–	Treat in pregnancy?
Assisted reproductive technology	Multiple implantations; IVF or ICSI?	+++/+	Y	Y	Counsel ↓ implants
Obstetric intervention	First is protective; risk of repeat?	+++/+	Y	Y	Appropriate delivery

adolescents, it is most likely due to social deprivation rather than physical limitations. At the other end of the reproductive life span, birth rates for women in their late 30s and 40s have risen, especially for first births resulting from assisted reproductive technologies (ARTs) [4–6].

Other trends in demographic characteristics may affect stillbirth rates but possibly not provide etiologic clues. These include decreased grand multiparity, decreased experience of prior perinatal loss, and temporal trends in maternal smoking [4–6]. As delivery by cesarean section has increased, its impact on stillbirth rates is complex. This is discussed later.

Overlapping and incompletely described maternal characteristics

Some exposures may be difficult to analyze separate from other exposures; for example, maternal age and multiparity are closely intertwined. A common—but perhaps less well recognized—problem in interpreting epidemiologic studies of demographics is that investigators may use something that can be measured with available data for a variable that they cannot measure but believe is etiologic. In countries with trends toward delaying childbearing, teenage childbearing may be a proxy for poverty, lack of social support from a married partner, adverse childhood experiences, and greater exposure to sexually transmitted diseases. Except for marital status, none of these factors is included in vital records which are often the main or sole data source. Thus, teenage childbearing in these settings may or may not represent maternal age-related risks independent of these other, unmeasured characteristics.

In the United States, race and education are proxies for income and wealth which are not reported in vital records. However, race and education are incomplete proxies for wealth and so may underestimate the impact of capital resources on stillbirth. Further, social status, psychological life course stress, other behaviors, and race often overlap considerably, so it may be difficult to separate the independent effects of each exposure on stillbirth risk unless all appropriate exposures are included in the study. Investigations that rely on large studies of vital records or medical records are missing these key exposure variables. Incomplete ascertainment of overlapping risk factors can lead to overestimate of effect for measured variables. For example, in a case–control study of socioeconomic status (SES) and stillbirth in Nova Scotia, Goy and colleagues [7] found that lower household income (but neither maternal education nor occupational status) was associated with increased risk of stillbirth. Further, maternal smoking (the one behavioral variable examined) reduced the odds ratio (OR) for SES by 18.5%, from 3.31 to 2.79.

Competing pregnancy outcomes

Stillbirth is just one of several potential adverse pregnancy outcomes. Some adverse outcomes occur early in pregnancy and may be difficult to study. As many as 10–30% of conceptions end in spontaneous abortions; many of these spontaneous abortions occur so soon after conception that they are not recognized as pregnancies by the woman. Recognized pregnancies may miscarry before the woman's first prenatal visit and escape medical attention. Ectopic and other extrauterine conceptions may be treated clinically and not reported in hospital discharge surveys. All these outcomes essentially "compete" with stillbirth, in that conceptions that terminate prior to 20 weeks gestation are not at risk of stillbirth.

Competing pregnancy outcomes may obscure the extent to which an exposure is a risk factor. In the extreme, an exposure such as a lethal gene that is a risk for spontaneous abortion may not be identified as a risk for stillbirth, as all affected conceptuses abort prior to 20 weeks. In less-extreme situations, an exposure might be incorrectly identified as a risk factor if it contributes to survival of a pregnancy into later gestation of a fetus that might not have survived to 20 weeks or later without the protective factor. In other words, the purported risk factor is actually a protective factor against early loss but not for incidence of the condition or ultimate survival of the affected fetus. Evidence for this phenomenon may be seen in the changing trend of birth defect-associated infant mortality for African-Americans compared with Caucasians in the United States. Among infants born in 1980, there was no increased first-year mortality risk attributed to birth defects for African-American infants [8]. However, by 1989 the infant mortality rate attributed to birth defects for African-American infants exceeded the rate for Caucasians, and the rates since then have continued to diverge [9]. It is instructive that the greatest racial difference is among deaths attributed to congenital heart and neural tube defects, as many of both types of defects are detectable through prenatal diagnosis. In 1980, these defects accounted for 59% of infant deaths attributed to birth defects. Since the 1980s, pregnancy terminations of prenatally diagnosed cases of congenital heart defects have affected reported rates of these causes of stillbirth and infant mortality (e.g., in Finland [10], France [11], and Northern England [12]). African-American women may be less likely to obtain prenatal diagnosis because of reduced access to early prenatal care. Also, they may be less likely to terminate a pregnancy that has been diagnosed with a birth defect [13]; as a result, stillbirths and infant deaths attributable to birth defects may be more common among African-American infants because the pregnancy was less likely to have been terminated and not because of an excess incidence of fatal malformations.

Competing adverse pregnancy outcomes are clearly apparent at delivery weights less than 500 g. This is a particular problem in the United States because it is the responsibility of each state to define vital events and provide quality control for vital records collection. Reported demographics and exposures for stillbirth may vary by the degree to which deliveries at the cusp of viability are classified as live births/early neonatal deaths or as stillbirths. For example, in a study of all reported deliveries in the United States from 1999 to 2002 with gestation of 20+ weeks, weighing <500 g and stillborn or dying within the first 24 h, the odds of the delivery being recorded as a live birth (vs. fetal death) ranged between states from 0.38 (95% confidence interval [CI] = 0.24–0.59) to 2.93 (95% CI = 2.26–3.78) and differed somewhat within states by maternal age and race and delivery year [14]. To avoid this issue, it may be preferable to examine perinatal mortality risks which incorporate both stillbirth and early neonatal mortality.

Definition of stillbirth

The gestational age or fetal weight at which intrauterine, spontaneous fetal deaths are termed stillbirths rather than spontaneous abortions or miscarriages has differed over time and, within the same time period, across geographic areas and among health care providers [15]. Part of the rationale for setting a minimum weight or gestational age limit for stillbirth reporting is to include statistics for deaths only of potentially viable fetuses. Gestational age of viability varies by the capability of newborn care facilities to resuscitate and care for frail newborns. To allow stillbirth rate comparisons across countries with different neonatal care capacities, international definitions of stillbirths begin at the higher limits of 28 weeks gestation or 1,000 g.

In high-resource areas, minimum gestational age limits may be as low as 16 weeks with no minimum fetal weight limit. This is to allow for lack of certainty in gestational age at delivery. Gestational age may be underestimated by up to 4 weeks due to early bleeding. For that reason, the minimum

gestational age for statistical reporting may be set about 4–6 weeks below viability so as to capture all possibly viable fetuses. In the United States, gestational age definitions for stillbirths vary from state to state and have a dramatic effect on reported stillbirth rates. For example, among reported stillbirths in 2005 (the latest year for which national data are available), the percentage of stillbirths at 20–27 weeks gestation (of all stillbirths of 20 weeks gestation or greater) varied from 50.5 to 57.2 depending on whether the lower gestational age for reporting fetal deaths was 20 weeks or 350 g (36 states), 16 weeks (1 state), or no gestational age limit (7 states) [15]. For the three states with the highest minimum fetal weight limit of 500 g (irrespective of gestational age), stillbirths at 20–27 weeks gestation comprised only 26.6% of reported stillbirths.

These differences in minimum reporting limits have a distinct impact on demographics and common exposures that vary by gestational age of the stillbirth. For example, exposures that increase preterm delivery (such as maternal infection) will appear to have a stronger effect in studies that have a lower reporting limit, while exposures that increase intrapartum death may appear to have a stronger effect in studies that have a higher reporting limit.

Control group selection

In determining whether a demographic characteristic or common exposure is a risk factor for stillbirth, we must compare the prevalence of the exposure among stillbirth cases with the exposure among controls. Thus, the definition of controls is a key to understanding risk. For example, if the risk being examined is fetal death at a certain gestational age, an appropriate control group would include all pregnancies continuing beyond that gestational age (irrespective of their ultimate outcome). This is sometimes called the prospective fetal mortality risk or rate; it is generally high at the extremes of gestation, to a certain extent reflecting causes related to antepartum (early) and intrapartum (late) stillbirths [15]. Figure 4.1 shows recent fetal mortality risk for the United States.

Alternatively, examination of risk of fetal death at any gestational age would call for a control group of all live births—or for a "rate," all live births plus

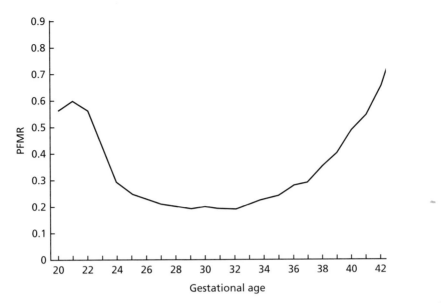

Figure 4.1 Prospective fetal mortality rate (PFMR) by single weeks of gestation: United States, 2005. Note: number of fetal deaths at a given gestational age per 1,000 live births and fetal deaths at a gestational age or greater. Data from CDC/NCHS, National Vital Statistics System.

fetal deaths. For example, in the United States in 2005 the fetal mortality rate for deliveries with maternal age less than 15 years was 12.2 per 1,000 deliveries, compared with 15.5 per 1,000 deliveries for women aged 45 or more and less than 6 per 1,000 deliveries for women aged 20–34 [15].

Finally, examination of survival at a given gestational age would require examination of potential risk factors between stillbirths and live births at that gestational age. For example, in 2005, the fetal mortality risk was 504.1 per 1,000 deliveries at 20–23 weeks of gestation; the risk declined sharply to a low of 0.86 per 1,000 deliveries at 40 weeks of gestation, and then increased to 1.66 per 1,000 deliveries for fetal deaths at 42 weeks of gestation or more [15].

Data availability and quality

Most information about demographic and other exposures derive from studies in the developed world, where vital registration is virtually universal and most women deliver in medical settings that are conducive to the conduct of epidemiologic investigations. These investigations vary in strengths and weaknesses, depending on whether they rely on existing vital registration systems, medical records,

maternal interviews, or prospective cohort studies. Table 4.2 provides a schematic for the general strengths and weaknesses of these data sources.

In the United States, the National Center for Health Statistics (NCHS) of the federal Centers for Disease Control and Prevention (CDC) periodically recommends modifications to standard certificates of live birth, fetal death, and other vital records. Priority is given to information that is needed for personal identification and documentation of the time and place of the event. Data that will provide valuable scientific information are added, with the caveat that data must be easily obtainable and not confer an undue burden on the reporters. In general, demographics and exposures are similar for both standard birth and fetal death certificates. In 1978, Apgar score was added to the standard birth certificate, and reporters were asked to fill in the blanks for maternal conditions and complications [16]. To make this information more uniform and of higher quality, check boxes for maternal complications such as preeclampsia, hemorrhage, and chronic hypertension were added in 1989, along with data on maternal smoking and alcohol consumption during pregnancy [17]. The 2003 revision included

Table 4.2 Relative strengths and weaknesses of epidemiologic studies of exposures associated with stillbirth.

Epidemiologic data source	Relative strength	Relative weakness
Vital records (unlinked)	Sample size	Data quality for maternal complications and procedures is generally weak
	Less selection bias	Number of relevant variables, including use of proxy data for SES
		Selective recall of some variables, including smoking, alcohol, pre-pregnant weight
Vital records (linked)	Sample size	No improvement for studies of primiparity
	Can improve data quality versus unlinked	Number of relevant variables is not increased over nonlinked vital records
	Some variables don't depend on selective recall	
Registries (including linked)	Possibly large sample size, less selection bias	Homogeneity of populations covered by registries
	Increased number of variables	Misclassification or misspecification because of secondary data analyses
	Some variables can be linked prospectively	Some important variables are not collected (e.g., depression, early adverse events)
Medical records-based studies	Maternal complications and treatments better captured	Generally small samples, possible selection biases
		Often missing key information on behavioral variables
Prospective studies (including in registries)	Variables of interest may be more precisely measured	Limited sample size
	Possibly less selective recall	Cost considerations may limit prospective exposure measurements
	Can be used to examine competing pregnancy outcomes	
Population-based case–control studies	Less selection bias	Selective recall
	Often better sample size than prospective studies	Cannot examine competing pregnancy outcomes
	Can examine for multiple exposures	

further refinements for maternal and infant conditions and complications, along with greater detail regarding obstetric procedures, method of delivery, and information on prior cesarean section [18].

States have the right to adopt the standard certificates or to develop their own certificates. By January 1, 2006, only 19 states had adopted the 2003 standard birth certificate [18]; other states had chosen to postpone or not to make the additional changes, primarily for cost considerations. However, there was also concern that the quality of reporting might not justify the additional effort

required. By the end of 2010, all but seven states may have modified their reporting requirements to comply with the 2003 standard certificates [18]. Another limitation with U.S. vital records is that data on maternal and fetal characteristics are often missing for fetal deaths—especially deaths at 20–27 weeks gestation—making it difficult to compare across states or, within states, between live births and fetal deaths [19].

Some states provide leadership in testing new data items before they are chosen for inclusion in the U.S. standard certificate. In particular, Missouri has been a vanguard for high-quality data collection, for example, having added a request for method of delivery, maternal smoking, height, and prepregnant weight in 1978. In addition, Missouri was one of the first states to develop a large database that linked birth, fetal death, and infant death events to the mother (if she were resident in Missouri for these events). As a result, much of what is known about demographics and exposures in the United States derives from analyses of this important resource that includes more than 8,000 stillbirth records and 1.4 million live birth records dating from 1978 to 1997 [20–34].

As previously mentioned, even in the best of circumstances, studies relying exclusively on vital records are limited to a small list of potential demographics and exposures. A study comparing stillbirth risk among younger versus older teens and women in their early 20s concluded that smoking has a greater impact if the woman is younger [22]; however, the investigators could not control for factors associated with beginning smoking at an early age, such as illicit drug use, increased risk of sexually transmitted diseases, and childhood traumas. All these factors have been associated with increased stillbirth risk in other studies. Further, information on behavioral factors is retrospectively obtained and may therefore be open to information bias. That is, parents with an adverse pregnancy outcome may be more likely than parents with a healthy baby to recall behaviors such as smoking and alcohol consumption. Information bias on smoking and alcohol consumption was not found in a validation study of 2,806 mothers in the Netherlands who gave birth between 1978 and 1979 except for cigarette consumption for mothers with a small-for-gestational-age child [35]. However, among white women in six U.S. states who gave birth between 1993 and 1995, smoking ascertainment ranged from 70.6% to 82.0% and was less complete for women with normal-weight births compared with women with births <2,500 g [36]. More recent validation studies have confirmed that demographic variables are highly accurate on birth certificates, but reports of alcohol consumption [37] and prepregnant body mass index (BMI) [38] have somewhat lower validity and may thus be more prone to information bias.

Many analyses utilizing vital records do not require maternally linked records [20–26, 28–29, 31–33]. However, for studies that do require linkage [27, 30] there may be biases associated with residential moves into and out of the state as well as incomplete records linkage. Incomplete linkage may be a particular problem for investigations of Hispanic populations in the United States [39]. Records linkage studies are much more complete and provide much richer sources of information in Scandinavian countries, where records can be linked through personal identification numbers and numerous registries are maintained. Examples of epidemiologic investigations of stillbirth include studies of previous adverse pregnancy outcomes and paternal contributions; maternal occupation; the effect of the sex of a previous child; and the effect of maternal mental disorders.

Scandinavian investigators have estimated the risk of stillbirth following pregnancies complicated by fetal growth restriction, abruptio placentae, preeclampsia, or live preterm birth and compared maternal and paternal contributions to these risks [40]. Among other important results, they found a six- to nine-fold excess risk of stillbirth in pregnancies following a preterm live birth (with gestational age less than 33 weeks) that had been complicated by preeclampsia and an OR of 2.4 (95% CI 1.1–5.5) for stillbirth in mothers whose partner had previously fathered a pregnancy by another woman, if that earlier pregnancy had been complicated by preterm preeclampsia.

Utilizing Finnish national registries, investigators determined that nurses but not midwives had a slightly elevated risk of stillbirth when compared with school teachers; however, women in these occupations had better pregnancy outcomes when compared with women in other occupations [41]. Examples of the use of Danish registries include a study of the sex of the previous-born child (with an 12% excess risk of stillbirth in the subsequent pregnancy following the birth of a boy) [42] and analysis of women with various psychiatric disorders that concluded that maternal behaviors associated with the disorders (such as unhealthy lifestyles) rather than the disorders themselves might explain observed differences in stillbirth risks [43].

While these examples illustrate that population registries have advantages in completeness and greater ease of linkage with diagnostic, occupational, and other registries, use of Scandinavian registries for stillbirth studies is limited in scope by the relatively homogeneous nature of Northern European populations as well as relatively sparse information on personal and behavioral risk factors of interest. To expand the capability of national registry data, in 1996 Olsen and colleagues [44] established a prospective cohort of pregnant women recruited through their prenatal care providers. By 2000, approximately 60,000 women had been enrolled. Enrolled women were interviewed by telephone twice during pregnancy and provided blood samples to bank for future studies. While voluntary participation in this Danish National Birth Cohort was low (30%), results of participants compared with registry data from the source population is reassuring with respect to exposures such as maternal smoking, in vitro fertilization (IVF), and prepregnancy body weight [45].

Researchers have begun to analyze the Danish National Birth Cohort for behavioral and sociodemographic etiologies of stillbirth [46–57]. The advantages to these investigations include prospective data collection on selected exposures such as conception through ART, over-the-counter drugs, obesity, psychosocial stress, caffeine consumption, smoking and alcohol [46–57], and linkage with genetic analyses [55]. Disadvantages of the research strategy include the necessity to prioritize among suspected etiologies so as to limit respondent burden, telephone-only interviews without environmental exposure measures, and the relatively homogeneous population of Danish citizens in the study. Also, there may be limited information on the cause of fetal death. The National Children's Study in the United States now being pilot tested is designed to improve on this strategy through environmental sampling of a large enough sample of pregnancies to represent the diverse U.S. population, in-depth interviews of women beginning for some before their conception, and extensive biological sampling.

The case–control study is another epidemiologic approach with complementary methodological strengths and weaknesses compared to these prospective cohort strategies. Advantages include a more detailed collection of exposure information for the specific exposures of interest and increased statistical power to assess exposures. Disadvantages generally include retrospective exposure assessment and limited capability to examine competing pregnancy outcomes. Several case–control studies in Great Britain and other developed countries have yielded important information. In the United States, the Stillbirth Collaborative Research Network (SCRN) study, sponsored by the *Eunice Kennedy Shriver* National Institute of Child Health and Human Development (NICHD), is a prospective, multicenter, population-based case–control study of all stillbirths (fetal deaths >20 weeks) and a representative sample of live births enrolled at delivery in five geographic areas at 59 hospitals averaging >80,000 deliveries/year. Figure 4.2 shows the states and locales where the SCRN study took place. SCRN participants underwent a standardized protocol including maternal interview, medical record abstraction, placental pathology, biospecimen testing, and, in stillbirths, postmortem examinations [58, 59]. Of 953 women with stillbirths eligible for the study, 126 were not approached, 164 refused, and 663 (70%) consented to participate. A total of 3,089 live birth controls were eligible, and 1,933 consented (63%) [58, 59]. To our knowledge, this is the largest population-based study of stillbirth with an extensive evaluation of both cases and controls. Compared to some other case–control studies, advantages of the SCRN include findings that are more generalizable than prior hospital-based studies or studies with small sample sizes, less complete ascertainment, non-standardized workup, or convenience sampling. In preliminary analyses, investigators have reported novel findings on maternal blood type (B or AB) [58] and a dose–response association between significant life events in the 12 months preceding delivery and risk of stillbirth [59].

In summary, while analyses of demographics and exposures can lead to a better understanding of the causes of stillbirth, all studies have methodological limitations and often may not adequately address potential overlap in characteristics or

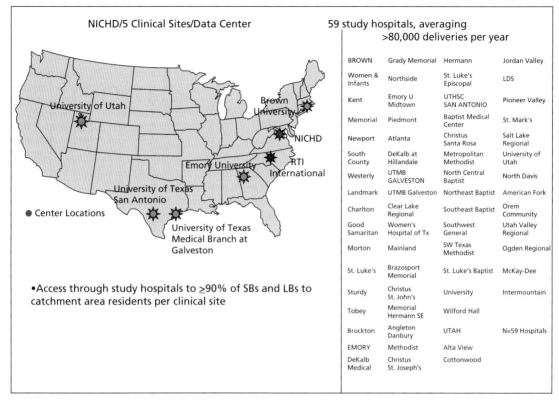

Figure 4.2 Stillbirth collaborative research network (SCRN) sites.

competing pregnancy outcomes to stillbirth. With these caveats in mind, let us review the literature on selected characteristics. For ease of presentation, characteristics are grouped into the following categories: age, race and ethnicity, pregnancy history, social environment, maternal substance use, maternal nutrition, maternal mental illness, and maternal health care.

Maternal age

In the United States, the percentage of births to women 35 years of age or older has risen steadily in this century, reaching 14.2% of live births in 2008, the latest year for which national data are available [60]. Older maternal age (generally 35+) has long been associated with increased risk of stillbirth [61]. Recent trends in postponing

childbearing into later ages, made possible in part by reliance on ART for subfecund couples, has changed the demographic stillbirth risk profile for older women, as proportionately more births to older women are first births of middle-class families rather than higher-order births of poorer families. Also, increased use of prenatal diagnosis and pregnancy termination has reduced stillbirth rates attributed to congenital anomalies. In Western Australia this changing demographic picture affected the relative risk for stillbirth for women aged 40 or older (compared with women 25–29 years) from 2.6 in the period 1984–1993 to 1.9 in the period 1994–2003 [62]. Using a somewhat different methodology for estimating stillbirth risks, in Missouri from 1989 to 1997, older maternal age was associated with antepartum, but not intrapartum, stillbirths among Caucasians but not African-Americans, after statistical control for lack of prenatal care and prepregnancy BMI [63].

Perhaps because of these trends, a recent examination of prospective stillbirth risk among 5.5 million pregnancies in the United States delivered between 2001 and 2002 found only a slightly elevated stillbirth risk for early fetal deaths (20–27 weeks gestation) for women aged 35+ compared with younger women [64]. The age-associated stillbirth risk rose dramatically after 33 weeks for women aged 40+ and after 37 weeks for women aged 35–39. Risk associated with advanced maternal age persisted after statistical control for race and ethnicity, parity, and mention of maternal complications on the certificates.

The studies summarized above pertain mainly to singleton deliveries. One intriguing analysis of quadruplets and quintuplets from the Missouri database suggests that older maternal age may be protective for these high-order multiple births [26]. However, much more research would be required before it is determined whether or by what means older maternal age decreases stillbirth risk for quadruplets and quintuplets.

While older maternal age appears to be an independent risk factor for stillbirth among singletons, it is not clear that younger maternal age is an independent risk factor. Rather, young maternal age may be a risk marker for unmeasured behavioral, social, and cultural factors that are not routinely captured by vital statistics databases. Perhaps extremely young maternal age less than 15 does confer an excess risk, as pregnancy within 2 years of menarche is known to increase maternal and infant complications. Fortunately there are very few such births in the United States. In 2008, there were just 5,775 births to mothers less than 15, which amount to less than 2 per 1,000 total births [60]. For births to teens of 15–19 years, there does not appear to be an independent effect of young maternal age.

Older paternal age has not been widely studied, and results are varied. In one analysis from the Danish National Birth Cohort, stillbirth risk increased with increasing paternal age after 45 [65]. Only 124 fathers of more than 20,000 studied were over 50. Compared with younger fathers, the stillbirth hazard ratio for these older fathers was

1.88 (95% CI = 0.93, 3.82) after statistical control for maternal age, reproductive history, and maternal lifestyle. Paternal lifestyle was not measured, as data about fathers came from record linkage to population registries. With increasing proportions of births to older women, further examination of the effect of older fathers is warranted.

Race and ethnicity

In many European countries, owing to historical issues of genocide, it is illegal to record an individual's race or ethnicity on a vital record. In Northern European countries capable of conducting high-quality record linkage studies, there is limited utility for examining the health of minority populations because many countries with the best registry systems have few residents who are members of racial or ethnic minorities. While this phenomenon is changing somewhat with increased migration from Africa, Asia, and the Middle East, most of the evidence for racial or ethnic differences in stillbirth risk derive from studies in the United States where race—and since 1989 Hispanic ethnicity—are recorded on vital records.

In the United States, phenotypic African-Americans' health reflects a complex combination of social determinants of health possibly interacting with genetic inheritance from several of the oldest continental populations [66–70]. Despite this complexity, "race" is often considered a strictly biological concept. For instance, in a review of published biomedical studies supported by the National Cancer Institute, Lee [66] found that authors rarely defined or operationalized the concepts of "race" and "ethnicity" adequately. She concluded that this "undertheorized and unspecified use of race or ethnicity and the biological conclusions drawn about health and difference have the potential to reify 'race' and to limit our thinking about what these biomedical differences suggest about health disparities and inequalities in general" [66, p. 1184].

Adequate conceptualization requires specifying a causal framework from which well-defined hypotheses can drive data collection of relevant variables [67]. A proposed causal framework for preterm birth among African-Americans [68] may be a good starting point for stillbirth studies comparing African-American and Caucasian pregnancies, as the excess stillbirth risk for African-Americans is greatest at earlier gestation ages [71]. This framework includes upstream measures of institutionalized and interpersonal discrimination; midstream measures of social environment including SES, residential neighborhood characteristics, and interpersonal social support; near-proximate measures of life course stress (early life, chronic, and acute), preconception health (including pre-pregnant weight, micronutrient deficiencies, infections, etc.), behavioral risk factors, and possible gene–environment interactions; and proximate measures of vascular dysfunction, hypothalamic-pituitary-adrenal (HPA) axis dysfunction, and inflammation [68]. To date, no published studies have yet tested this framework, but the SCRN study may have sufficient power and measures to perform such a test.

It is important to understand racial disparity in stillbirth risk, as African-Americans have a higher overall risk when compared to Caucasians. In 2005, the stillbirth rate for non-Hispanic African-Americans was 11.13 per 1,000 deliveries—a 2.3-fold excess compared to the non-Hispanic Caucasian rate of 4.79 [15]. Other minority groups also had elevated rates: 5.44 among Hispanic women and 6.17 among American Indian and Alaska Native women. Overall, fetal mortality has not declined from 2003, and early fetal mortality (20–27 weeks gestation) has not declined since 1990. The racial disparity is less for twins and triplets than for singleton births [28]. Stillbirth risk is particularly high among women with a previous stillbirth, but even in this high-risk group African-American women have been found to be more than twice as likely as Caucasian women to experience a second stillbirth [27]. Given the trend toward increasing cesarean deliveries, a troubling finding is that African-American women may have 1.4 times the risk of stillbirth in a pregnancy following a cesarean delivery when compared with African-American women with a previous vaginal delivery [30].

Hypotheses regarding the cause for excess preterm birth risk among African-Americans include nutritional deficiencies in iron, folic acid, zinc, and vitamin D, and lower levels of n–3 polyunsaturated fatty acids (PUFA) intake and higher n–6 PUFA intake [72]. African-American women are more likely to be deficient in these nutritional factors, but whether these factors account for any excess in preterm live birth or stillbirth has yet to be established. Moderate anemia was associated with late fetal death (28+ weeks gestation) in the United States. National Maternal and Infant Health Study of 1988 among non-Hispanic Caucasian women (adjusted hazard ratio 4.4 [95% CI 1.02–19.01]), but not among the smaller number of non-Hispanic African-American women [73]. Thus, if iron deficiency has an impact, it may be small and/or limited to early fetal loss.

The role of obesity is much clearer, as African-American women are more likely to be overweight or obese before pregnancy, and obesity is a known risk factor for stillbirth (although the mechanism of effect is unknown—see later). In one study in which BMI was divided into three levels of severity, stillbirth risk increased as severity level increased. Stillbirth risk for African-Americans exceeded the risk for Caucasians at each level [29]. For underweight women, there was no increased stillbirth risk among African-Americans [31].

Increasingly, parents in the United States are of different races. Studies of mixed-race parents in the United States from 1995 to 2001 [74] and in California from 1998 to 2002 [75] had similar findings. From highest to lowest stillbirth risk, combinations were: African-American/African-American parents; African-American mother/Caucasian father; Caucasian mother/African-American father; and Caucasian/Caucasian parents. As data for these studies came from vital records, investigators were unable to examine many potential risk factors; however, it was possible to conclude that the observed excess stillbirth risk for all parent combinations was a result of excess preterm delivery or low birthweight after other measurable risk factors were statistically controlled [75].

In summary, stillbirth risk is higher for African-Americans and may be higher for certain other minority populations. For African-Americans, excess stillbirth risk is associated with preterm delivery, but the underlying causes of both preterm live births and preterm stillbirths remain obscure. Infections (the subject of chapter 5) are higher among African-Americans, but this is a proximate cause of premature delivery and does not address the upstream and social determinants of increased infection or increased inflammation resulting from infection [76–78]. Answers to these questions will depend on studies that go beyond data available on vital records.

Pregnancy history

Nulliparity is a known risk factor for antepartum stillbirth [79] and has been reported to account for the excess prospective stillbirth mortality of pregnancies lasting 41 weeks or more in England [80], prompting a recommendation to limit obstetric intervention in prolonged pregnancies to nulliparous women. However, others have pointed to the increasing risk of stillbirth for all prolonged pregnancies as an argument for elective cesarean section [3, 81]. Grand multiparity is also associated with increased stillbirth risk, although this may be related to physical conditions associated with advanced maternal age or factors associated with poverty, especially in the developed world where families tend to be smaller in number.

Women with a history of pregnancy complications in a prior pregnancy are at increased risk of stillbirth in the current pregnancy [82, 83]. While a majority of women experiencing stillbirth will have a healthy subsequent pregnancy, there is a documented elevated risk of stillbirth recurrence from 20% [82] to 500% [27] and may be even higher for some women, such as African-Americans.

One way to reduce the risk of subsequent stillbirth is to space pregnancies at least 18 months apart from the culmination of one to the conception of the next. Numerous studies have found that an ideal length of time from the previous delivery to the next conception—known as the interpregnancy interval—is between 18 and 23 months [76]. Either shorter or longer interpregnancy intervals are more likely to result in poor pregnancy outcomes. However, the association between longer interpregnancy intervals and poor pregnancy outcomes is likely related to maternal subfecundity and other morbidities that affect the woman's ability to conceive.

It is widely recognized that women who experience miscarriage, late fetal death, or neonatal loss are motivated to "replace" the loss quickly [84, 85]. For instance, in a study in Sweden from 1983 to 1997, 31.9% of women who experienced a stillbirth were pregnant within 3 months, and 59.6% were pregnant in less than 8 months, compared with 1.5% and 8.1%, respectively, of women with live births [85]. Also, women who are at risk of poor pregnancy outcomes because of socioeconomic factors are more likely to experience a shorter interpregnancy interval because of an unplanned pregnancy. However, results of studies that limit analyses to women with no poor prior pregnancy outcomes and that control for maternal age, parity, social factors, and other hypothesized confounders show a consistent residual effect of the short interval. For example, after controlling for these variables in a study of Scottish women delivering from 1992 to 1998, Smith and colleagues [84] estimated the population attributable risk for interpregnancy intervals less than 6 months to be 6.1% for very preterm birth (24–32 weeks) and 3.9% for moderate preterm birth (33–35 weeks) among women with a previous healthy infant.

A causal hypothesis for the effect of short interpregnancy interval is that women are nutritionally depleted by pregnancy and require a certain amount of time to replenish their nutritional stores [86–88]. In particular, folate [88] or iron [87] stores may require longer than 6 months to become replenished postdelivery. The association between short interpregnancy intervals and U.S. racial groups may help to explain why African-American women enter pregnancy with a higher risk of reduced essential nutrients [72].

In summary, the following characteristics pose extra risks for stillbirth: the first delivery, a pregnancy subsequent to an adverse pregnancy outcome, and a pregnancy conceived within 18 months of a previous pregnancy outcome. Women having these characteristics may need to be followed more closely.

Social environment

Lower maternal education is consistently associated with increased risk of stillbirth [3, 89]. Neighborhood context may somewhat mitigate social disadvantage associated with lower maternal education. In Quebec, Canada, women with lower educational attainment who also reside in lower-income neighborhoods have higher stillbirth rates than women with lower educational attainment living in higher-income neighborhoods [89]. While it is relatively easy to establish the association between poorer social environment and stillbirth, it is much more difficult to understand the underlying mechanisms for this association. As discussed earlier, a causal framework for the effect of social environment on poor pregnancy outcomes involves biological and environmental factors related to social position and interpersonal relationships throughout the life course [68]. In addition, poor social environment is correlated with environmental exposures such as to a toxic neighborhood environment, dangerous occupation, etc. Further, in some countries such as the United States, lack of access to good health care is associated with poor social environment. Also, women may adjust to reduced social circumstances through behaviors that may be toxic, for example, overeating leading to obesity, smoking, binge drinking, and illicit drug use, as well as risky sexual behavior. For example, in one study of women who received no prenatal care prior to delivery in Louisiana, correlations were found with lower maternal education and lack of health insurance, smoking, cocaine use, prior substance abuse, syphilis, and HIV infection, as well as with poor pregnancy outcomes including stillbirth [90].

It would be highly desirable to distinguish among the many purported social environmental factors those that may be underlying causes, amenable to intervention and prevention of stillbirth (e.g., smoking), from those that are risk markers

for yet-to-be-identified causes. However, the social environment is complex, with correlated variables that make it difficult to isolate on one or another potential cause. This and subsequent sections on behavioral risk factors and nutrition include illustrative examples of studies that attempt to isolate on single social environmental variables.

Social position

Stephansson and colleagues [91] estimated the effect of social position (as measured by occupation) while controlling for associated factors in a population-based matched case–control study of Swedish stillbirths from 1987 to 1996. After adjusting for maternal age, BMI, smoking, and country of origin, the investigators found a significant association between stillbirth risk and occupation. Compared with high-level white-collar workers, unskilled blue-collar workers had an adjusted relative risk of 2.2 (95% CI 1.3–3.7); skilled blue-collar workers, 2.4 (95% CI 1.3–4.1); low-level white-collar workers, 1.9 (95% CI 1.2–3.2); and intermediate-level white-collar workers 1.4 (95% CI 0.9–2.4). Results were similar after further adjustment for level of prenatal care, prior pregnancy history, and after limiting the analysis to women with no maternal conditions or complications. Stillbirth risk was greatest for term antepartum fetal deaths and intrapartum stillbirths. This study points to the potential for further investigation of factors that cause both a reduction in social position and increased risk of stillbirth. One such mechanism could be activation of the HPA axis through early adverse life events, or early or current life stressors that may lead to posttraumatic stress disorder (PTSD).

Occupation

While Stephansson et al. [91] used occupational category to define social position, in a small number of unrelated studies, others have suggested that the occupation itself may incur risk of stillbirth, perhaps through exposure to toxic agents. For example, women's agricultural exposure to pesticides has been suggested to increase of stillbirth [92]. In the United Kingdom, men's (but not women's) exposures as commercial flight crews, compared with ground traffic controllers, was associated with higher reported risk of stillbirth in a retrospective study of pregnancy outcomes [93]. On the other hand, in a small study of 350 cosmetologists and 397 women in other occupations, no excess risk of stillbirth was reported [94]. In a larger, retrospective National Maternal and Infant Health Survey of 1988 in the United States, Savitz and colleagues [95] compared women by occupation categories, with clerical workers as the referent group. Elevated risks for stillbirth were found among textile workers, food service workers, and janitors, while teachers and librarians had reduced risks of adverse pregnancy outcomes. No specific causal agents for stillbirth have been identified, as yet, and none of the scattered studies of occupational exposure has controlled for potential confounding associated with the correlation of occupation, social position, and stress.

Marital status

In the United States, if the mother is unmarried at the time of delivery, especially if the father is not identified on the birth certificate, her delivery is more likely to be a stillbirth, preterm live birth, or a live-born infant who dies before the first birthday. While associations with unmarried status and poor pregnancy outcome are reported in other developed countries as well, it has not been established that unmarried status is an independent risk factor or rather a marker for poor social or economic circumstances. Arntzen and colleagues [96] studied 93,800 firstborn infants of mothers delivering from 1978 to 1982 in Norway, which is a welfare state with substantial economic support for lower-income families. After controlling for maternal age, education, and SES, investigators found no additional increased risk for stillbirth attributable to unmarried status. This finding may or may not reflect the current relationship between marital status and stillbirth in Norway or other developed countries, as social mores and social status associated with marriage have shifted over time. Also, societal support for unmarried parents varies from country to country. Marital status is reported on vital records in the United States, but other social characteristics such as income and social support

are not. Thus, whether unmarried status confers an independent association with stillbirth in the United States—and if so, what are the underlying risk(s) associated with unmarried status—remain unanswered research questions.

Unmarried status is one type of potential chronic stressor for pregnant women. Married women tend to be wealthier than unmarried women, to have stronger social networks, and to have more stable home environments; such social support may buffer both chronic and acute stresses that otherwise would increase their risk of poor pregnancy outcomes. Also, compared with married women, unmarried women may experience more chronic and acute stressors that are directly related to their marital status. For example, unmarried partners may be more prone to physical violence which has been linked with increased risk of stillbirth in two studies [97]. In a recent study, Coker and colleagues conducted a cross-sectional survey of pregnancy history and history of partner violence among 755 women. After controlling for maternal age, race, smoking, insurance status, and marital status, they found an adjusted OR for perinatal mortality (stillbirths plus neonatal deaths in the first 28 days) of 2.1 (95% CI 1.3–3.4) for women who reported being a victim of violence in that pregnancy, compared with women who reported no violence in that pregnancy. As the authors point out, if this association reflects a real risk it may be a direct result of blunt force trauma, a concomitant association with maternal infection, or an indirect result of stress.

Psychosocial stress

Stress exposure is difficult to quantify in epidemiologic research because it can be categorized in a number of different ways, each of which may be open to measurement errors [98]. Stress may be categorized as a type of personality trait (anxiety, primarily), or experience of major acute life events such as divorce or the death of a spouse, or a life course filled with chronic and persistent hassles. Each of these is a valid construct, but with potentially different physiologic effects and impacts on pregnancy outcome.

To date, studies of maternal stress and perinatal outcomes have tended to focus on preterm birth as an outcome. Recent literature reviews [68, 99] have concluded that perceived general stress may increase preterm birth risk by 20–80%. The literature is inconclusive with respect to whether major acute life events increase preterm birth risk. Further, studies suggest that preterm birth risks may differ between non-Hispanic white and black women, with white women being more susceptible to anxiety and black women being more susceptible to depression and PTSD—which may reflect their increased exposure to life course and chronic stressors.

There is a small, but growing body of evidence that stress may also affect stillbirth risk. In the SCRN study, participants were asked whether they had experienced 13 stressful life events (SLEs) in the 12 months leading up to their delivery: a close family member was hospitalized or died; the woman or her partner lost employment or had money problems; she or her partner were in jail; she fought with her partner or others or became divorced; her family had drugs or alcohol issues; she moved or became homeless; or her pregnancy had been unwanted by her partner [59]. Of 953 women with stillbirth eligible for the study, 126 were not approached, 164 refused, and 663 (70%) consented to participate. A total of 3,089 live birth controls were eligible, and 63% consented. Analyses comparing stillbirth and live birth were weighted to account for oversampling in the design and percentage consenting within subgroups.

SLEs ranged from 0 to 12 per woman. Compared to 0 SLEs, $\geq$1 SLE was associated with stillbirth (OR 1.6, 95% CI 1.2–2.0). As the number of SLEs increased, the OR increased from 1.2 (95% CI 0.9–1.6) for 1 to 2.5 (95% CI 1.8–3.5) for $\geq$5 SLEs. This dose–response relationship remained unchanged and significant ($p < 0.0001$) after control for clinic site, mother's age (<20, 20–34, 35–39, >39 years), race/ethnicity, pregnancy history (including previous spontaneous abortions or stillbirth), education (<12, 12, $\geq$13 years), marital status, insurance status, reported drug use during pregnancy, and prepregnancy smoking. No covariates interacted statistically with the association of SLE with stillbirth. Three of the SLEs were not individually associated with stillbirth risk (moving to a new address,

husband or partner lost his job, someone close to the mother died). This specificity of effect suggests that selective recall may not explain the observed association. Results of the SCRN study were similar to Wisborg's findings among Danish women [48]. The measure of acute stressors in this study was the 12-item General Health Questionnaire (GHQ) which measures psychological distress. Pregnant women were administered the GHQ prospectively at 30 weeks gestation. Compared with women with a subsequent live birth, women whose pregnancy ended in stillbirth had an elevated GHQ score (adjusted OR 1.9 [1.1–3.2]).

Major adverse childhood events (ACEs) (physical or sexual abuse, death of a parent) are associated with a number of health problems arising later in life. In one study, ACEs were associated in a dose–response relationship with experience of a stillbirth [100]. Respondents were asked to recall eight adverse experiences: household substance abuse (prevalence of reporting 29.7%); physical abuse (27.25%); sexual abuse (24.9%); parental separation or divorce (24.6%); mental illness in household (23.5%); intimate partner violence among parents or guardians (13.8%); verbal abuse (13.3%); and incarcerated household member (5.2%). Scores ranged from 0 to 8, with 34.1% reporting no ACE and 1.5% reporting 7 or 8 ACE. Compared with women who reported no ACE, and after adjustment for age, race, education, and experience of an adolescent pregnancy, adjusted ORs for stillbirth ranged from 1.2 (95% CI 0.96–1.4) for 1–2 ACE to 1.8 (95% CI 1.3–2.3) for 5 or more ACE. This study has several methodological limitations, including the retrospective recall of stillbirth, and the age of respondents which ranged from young adults to women in their 50s. However, the strength of the association and dose–response relationship justify a more methodologically rigorous study. The SCRN has endeavored to partially fill this gap with a follow-up study of women with stillbirth and live birth. The follow-up questionnaire included an assessment of adverse childhood experiences. This study is currently in the analysis phase.

The most proximate mechanisms commonly used to explain the effects of maternal stress on perinatal outcomes are dysfunction of the maternal-placental-fetal HPA axis or alteration of maternal susceptibility and immune response to infection. A broader explanation first articulated by Geronimus [101] is termed the "weathering" hypothesis. Geronimus posits that chronic exposures to psychosocial and environmental stressors prematurely age exposed women, shifting age-related risk to the peak of reproductive activity. It is possible that early life experiences incur a heavier stress–age effect than later experiences incur, possibly because of increased susceptibility to depression or PTSD at young ages or the chronic impact of early-onset depression and PTSD on the life course [102].

In summary, it is possible that severe, recent acute adverse experiences increase stillbirth risk. It is also possible that chronic or early life experiences are risk factors for stillbirth. Early and cumulative life course stress may prematurely age a woman or increase her risk of PTSD or depression. While few studies have addressed these issues, it is anticipated that more information will become available in the near future.

Maternal substance use

Caffeine, smoking, and alcohol

Commonly consumed chemicals in cigarettes as well as caffeine (through coffee, tea, soft drinks, high-powered drinks, pills, etc.) and alcohol consumption have been found to be associated with increased risk of stillbirth in some, but not all, studies. The strength of the association varies by type of exposure as well as quality of exposure measurement. Also, as mentioned earlier women who smoke, drink alcohol, or consume caffeine in large quantities may have other characteristics that place them at elevated risk of stillbirth, and determining the causal impact of commonly consumed drugs is difficult to separate from these other factors.

A systematic review of epidemiologic studies of caffeine consumption and stillbirth published in 2005 concluded that caffeine consumption cannot be declared a risk factor with certainty because of the paucity of studies, relatively modest effects reported, and possibility of publication bias [103].

More recently, a prospective cohort study in the United Kingdom of 2,643 pregnant women beginning in their first trimester, using a validated tool for estimating caffeine intake and controlling for potential confounders (including smoking with salivary cotinine measures), reported a significant risk of late miscarriage and stillbirth with increasing caffeine consumption during the first trimester [104]. More such studies are needed before there would be conclusive evidence of effect. Nevertheless, caution in caffeine consumption during pregnancy is warranted.

Smoking is not recommended for anyone, and women who smoke are counseled to stop when they become pregnant to avoid the well-established effects on their fetus associated with hypoxia and placental abruption [105]. Smoking may increase risk of stillbirth by 20% or more [34], and in populations where smoking is common, smoking may account for much of the difference observed between populations. For example, women who reported smoking accounted for 38% of the difference in stillbirth risk across socioeconomic categories in Scotland during the period 1994–2003 [106]. Smoking also exacerbates the already-high stillbirth risk among older women [23]. Preventing smoking during pregnancy should reduce stillbirth incidence among smokers. Stillbirth risk is not elevated if women stop smoking prior to pregnancy [107] or in the first trimester [51], and nicotine replacement therapy appears not to be a risk factor for stillbirth [57].

Binge drinking may increase stillbirth risk, although recent systematic reviews disagree on the strength of the evidence linking heavy alcohol consumption to stillbirth [108, 109]. Data from the Missouri vital statistics study [33] and the Danish National Birth Cohort [53] report significant, but weak effects of high levels of alcohol consumption. Because women who binge drink are likely to differ in many respects that are difficult or impossible to measure in these registry-based studies, the question of the impact of binge drinking on stillbirth remains unanswered.

Illicit drug use

It is extremely difficult to study the impact of illicit drug use on stillbirth, because of selective recall as well as major differences in populations who do and do not use illicit drugs. Biomarkers of drug use at delivery cannot document drug use early in pregnancy, and prospective studies with biomarkers are lacking. Cocaine has pharmacologic effects in experimental studies that mirror case reports of restricted fetal growth and placental abruption [110], and small studies of acknowledged cocaine users report an increased risk of stillbirth [111, 112]. Self-reported marijuana (cannabis) use has been associated with placental abruption [113] but has not been associated with increased stillbirth risk in some research [114]. In a large South Australian study, only 707 of 89,080 women delivering from 1998 to 2002 self-reported illicit drug use (including marijuana, methadone, amphetamines, and heroin) [115]. Among these women, after statistical control for some confounding factors the OR for stillbirth was 2.5, mostly attributable to placental abruption or other causes of antepartum hemorrhage. In general, the few human studies reported to date are too sparse and flawed to develop a definitive measure of effect for any specific illicit drug use.

Maternal nutrition

Obesity (also see Chapter 8)

The worldwide obesity epidemic has serious consequences for maternal and infant health. In most epidemiologic studies, women are defined as overweight or obese by BMI (or weight in km divided by height in m^2) of 25.0–29.9 or 30.0+, respectively. Maternal obesity is associated with hypertension, diabetes, and other chronic conditions related to poor pregnancy outcome. Obesity is also associated with prolonged gestation which, without obstetric intervention, is related to higher risk of intrapartum stillbirth. For these reasons, higher prepregnant BMI has been associated with an increased risk of stillbirth in most published studies [29, 116–118]. In Missouri, the adjusted hazards ratio for stillbirth among obese mothers was 1.4 (95% CI 1.2–1.4) [29], and the hazards rose with rising BMI to 1.9 (95% CI 1.6–2.1) for women with BMI of 40+. In Sweden, women

who gained as much as 3 BMI units between the first and second pregnancy had a stillbirth OR of 1.6 (95% CI 1.2–2.2) in their second pregnancy when compared with women who lost weight or gained less than 0.9 BMI units [119]. Overweight and obesity may exacerbate already-high risks of stillbirth associated with type 2 diabetes [120], multiple pregnancies [32], and African-American race [29].

However, in some large population-based studies in Argentina [121] and China [122] in which obesity was associated with increased risks of preeclampsia, gestational diabetes, and preterm delivery, no significant elevation in stillbirth risk was found. It is possible that in populations where cesarean section is more common for obese women or women with prolonged gestation [121–123], obesity-associated stillbirth rates might have been mitigated by earlier obstetric intervention for obesity. More careful monitoring of obese women throughout pregnancy may help to identify those who need early intervention. Nevertheless, primary prevention of obesity-associated stillbirth will require effective interventions to prevent excessive weight gain prior to pregnancy.

Iron

Iron deficiency is frequently associated with poor pregnancy outcomes in developing countries, where interference of the mechanism of iron homeostasis may help to explain differences in the impact of iron supplementation in various randomized trials [124]. Altitude may also have an impact on hemoglobin-associated stillbirth. In Peru, low hemoglobin (<7 g/dl) was associated with higher stillbirth risk in both low-altitude and high-altitude environments, while high hemoglobin (>15.5 g/dl) was associated with stillbirth only at high elevations [125]. In developed countries, studies of the effect of maternal hemoglobin concentration in the first or second trimester on stillbirth risk have reported mixed results. Among U.S. deliveries in 1988, adjusted hazards ratio of stillbirth at 28+ weeks gestational age was 4.4 (95% CI 1.0–19.0) for women with moderate prenatal anemia (8.5 to <9.5 g/dl) compared to women with normal hemoglobin levels (9.5–14.5 g/dl) prior to 28 weeks gestation [73]. On the other hand, a high hemoglobin level (>14.6 g/dl)—but not anemia—was associated with stillbirth risk in a Swedish study conducted from 1987 to 1996 [126]. Across all studies, however, the lowest stillbirth risk occurred among women with normal prenatal hemoglobin levels (generally in the range of 12.6–13.5 g/dl before the third trimester). Whether monitoring of hemoglobin throughout pregnancy and maintenance within that range will alter stillbirth rates has yet to be determined.

Maternal mental illness

Little is known about the impact of maternal mental disorders and stillbirth risk. A meta-analysis published in 2005 concluded that most relevant studies were of schizophrenia, but were generally small, clinic-based studies subject to bias and with little statistical power [127].

More recently, substance abuse disorders were examined in the U.S. National Comorbidity Study (NCS) [128]. The adjusted OR of 1.4 for women with substance abuse disorders is comparable to the elevated risks associated with self-reported illicit drug use (see earlier). At this time it is not possible to separate the relative impact of the substance or the disease that leads to substance abuse.

Also in the NCS, any mental disorder was associated with an adjusted OR of 1.8, and for affective disorders, with an OR of 1.6 [128]. Affective disorder was also associated with stillbirth in Sweden [129], but the observed difference was not statistically significant (OR 2.2, 95% CI 0.55–8.76). More study is warranted to assess whether mental disorders are associated with increased etiology of stillbirth (and if so, how) and whether there is an impact of prenatal treatment of schizophrenia and affective disorders on stillbirth risk.

Maternal health care

Since the mid-twentieth century, two obstetric practices—ARTs and cesarean section—have contributed to alterations in the epidemiology of stillbirth in the developed world.

Assisted reproductive technologies

As an increasing number of women who could not conceive without assistance have been successful through ART, there is a growing concern that ART may increase stillbirth risk among pregnancies conceived through ART [130]. Possible reasons for this risk include greater risk of multiple conceptions that are inherently at greater risk of stillbirth [131]; older maternal age at delivery with concomitant higher, age-related maternal morbidity, or conception by subfertile women whose pregnancies would be at risk irrespective of how they were conceived [52, 132, 133]; and differential effects of different assistance modalities, such as IVF or intracytoplasmic sperm injection (ICSI) and non-IVF ART [52]. While it is clear that ART is associated with increased multiple conceptions that are at greater intrinsic risk of stillbirth, improved ART methods that reduce multiple conceptions may not eliminate the impact of ART on stillbirth. In the Danish Aarhus Birth Cohort study, from 1989 to 2006, among 20,166 singleton pregnancies, the adjusted stillbirth OR for pregnancies conceived by IVF/ICSI was 4.1 (95% CI 2.11–7.93), while pregnancies conceived by non-IVF ART, pregnancies of subfertile women without ART, and pregnancies of fertile women had similar stillbirth risks [52].

Induction of labor and elective cesarean section

In recent decades, deliveries by cesarean section have increased dramatically as a proportion of all live birth deliveries. In the United States, for example, 31.1% of deliveries were by cesarean section in 2006, a 50% increase since 1996 [134]. Many cesarean deliveries are planned, either with or without a trial of labor. It is now well established that elective obstetric intervention including labor induction and cesarean deliveries at 39 weeks gestation or whenever labor is established reduce both antepartum and intrapartum stillbirths associated with fetal hypoxia [81, 135]. In a meta-analysis, Hankins and colleagues [81] estimated that elective delivery at 39 weeks would prevent two fetal deaths per 1,000 fetuses alive at 39 weeks; this amounts to as many as 6,000 stillbirths in the United States each year. Increased obstetric intervention of term singleton pregnancies in Scotland is credited with most of an observed 20-year decrease in stillbirths among fetuses without anomalies and with cephalic presentation at term, from 1988 to 2007 [135]. Similarly, more than half of a 48% decline in twin stillbirth rates in Missouri from 1989 to 1989 was attributed to increased labor induction and cesarean delivery, particularly for gestational ages at 32 weeks and above [136]. Responding to this evidence, some have called for all women to be scheduled for elective labor or cesarean section (depending on the woman's desires [137] as well as her physician's recommendation) when they attain 39 weeks gestation. A more conservative recommendation, which is designed to avoid unnecessary neonatal morbidity and mortality associated with inaccurate gestational age assessments leading to late preterm deliveries, is to induce labor for women at 41 weeks gestation. A recent meta-analysis of trials of elective induction of labor concluded that elective induction of labor at 41 weeks gestation or later may decrease both the risk of emergency cesarean delivery and fetal morbidity such as meconium-stained amniotic fluid, whereas the evidence regarding elective labor induction prior to 41 weeks gestation is insufficient to draw any conclusion [138]. The authors concluded that there is a great need for translational research of these research findings into routine obstetric practice [138].

While increasing primary cesarean sections in the United States and elsewhere may have contributed to reducing stillbirth risk in the primary pregnancy, there is considerable controversy about the impact of prior cesarean section on stillbirth risk of the next pregnancy [30, 139–142]. In a study of 120,633 singleton second births in Scotland from 1980 to 1998, the adjusted hazards ratio for stillbirth at 34+ weeks gestation in a pregnancy following primary cesarean section (compared with vaginal delivery of the first birth) was 2.7 (95% CI 1.7–4.3) [139]. However, over approximately the same time period (i.e., 1978–1997) in Missouri, stillbirth in the second pregnancy following cesarean section of the first pregnancy was not statistically elevated for all women or for white women, but was elevated for African-American women, with an adjusted relative risk of 1.4 (95% CI 1.1–1.7) [30]. Subsequent

investigators have reported mixed results [140–142]. Since all studies are observational, it is difficult to separate medical and other reasons for the mode of delivery from an effect of the mode of delivery itself. Controlling for possible confounding variables is incomplete, and the underlying reasons for choice of cesarean section in the first and second pregnancies may have an impact on pregnancy risk in the second pregnancy. Because cesarean deliveries continue to comprise a large percentage of births, continued and improved research into the question of stillbirth risk in pregnancies following cesarean section deliveries is warranted.

Summary and conclusions

The overview provided in this chapter briefly reviews the literature for more than 20 common exposures or demographic characteristics that have been associated with different stillbirth rates. In a few instances, stillbirth should be declining because certain characteristics are becoming less common in the United States (e.g., prolonged gestations, very young maternal age, grand multiparity, and multiple gestations from ART). Other characteristics are increasing in prevalence and may be stalling improvements in stillbirth rates. Most notably, these include older maternal age and obesity. Increasing age at first delivery contributes to increased resort to ART, as fertility declines with increasing age. It is important to determine whether further progress can be made in limiting ART-associated gestations to singletons. Also, ART methods should be further investigated to determine if some create greater stillbirth risks than others. It is also important to improve vital records data quality so that trends can be better tracked in the future.

Evidence of a consistent relationship is limited for many factors that have been identified in one or more studies. These factors are noted in Table 4.1 with a single plus (+) in the column for level of evidence. For example, while it is clear that obstetric intervention to avoid postterm delivery reduces stillbirth risk in those pregnancies, many of these interventions result in primary cesarean deliveries. It is

> **Box 4.1 Research priorities for increasing knowledge of why common exposures are associated with stillbirth and of how to mitigate their effect through primary or secondary prevention**
>
> **For etiologic investigation, mount prospective epidemiologic studies beginning in early pregnancy.**
> Conduct large-scale studies of African-Americans, with measurement of multiple possible causes of preterm live- and stillbirth.
> Conduct large-scale studies, with serial biomarkers of caffeine, alcohol, stress, etc. to determine etiologic fraction and interactions.
> A targeted investigation of infertility treatments should address the question of whether treatment type affects pregnancy outcome.
> **For clinical effectiveness, mount randomized trials preconception of potential interventions.**
> Can a targeted weight loss intervention begun postpartum and continued to the next conception reduce weight-associated stillbirth risk?
> Can women be counseled and provided effective interventions to achieve interpregnancy intervals of 18–23 months?
> Can targeted, preconception support for socioculturally based risk factors reduce poor pregnancy outcomes for first and higher-order births?
> Does screening and treatment preconceptionally for PTSD, depression, and other mental disorders reduce risk of poor pregnancy outcomes?
> Does preconception provision of iron supplementation reduced stillbirth risk?
> Can infertility care be enhanced to reduce multiple embryo implantations and risk of multiple gestations?
> **For clinical effectiveness, mount randomized trials of pregnant women to test potential interventions.**
> Does frequent monitoring and delivery intervention decrease stillbirth risk among women identified as high risk because of behavioral/sociocultural factors?
> Can prenatal care be improved to reduce iatrogenic preterm delivery and provide appropriate mode of delivery—to reduce risks associated with interventions?
> Will a patch for smokers reduce smoking-associated poor pregnancy outcomes, including stillbirth?
> Does biomarker screening and treatment for alcohol, smoking, and substance abuse reduce risk of poor pregnancy outcomes?
> Does nonpharmaceutical treatment in pregnancy of PTSD, depression, and other mental disorders reduce risk of poor pregnancy outcomes?

not clear whether stillbirth risk is increased in subsequent pregnancies with repeat cesareans.

Box 4.1 lists some priority areas for future research. Two of the strongest observed associations of increased stillbirth risk are with African-American race and with lower SES or social position. What contributes to these associations, however, has yet to be determined. Multiple causation, complex interactions, and possible gene–environment interactions with many other factors that covary with these populations will require that future research be more comprehensive, in comparison with past studies that have relied heavily on vital records and medical records. The National Children's Study is currently targeted to begin in 2012. This prospective study of environmental exposures of at least 100,000 children from preconception or prenatal status to age 21 can serve as a platform for many epidemiologic questions. It could be enhanced with oversampling of minority populations to address questions about stillbirth, which is a relatively rare condition.

Evidence from epidemiologic studies of demographics and common exposures can help prioritize intervention research. Box 4.1 lists several priorities for randomized trials in both preconception and prenatal care. It is not feasible to measure stillbirth per se for most clinical trials, owing to its rarity. However, as stillbirth shares many risk factors with more common outcomes such as preterm birth, randomized trials of improving pregnancy outcome in general should shed light on the impact on stillbirth.

Finally, it is worth noting that stillbirth rates declined dramatically over several decades from the mid-twentieth century. The slow decline in recent years reflects the difficulty of attacking the remaining causes. Some causes, such as obesity, require political will and social action outside medical care, as well as improved methods of primary and secondary prevention. Progress can be made in the twenty-first century, with adequate attention to effective means to intervene.

References

1. McClure EM, Saleem S, Pasha O, et al. Stillbirth in developing countries: a review of causes, risk factors and prevention strategies. J Matern Fetal Neonatal Med 2009;22:183–90.
2. Lawn JE, Gravett MG, Nunes TM, et al. Global report on preterm birth and stillbirth (1 of 7): definitions,

description of the burden and opportunities to improve data. BMC Pregnancy Childbirth 2010;10 (Suppl. 1):1–22.

3. Fretts RC. Etiology and prevention of stillbirth. Am J Obstet Gynecol 2005;193:1923–35.

4. Joseph KS, Fahey J, Dendukuri N, et al. Recent changes in maternal characteristics by socioeconomic status. J Obstet Gynaecol Can 2009;31:422–33.

5. Glinianaia SV, Rankin J, Pless-Mulloli T, et al. Temporal changes in key maternal and fetal factors affecting birth outcomes: a 32-year population-based study in an industrial city. BMC Pregnancy Childbirth 2008;8:39.

6. Sipila P, Hartikainen AL, von Wendt L, et al. Changes in risk factors for unfavorable pregnancy outcome among singletons over twenty years. Acta Obstet Gynecol Scand 1994;73:612–18.

7. Goy J, Dodds L, Rosenberg MW, et al. Health-risk behaviours: examining social disparities in the occurrence of stillbirth. Paediatr Perinat Epidemiol 2008; 22:314–20.

8. Berry RJ, Buehler JW, Strauss LT, et al. Birth weight-specific infant mortality due to congenital anomalies, 1960 and 1980. Public Health Rep 1987;102:171–81.

9. Yang Q, Chen H, Correa A, et al. Racial differences in infant mortality attributable to birth defects in the United States, 1989–2002. Birth Defects Res A Clin Mol Teratol 2006;76:706–13.

10. Gissler M, Ollila E, Teperi J, et al. Impact of induced abortions and statistical definitions on perinatal mortality figures. Paediatr Perinat Epidemiol 1994;8:391–400.

11. Khoshnood B, De Vigan C, Vodovar V, et al. Trends in prenatal diagnosis, pregnancy termination, and perinatal mortality of newborns with congenital heart disease in France, 1983–2000: a population-based evaluation. Pediatrics 2005;115:95–101.

12. Dadvand P, Rankin J, Shirley MDF, et al. Descriptive epidemiology of congenital heart disease in Northern England. Paediatr Perinat Epidemiol 2009;23:58–65.

13. Siffel C, Correa A, Cragan J, et al. Prenatal diagnosis, pregnancy terminations and prevalence of Down Syndrome in Atlanta. Birth Defects Res A Clin Mol Teratol 2004;70:565–71.

14. Ehrenthal DB, Wingate MS, Kirby RS. Variation by state in outcomes classification for deliveries less than 500 g in the United States. Matern Child Health J 2010; DOI 10.107/s 10995-010-0716-2. Published online: November 2010.

15. MacDorman MF, Kirmeyer S. Fetal and perinatal mortality, United States, 2005. Natl Vital Stat Rep 2009;57:1–19.

16. Dundon ML, Gay GA, George JL. The 1978 revision of the U.S. standard certificates. Vital and Health Statistics, Series 4, No. 23. DHHS Pub. No. (PHS) 83–1460;1983:1–64.

17. Freedman MA, Gay GA, Brockert JE, et al. The 1989 revisions of the US standard certificates of live birth and death and the US standard report of fetal death. Am J Public Health 1988;78:168–72.

18. Osterman MJK, Martin JA, Menacker F. Expanded health data from the new birth certificate, 2006. Natl Vital Stat Rep 2009;58(5):1–24.

19. Barfield WD, Tomashek KM, Flowers LM, et al. Contribution of late fetal deaths to US perinatal mortality rates, 1995–1998. Semin Perinatol 2002;26:17–24.

20. Aliyu MH, Salihu HM, Wilson RE, et al. Prenatal smoking and risk of intrapartum stillbirth. Arch Environ Occup Health 2007;62:87–92.

21. Wilson RE, Alio AP, Kirby RS, et al. Young maternal age and risk of intrapartum stillbirth. Arch Gynecol Obstet 2008;278:231–6.

22. Aliyu HM, Salihu HM, Alio AP, et al. Prenatal smoking among adolescents and risk of fetal demise before and during labor. J Pediatr Adolesc Gynecol 2010;23:129–35.

23. Aliyu MH, Salihu HM, Wilson RE, et al. The risk of intrapartum stillbirth among smokers of advanced maternal age. Arch Gynecol Obstet 2008;278: 9–45.

24. Aliyu MH, Salihu HM, Keith LG, et al. Extreme parity and the risk of stillbirth. Obstet Gynecol 2005;106:446–53.

25. Salihu HM, Aliyu MH, Rouse DJ, et al. The association of parity with mortality outcomes among triplets. Am J Obstet Gynecol 2004;190:784–9.

26. Salihu HM, Aliyu MH, Kirby RS, et al. Effect of advanced maternal age on early mortality among quadruplets and quintuplets. Am J Obstet Gynecol 2004;190:383–8.

27. Sharma PP, Salihu HM, Oyelese Y, et al. Is race a determinant of stillbirth recurrence? Obstet Gynecol 2006;107:391–7.

28. Salihu HM, Kinniburgh BA, Aliyu MH, et al. Racial disparity in stillbirth among singleton, twin, and triplet gestations in the United States. Obstet Gynecol 2004;104:734–40.

29. Salihu HM, Dunlop AL, Hedayatzadeh M, et al. Extreme obesity and risk of stillbirth among black and white gravidas. Obstet Gynecol 2007;110:552–7.

30. Salihu HM, Sharma PP, Kristensen S, et al. Risk of stillbirth following a cesarean delivery: black-white disparity. Obstet Gynecol 2006;107:383–90.

31. Salihu HM, Mbah AK, Alio AP, et al. Maternal pre-pregnancy underweight and risk of early and late stillbirth in black and white gravidas. J Natl Med Assoc 2009;101:582–7.

32. Russell Z, Salihu HM, Lynch O, et al. The asso-ciation of prepregnancy body mass index with pregnancy outcomes in triplet gestations. Am J Perinatol 2010;27:41–6.

33. Aliyu MH, Wilson RE, Zoorob R, et al. Alcohol con-sumption during pregnancy and the risk of early still-birth among singletons. Alcohol 2008;42:369–74.

34. Salihu HM, Sharma PP, Getahun D, et al. Prenatal tobacco use and risk of stillbirth: a case-control and bidirectional case-crossover study. Nicotine Tob Res 2008;10:159–66.

35. Verkerk PH, Buitendijk SE, Verloove-Vanhorick SP. Differential misclassification of alcohol and ciga-rette consumption by pregnancy outcome. Int J Epidemiol 1994;23:1218–25.

36. Dietz PM, Adams MM, Kendrick JS, et al., and the PRAMS Working Group. Completeness of ascertain-ment of prenatal smoking using birth certificates and confidential questionnaires. Am J Epidemiol 1998;148:1048–54.

37. Vinikoor LC, Messer LC, Laraia BA, et al. Reliability of variables on the North Carolina birth certifi-cate: a comparison with directly queried values from a cohort study. Paediatr Perinat Epidemiol 2010;24:102–12.

38. Park S, Sappenfield WM, Bish C, et al. Reliability and validity of birth certificate prepregnancy weight and height among women enrolled in prenatal WIC program: Florida, 2005. Matern Child Health J 2009; DOI 10.1007/s 10995-009-0544-4. Published online: November 2009.

39. Liess JK, Giles D, Sullivan KM, et al. U.S. mater-nally linked birth records may be biased for Hispanics and other population groups. Ann Epidemiol 2010;20:23–31.

40. Rasmussen S, Irgens LM, Skjaerven R, et al. Prior adverse pregnancy outcome and the risk of still-birth. Obstet Gynecol 2009;114:1259–70.

41. Quansah R, Gissler M, Jaakkola JJK. Work as a nurse and a midwife and adverse pregnancy out-comes: a Finnish nationwide population-based study. J Women's Health 2009;18:2071–6.

42. Nielsen HS, Mortensen LH, Nygaard U, et al. Sex of prior children and risk of stillbirth in subsequent pregnancies. Epidemiology 2010;21:114–17.

43. King-Hele S, Webb RT, Mortensen PB, et al. Risk of stillbirth and neonatal death linked with maternal mental illness: a national cohort study. Arch Dis Child Fetal Neonatal Ed 2009;94:F105–10.

44. Olsen J, Melbye M, Olsen SF, et al. The Danish national birth cohort—its background, structure and aim. Scand J Public Health 2001;29:300–7.

45. Nohr EA, Frydenberg M, Henriksen TB, et al. Does low participation in cohort studies induce bias? Epidemiology 2006;17:413–18.

46. Nohr EA, Bech BH, Davies MJ, et al. Prepregnancy obesity and fetal death: a study within the Danish National Birth Cohort. Obstet Gynecol 2005;106:250–9.

47. Bech BH, Nohr EA, Vaeth M, et al. Coffee and fetal death: a cohort study with prospective data. Am J Epidemiol 2005;162:983–90.

48. Wisborg K, Barklin A, Hedegaard M, et al. Psychological stress during pregnancy and stillbirth: prospective study. BJOG 2008;115:882–5.

49. Wisborg K, Kesmodel U, Bech BH, et al. Maternal consumption of coffee during pregnancy and still-birth and infant death in first year of life: prospec-tive study. BMJ 2003;326:420.

50. Kesmodel U, Wisborg K, Olsen SF, et al. Moderate alcohol intake during pregnancy and the risk of stillbirth and death in the first year of life. Am J Epidemiol 2002;155:305–12.

51. Wisborg K, Kesmodel U, Henriksen TB, et al. Exposure to tobacco smoke in utero and the risk of stillbirth and death in the first year of life. Am J Epidemiol 2001;154:322–7.

52. Wisborg K, Ingersley HJ, Henriksen TB. IVF and stillbirth: a prospective follow-up study. Hum Reprod 2010;25:1312–16.

53. Strandberg-Larsen K, Nielsen NR, Gronboek M, et al. Binge drinking in pregnancy and risk of fetal death. Obstet Gynecol 2008;111:602–9.

54. Zhu JL, Hjollund NH, Andersen AMN, et al. Shift work, job stress, and late fetal loss: the national birth cohort in Denmark. J Occup Environ Med 2004;46:1144–9.

55. Bech BH, Autrup H, Nohr EA, et al. Stillbirth and slow metabolizers of caffeine: comparison by geno-types. Int J Epidemiol 2006;35:948–53.

56. Rebordosa C, Kogevinas M, Bech BH. Use of aceta-minophen during pregnancy and risk of adverse pregnancy outcomes. Int J Epidemiol 2009;38:706–14.

57. Strandberg-Larsen K, Tinggaard M, Andersen AMN, et al. Use of nicotine replacement therapy dur-ing pregnancy and stillbirth: a cohort study. BJOG 2008;115:1405–10.

58. Saade G, for the Eunice Kennedy Shriver National Institute of Child Health Stillbirth Collaborative Research Network. Demographic and pre-pregnancy risk factors for stillbirth: a population-based study. MFM abstract 2009.

59. Hogue CJR, for the Eunice Kennedy Shriver National Institute of Child Health Stillbirth Collaborative Research Network. Association of significant life events with risk of stillbirth. SGI abstract 2010.

60. Hamilton BE, Martin JA, Ventura SJ. Births: preliminary data for 2008. Natl Vital Stat Rep 2010;58: 1–18.

61. O'Leary CM, Bower C, Knuiman M, et al. Changing risks of stillbirth and neonatal mortality associated with maternal age in Western Australia 1984–2003. Paediatr Perinat Epidemiol 2007;21:541–9.

62. Usta I, Nassar AH. Advanced maternal age. Part I: obstetric complications. Am J Perinatol 2008;25: 521–34.

63. Getahun D, Ananth CV, Kinzler WL. Risk factors for antepartum and intrapartum stillbirth: a population-based study. Am J Obstet Gynecol 2007; 196:499–507.

64. Reddy UM, Ko CW, Willinger M. Maternal age and the risk of stillbirth throughout pregnancy in the United States. Am J Obstet Gynecol 2006;195:764–70.

65. Andersen AMN, Hansen KD, Andersen PK, et al. Advanced paternal age and risk of fetal death: a cohort study. Am J Epidemiol 2004;160:1214–22.

66. Lee C. "Race" and "ethnicity" in biomedical research: how do scientists construct and explain differences in health? Soc Sci Med 2009;68:1183–219.

67. James S. Epidemiologic research on health disparities: some thoughts on history and current developments. Epidemiol Rev 2009;31:1–6.

68. Kramer MR, Hogue CR. What causes racial disparities in very preterm birth? Epidemiol Rev 2009;31:84–98.

69. Gee GC, Ro A, Shariff-Marco S, et al. Racial discrimination and health among Asian Americans: evidence, assessment, and directions for future research. Epidemiol Rev 2009;31:130–51.

70. Hogue CJR. Towards reducing disparities in disparities research. Am J Epidemiol 2009;170:1195–6.

71. Willinger M, Ko CW, Reddy UM. Racial disparities in stillbirth risk across gestation in the United States. Am J Obstet Gynecol 2009;201:469.e1–8.

72. Dunlop AL, Kramer M, Hogue CJR, et al. The association of nutritional factors and racial disparities in preterm birth rates. Acta Obstet Gynecol 2010.

73. Tomashek KM, Ananth CV, Cogswell ME. Risk of stillbirth in relation to maternal haemoglobin concentration during pregnancy. Matern Child Nutr 2006;2:19–28.

74. Getahun D, Ananth CV, Selvam N, et al. Adverse perinatal outcomes among interracial couples in the United States. Obstet Gynecol 2005;106:81–8.

75. Gold KJ, Lantz SM, Hayward PM, et al. Prematurity and low birth weight as potential mediators of higher stillbirth risk in mixed black/white race couples. J Women's Health 2010;19:767–73.

76. Hogue CJ, Menon R, Dunlop AL, et al. Racial disparities in preterm birth rates and short interpregnancy interval. An overview. Acta Obstet Gynecol; in press (2011).

77. Menon R, Dunlop AL, Kramer MR, et al. An overview of racial disparities in preterm birth rates: caused by infection or inflammatory response? Acta Obstet Gynecol; in press (2011).

78. Kramer MR, Hogue CJ, Dunlop AL, et al. Preconceptional stress and racial disparities in preterm birth: an overview. Acta Obstet Gynecol 2010.

79. Smith GC, Gordon CS. Predicting antepartum stillbirth. Curr Opin Obstet Gynecol 2006;18:625–30.

80. Hilder L, Sairam S, Thilaganathan B. Influence of parity on fetal mortality in prolonged pregnancy. Eur J Obstet Gynecol Reprod Biol 2007;132:167–70.

81. Hankins GD, Clark SM, Munn MB. Cesarean section on request at 39 weeks: impact on shoulder dystocia, fetal trauma, neonatal encephalopathy, and intrauterine fetal demise. Semin Perinatol 2006; 30:276–87.

82. Black M, Shetty A, Bhattacharya S. Obstetric outcomes subsequent to intrauterine death in the first pregnancy. BJOG 2008;115:269–74.

83. Smith GC, Shah I, White IR, et al. Previous preeclampsia, preterm delivery, and delivery of a small for gestational age infant and the risk of unexplained stillbirth in the second pregnancy: a retrospective cohort study, Scotland, 1992–2001. Am J Epidemiol 2007;165:194–202.

84. Smith GC, Pell JP, Dobbie R. Interpregnancy interval and risk of preterm birth and neonatal death: retrospective cohort study. BMJ 2003;327:313.

85. Stephansson O, Dickman PW, Cnattingius S. The influence of interpregnancy interval on the subsequent risk of stillbirth and early neonatal death. Obstet Gynecol 2003;102:101–8.

86 Winkvist A, Rasmussen K, Habicht J-P. A new definition of maternal depletion syndrome. Am J Public Health 1992;82:691–4.

87. Singh K, Fong YF, Arulkumaran S. Anaemia in pregnancy—a cross-sectional study in Singapore. Eur J Clin Nutr 1998;52:65–70.

88. Smits LJM, Essed GGM. Short interpregnancy intervals and unfavourable pregnancy outcome: role of folate depletion. Lancet 2001;358:2074–7.

89. Luo ZC, Wilkins R, Kramer MS. Effect of neighbourhood income and maternal education on birth outcomes: a population-based study. CMAJ 2006; 174:1415–20.

90. Maupin R Jr, Lyman R, Fatsis J, et al. Characteristics of women who deliver with no prenatal care. J Matern Fetal Neonatal Med 2004;16:45–50.

91. Stephansson O, Dickman PW, Johansson AL, et al. The influence of socioeconomic status on stillbirth risk in Sweden. Int J Epidemiol 2001;30:1296–301.

92. Hanke W, Jurewicz J. The risk of adverse reproductive and developmental disorders due to occupational pesticide exposure: an overview of current epidemiological evidence. Int J Occup Med Environ Health 2004;17:223–43.

93. dos Santos Silva I, Pizzi C, Evans A, et al. Reproductive history and adverse pregnancy outcomes in commercial flight crew and air traffic control officers in the United Kingdom. J Occup Environ Med 2009;51:1298–305.

94. Gallicchio L, Miller S, Greene T, et al. Cosmetologists and reproductive outcomes. Obstet Gynecol 2009; 113:1018–26.

95. Savitz DA, Olshan AF, Gallagher K. Maternal occupation and pregnancy outcome. Epidemiology 1996;7:269–74.

96. Arntzen A, Moum T, Magnus P, et al. Marital status as a risk factor for fetal and infant mortality. Scand J Soc Med 1996;24:36–42.

97. Coker AL, Sanderson M, Dong B. Partner violence during pregnancy and risk of adverse pregnancy outcomes. Paediatr Perinat Epidemiol 2004;18: 260–9.

98. O'Campo P, Schempf A. Racial inequalities in preterm delivery: issues in the measurement of psychological constructs. Am J Obstet Gynecol 2005;192:S56–63.

99. Behrman RE, Butler AS (eds). Preterm birth: causes, consequences, and prevention. Washington, DC: National Academy Press, Institute of Medicine; 2007.

100. Hillis SD, Anda RF, Dube SR, et al. The association between adverse childhood experiences and adolescent pregnancy, long-term psychosocial consequences, and fetal death. Pediatrics 2004; 113:320–7.

101. Geronimus AT. The weathering hypothesis and the health of African-American women and infants: evidence and speculations. Ethn Dis 1992;2:207–21.

102. Hogue CJ, Bremner JD. Stress model for research into preterm delivery among black women. Am J Obstet Gynecol 2005;192:S47–55.

103. Matijasevich A, Santos IS, Barros FC. Does caffeine consumption during pregnancy increase the risk of fetal mortality? A literature review. Cad Saude Publica 2005;21:1676–84.

104. Greenwood DC, Alwan N, Boylan S, et al. Caffeine intake during pregnancy, late miscarriage and stillbirth. Eur J Epidemiol 2010;25:275–80.

105. Salihu HM, Wilson RE. Epidemiology of prenatal smoking and perinatal outcomes. Early Hum Dev 2007;83:713–20.

106. Gray R, Bonellie SR, Chalmers J, et al. Contribution of smoking during pregnancy to inequalities in stillbirth and infant death in Scotland 1994–2003: retrospective population based study using hospital maternity records. BMJ 2009;339:b3754.

107. Hogberg L, Cnattingius S. The influence of maternal smoking habits on the risk of subsequent stillbirth: is there a causal relation? BJOG 2007;114:699–704.

108. Gray R. Systematic review of the fetal effects of prenatal binge drinking. J Epidemiol Community Health 2007;61:1069–73.

109. Burd L, Roberts D, Olson M, et al. Ethanol and the placenta: a review. J Matern Fetal Neonatal Med 2007;20:361–75.

110. Kain ZN, Rimar S, Barash PG. Cocaine abuse in the parturient and effects on the fetus and neonate. Anesth Analg 1993;77:835–45.

111. Bingol N, Fuchs M, Diaz V, et al. Teratogenicity of cocaine in humans. J Pediatr 1987;110:350.

112. Loebstein R, Koren G. Pregnancy outcome and neurodevelopment of children exposed in utero to psychoactive drugs: the Motherisk experience. J Psychiatry Neurosci 1997;22:192–6.

113. Williams MA, Lieberman E, Mittendorf R, et al. Risk factors for abruptio placentae. Am J Epidemiol 1991;134:965–72.

114. Fergusson DM, Horwood LJ, Northstone K, for the ALSPAC Study Team. Maternal use of cannabis and pregnancy outcome. BJOG 2002;109:21–7.

115. Kennare R, Heard A, Chan A. Substance use during pregnancy: risk factors and obstetric and perinatal outcomes in South Australia. Aust N Z J Obstet Gynaecol 2005;45:220–5.

116. Chu SY, Kim SY, Lau J, et al. Maternal obesity and risk of stillbirth: a metaanalysis. Am J Obstet Gynecol 2007;197:223–8.

117. Arendas K, Qiu Q, Gruslin A. Obesity in pregnancy: pre-conceptional to postpartum consequences. J Obstet Gynaecol Can 2008;30:477–88.

118. Denison FC, Price J, Graham C, et al. Maternal obesity, length of gestation, risk of postdates pregnancy and spontaneous onset of labour at term. BJOG 2008;115:720–5.

119. Villamor E, Cnattingius S. Interpregnancy weight change and risk of adverse pregnancy outcomes: a population-based study. Lancet 2006;368:1164–70.

120. Yogev Y, Visser GH. Obesity, gestational diabetes and pregnancy outcome. Semin Fetal Neonatal Med 2009;14:77–84.

121. Hauger MS, Gibbons L, Vik T, et al. Prepregnancy weight status and the risk of adverse pregnancy outcome. Acta Obstet Gynecol Scand 2008;87:953–9.

122. Leung TY, Leung TN, Sahota DS, et al. Trends in maternal obesity and associated risks of adverse pregnancy outcomes in a population of Chinese women. BJOG 2008;115:1529–37.

123. Khashan AS, Kenny LC. The effects of maternal body mass index on pregnancy outcome. Eur J Epidemiol 2009;24:697–705.

124. Schumann K, Ettle T, Szegner B, et al. On risks and benefits or iron supplementation recommendations for iron intake revisited. J Trace Elem Med Biol 2007;21:147–68.

125. Gonzales GF, Steenland K, Tapia V. Maternal hemoglobin level and fetal outcome at low and high altitudes. Am J Physiol Regul Integr Comp Physiol 2009;297:R1477–85.

126. Stephansson O, Dickman PW, Johansson A, et al. Maternal hemoglobin concentration during pregnancy and risk of stillbirth. JAMA 2000;284:2611–17.

127. Webb R, Abel K, Pickles A, et al. Mortality in offspring of parents with psychotic disorders: a critical review and meta-analysis. Am J Psychiatry 2005;162:1045–56.

128. Gold KJ, Dalton VK, Schwenk TL. What causes pregnancy loss? Preexisting mental illness as an independent risk factor. Gen Hosp Psychiatry 2007;29:207–13.

129. MacCabe JH, Martinsson L, Lichtenstein P, et al. Adverse pregnancy outcomes in mothers with affective psychosis. Bipolar Disord 2007;9:305–9.

130. Dodds L, King WD, Fell DB, et al. Stillbirth risk factors according to timing of exposure. Ann Epidemiol 2006;16:607–13.

131. Oakley L, Doyle P. Predicting the impact of in vitro fertilisation and other forms of assisted conception on perinatal and infant mortality in England and Wales: examining the role of multiplicity. BJOG 2006;113:738–41.

132. Zuppa AA, Scorrano A, Cota F, et al. Neonatal outcomes in triplet pregnancies: assisted reproduction versus spontaneous conception. J Perinat Med 2007;35:339–43.

133. Sun LM, Walker MC, Cao HL, et al. Assisted reproductive technology and placenta-mediated adverse pregnancy outcomes. Obstet Gynecol 2009;114:818–24.

134. Martin JA, Hamilton BE, Sutton PD, et al. Births: final data for 2006. Natl Vital Stat Rep 2009;57(7):1–202.

135. Pasupathy D, Wood AM, Pell JP, et al. Rates of and factors associated with delivery-related perinatal death among term infants in Scotland. JAMA 2009;302:660–8.

136. Ananth CV, Joseph KS, Kinzler WL. The influence of obstetric intervention on trends in twin stillbirths: United States, 1989–99. J Mater Fetal Neonatal Med 2004;15:380–7.

137. National Institutes of Health state-of-the-science conference statement. Obstet Gynecol 2006;107:1386–97.

138. Caughey AB, Sundaram V, Kaimal AJ. Maternal and neonatal outcomes of elective induction of labor. Evidence Report/Technology Assessment No. 176. (Prepared by the Stanford University-UCSF Evidence-based Practice Center under contract No. 290-02-0017.) AHRQ Publication No. 09-E005. Rockville, MD: Agency for Healthcare Research and Quality; 2009.

139. Smith GC, Pell JP, Dobbie R. Caesarean section and risk of unexplained stillbirth in subsequent pregnancy. Lancet 2003;62:1779–84.

140. Gray R, Quigley MA, Hockley C, et al. Caesarean delivery and risk of stillbirth in subsequent pregnancy: a retrospective cohort study in an English population. BJOG 2007;114:264–70.

141. Kennare R, Tucker G, Heard A, et al. Risks of adverse outcomes in the next birth after a first cesarean delivery. Obstet Gynecol 2007;109:270–6.

142. Wood SL, Chen S, Ross S, et al. The risk of unexplained antepartum stillbirth in second pregnancies following caesarean section in the first pregnancy. BJOG 2008;115:726–31.

CHAPTER 5
Infection

Robert L. Goldenberg, MD and Elizabeth M. McClure, MEd

Department of Obstetrics and Gynecology, Drexel University College of Medicine, Philadelphia, PA, USA
Department of Statistics and Epidemiology, RTI International, Research Triangle Park, NC, USA

Stillbirth, defined as a newborn having no sign of life at delivery, is one of the most common adverse outcomes of pregnancy. Three million or more occur worldwide each year with 98% or more occurring in low- and middle-income countries. In high-income countries, stillbirth rates generally range from 3 to 7 per 1,000 births when compared to 20–40 per 1,000 births in many low- and middle-income countries, which may have rates as high as 100 per 1,000 in some areas [1–3]. In the United States, the stillbirth rate is about 6–7 per 1,000 births and about 28,000 stillbirths occur each year.

A number of maternal and fetal conditions may cause stillbirth, with the major causes being similar, though with different attribution, across countries worldwide. Of the various conditions contributing to stillbirth, infection may be among the most important numerically. In high-income countries, 10–25% of stillbirths are attributed to maternal or fetal infections [4–6]. In many low- and middle-income countries, infections appear to account for about 50% of stillbirths [2]. In an analysis of stillbirth etiology in low- and middle-income countries, of the five factors identified as having a very strong relationship with stillbirth, two—syphilis and chorioamnionitis—were infection related [3]. Furthermore, the etiology of most stillbirths is multifactorial and thus infection may contribute to many more. Infection is more clearly associated with early stillbirth (<28 weeks) when compared with late stillbirth (≥28 weeks) and

with lower birthweight. Since the lower limits of gestational age and birthweight used to define stillbirth vary across geographic areas and have ranged from 20 to 28 weeks and from 350 to 1,000 g, respectively [3, 5–7], studies including only late fetal deaths (i.e., ≥28 weeks) miss much of the large contribution of infection to stillbirths.

Mechanisms of infection leading to fetal death

Stillbirth may result from maternal or fetal infection through a variety of mechanisms, including direct infection, placental damage, and severe maternal illness. First, the fetus may be directly infected via the placenta or membranes, with the organisms damaging a vital organ such as the lung or heart. Group B streptococcal fetal pneumonitis is an example of this type of infection. Second, the placenta may be directly infected without fetal involvement, resulting in reduced blood flow to the fetus. Malaria and, at times, syphilis may kill the fetus by this mechanism. When early infection occurs, the fetus may develop a congenital anomaly or fetal condition such as hydrops with a subsequent fetal death due to the anomaly or condition. Rubella and parvovirus are examples of this type of infection. Third, maternal infection may lead to a severe maternal illness. Due to high maternal fever, poor oxygenation, or systemic reactions to the illness, the fetus may die without transmission of organisms to the placenta or fetus. Maternal influenza and polio are examples of this type of infection. Finally, maternal infection may precipitate preterm labor, with the fetus unable to tolerate delivery resulting in stillbirth. Ureaplasma and mycoplasma infections frequently cause early preterm labor leading to fetal death.

Stillbirths have been associated with almost every type of infection, including those caused by bacteria, viruses, fungi, and many parasites (Table 5.1). Nevertheless, of the thousands of infectious agents in the environment, relatively few have been proven causal for stillbirth. Moreover, as with many purported causes of stillbirth, a key question is why some women with common infections suffer stillbirth, while other women with similar infections will achieve a normal pregnancy outcome.

Reasons for the apparent lack of association between infection and stillbirth

The relationships between maternal or fetal infection and stillbirth may not become apparent for several reasons. First, the presence of infection is often not easily identified based on the case history or physical examination of the mother or the fetus. Routine histologic evaluations of the placenta and fetal autopsies may miss organisms that contribute to fetal death. Neither positive serologic tests nor organisms cultured from the placenta or even the fetus prove causality. Even when there is evidence of an infection, understanding precisely why a specific stillbirth occurred is difficult. For example, a fetal autopsy and histologic study of the placenta may suggest other etiologies in addition to the presence of infection. In these cases, whether the death should be attributed to the infection is often uncertain. Finally, infection may initiate the events leading to stillbirth, and its contribution to the fetal death may not be recognized (e.g., parvovirus infection causing hydrops or early rubella infections causing congenital anomalies).

Which cases of stillbirth are attributed to infection depends, in part, upon the extent of the evaluation, the clinical judgment of the examiner, and the classification system used [8]. In high-income countries, placental histologic examination, culture, and fetal autopsies are generally available though they are not routinely performed. In low- and middle-income countries, where most stillbirths occur, these tests are usually unavailable. Thus, because confirming an infectious etiology of stillbirth generally requires use of these techniques, we believe that the causal contribution of infections for stillbirth is significantly underdiagnosed in both types of settings. If routine bacterial and viral cultures were supplemented by more sophisticated molecular techniques and were widely used, it is likely that the apparent contribution of infection to stillbirth would rise still further.

Bacterial infections

More than 130 different bacteria causing intrauterine infections have been described. Many of these have also been associated with stillbirth [4, 6]. The types of organisms and the mechanisms by which they contribute to fetal death are generally similar across geographic areas. However, the proportion of pregnancies affected by bacterial infection is often much higher in low- and middle-income countries than high-income countries [3, 9]. Bacterial infections may reach the fetus and lead to stillbirth by two routes: (1) those that reach the fetal compartment through the placenta, and (2) infections that ascend from the vagina through the cervix (Figure 5.1). In transplacental infections, the placental villi often show evidence of infection. Also, since the organisms enter the fetus through the umbilical vein, the liver is the organ most commonly infected. We first describe fetal infections that are transmitted transplacentally.

Syphilis

Treponema pallidum is the spirochete responsible for syphilis. Of all the potential infectious causes of stillbirth worldwide, syphilis is of special interest because it causes a large number of stillbirths which are nearly always preventable through

Table 5.1 Maternal infections and stillbirths.

Organism	Maternal disease	Comment
Bacteria		
Ascending infections		
Ureaplasma urealyticum	Generally asymptomatic	Confirmed as a cause of stillbirth
Mycoplasma hominus	Generally asymptomatic	Confirmed as a cause of stillbirth
E. coli	Generally asymptomatic	Confirmed as a cause of stillbirth
Group B *Streptococcus*	Generally asymptomatic	Confirmed as a common cause of stillbirth
Klebsiella	Generally asymptomatic	Confirmed as a common cause of stillbirth
Enterococcus	Generally asymptomatic	Confirmed as a cause of stillbirth
Bacteroidaceae	Generally asymptomatic	Confirmed as a cause of stillbirth
Neisseria gonorrhoeae	Pelvic infection	Suggested as cause of stillbirth by case reports
Chlamydia trachomatis	Pelvic infection	Suggested as cause of stillbirth by case reports
Transplacental infections		
Treponema pallidum	Syphilis	Major cause of stillbirth when maternal prevalence is high
Borrelia burgdorferi	Lyme disease	Tick-borne infection and a confirmed but not common cause of stillbirth
Borrelia recurrentis	Relapsing fever	Tick-borne infection common in the western United States and a confirmed but rare cause of stillbirth
Borrelia duttonii	Relapsing fever	Tick-borne infection common in sub-Saharan Africa and probably an important cause of stillbirth
Leptospira interrogans	Leptospirosis	Confirmed as a cause of stillbirth but not common
Listeria monocytogenes	Listeriosis	Confirmed as a cause of stillbirth; generally transmitted transplacentally
Other bacterial infections usually transmitted transplacentally*		Each organism has been implicated as causal for stillbirth by case reports
Viruses		
Parvovirus (B19)	Erythema infectiosum	Confirmed as cause of stillbirth and likely is the most common viral etiologic agent
Coxsackie A and B	Various presentations	Confirmed as causes of stillbirth and may be an important contributor to overall stillbirth rate
Echovirus	Various presentations	Confirmed as cause of stillbirth but of unknown importance
Enterovirus	Various presentations	Confirmed as cause of stillbirth but of unknown importance
Hepatitis E virus	Fulminant hepatic failure	Probable cause of stillbirth especially in geographic areas with epidemic outbreaks
Polio virus	Polio	Historically likely cause of stillbirth but since routine vaccination is rarely seen in developed countries
Varicella zoster	Chickenpox	Confirmed as a rare cause of stillbirth but with routine vaccination almost never seen
Rubella	German measles	Confirmed as a cause of stillbirth but rarely reported as a cause of stillbirth in developed countries
Mumps	Parotitis	Possibly a cause of stillbirth historically but rarely reported as a cause of stillbirth in developed countries
Rubeola	Measles	A probable cause of stillbirth historically but rarely reported as a cause of stillbirth in developed countries
CMV	Generally asymptomatic in adults	Reported as a cause of stillbirth in case reports but overall contribution is unknown
Variola	Smallpox	Historically a cause of stillbirth but with vaccination no longer seen

Organism	Maternal disease	Comment
Ljungan virus	Diabetes, neurological disease, myocarditis, and deaths	Carried by wild rodents, it is associated with several cases of stillbirth in a single report
Dengue virus	Dengue fever	Carried by mosquitoes and confirmed as a cause of stillbirth
Lymphocytic choriomeningitis virus	Lymphocytic choriomeningitis	A possible cause of stillbirth but of unknown importance
HIV	Acquired immunodeficiency syndrome	Associated with stillbirth due to maternal cachexia and comorbidities, but fetal infection is not likely causative
Influenza virus	Influenza	Associated with stillbirth with severe illness
Influenza virus (H1N1)	Severe maternal influenza	At times kills both mother and fetus
Protozoa		
Trypanosoma brucei	Trypanosomiasis	Carried by tsetse fly; a likely cause of stillbirth in southern Africa, but overall contribution is unknown
Trypanosoma cruzi	Chagas disease	Carried by the Triatomine (kissing bug) and a confirmed cause of stillbirth in South America but overall contribution is unknown
Plasmodium falciparum	Malaria	Carried by mosquitoes and likely an important cause of stillbirth in newly endemic areas or in newly infected women
Plasmodium vivax	Malaria	Carried by mosquitoes and a possible cause of stillbirth but likely less important than with *Plasmodium falciparum*
Toxoplasmosis gondii	Toxoplasmosis	Confirmed as a rare cause of stillbirth
Coxiella burnetti	Q fever	Confirmed as cause of stillbirth but of unknown importance
Fungi		
Candida albicans	Thrush, vaginitis	Confirmed as cause of stillbirth by case reports
Candida glabrata	Vaginitis	Case reports of stillbirth associated with IVF
Helminths		Deworming has been associated with a decrease in stillbirths

*Include Tularemia, Tuberculus, Brucellosis, Clostridia, Typhoid, Anthrax, *Streptococcus pseudoporcinus*, *Agrobacterium radiobacter*, *Pseudomonas*, etc.

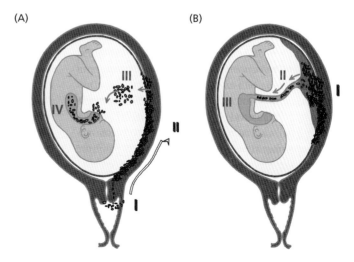

Figure 5.1 Pathways to placental and fetal infection: (A) ascending infection and (B) hematogenously spread infection.

screening for and treatment of syphilis in pregnancy. The rate of active syphilis infection among women of reproductive age varies from as high as 20% among some African populations to about 0.02% in many high-income countries [10–14]. Spirochetes can cross the placenta and infect the fetus, with risk of fetal infection related to maternal syphilis stage. If the mother is infected but untreated, about 40% of fetuses will die in utero and another 30–40% will be born alive but have congenital syphilis. More than one million cases of congenital syphilis occur worldwide each year [15]. The most common cause of fetal death appears to be placental infection with decreasing blood flow to the fetus, although direct fetal infection also occurs [16]. Most studies report women with syphilis to have a relative risk for stillbirth in the range of 2–5; however, a relative risk of 18 was reported for Tanzanian women with active syphilis [17]. In some areas of sub-Saharan Africa, between 25% and 50% of all stillbirths have been associated with syphilis [12]. Syphilis also contributes to a significant proportion of the stillbirths in other areas of the world including Russia, Asia, and South America [18–20].

Stillbirths due to syphilis should be easy to eradicate. Within a functioning health system, it is feasible to screen pregnant women for syphilis and once diagnosed, easy and inexpensive to treat. Women who have been treated for syphilis during pregnancy have a similar or only slightly greater stillbirth risk compared to noninfected women [21, 22]. The failure to eliminate congenital syphilis—especially in sub-Saharan Africa—appears to be due to the fact that many women do not have access to or utilize prenatal care which includes syphilis testing and treatment. Because of lack of resources, a poorly functioning supply system, and other priorities such as human immunodeficiency virus (HIV) screening and treatment, appropriate syphilis-related care is often not provided in these settings. To address some of these issues, a recent study suggested that point-of-care rapid testing and treatment is the most cost-effective method to reduce adverse pregnancy outcomes associated with syphilis [23]. Schmid et al. converted the fetal/neonatal consequences of maternal syphilis into disability-adjusted life years

(DALYs). They estimated that when stillbirth is included, the cost of one DALY saved was about US $10 and was 25 times less expensive than the cost of one DALY saved among infants born to HIV-positive women [24]. Based on these and other data, the World Health Organization has launched a program to eliminate congenital syphilis worldwide [25].

Other spirochetal infections

Another spirochetal infection associated with stillbirth is Lyme disease, a systemic illness caused by the tick-borne spirochete *Borrelia burgdorferi*. The first case of stillbirth associated with Lyme disease was described in 1987 [26]. In that case, the mother acquired the disease in the first trimester, and at 34 weeks delivered a stillborn infant who had *B. burgdorferi* in the placenta and internal fetal organs. In other reports, after first-trimester infection and subsequent fetal death, spirochetes were found in fetal liver, spleen, kidney, and brain. Subsequently, small series of stillbirths after maternal Lyme disease have been described, with most deaths occurring in the mid-trimester. In Tanzania, more than 30% of adults are seropositive for *B. burgdorferi* [27] compared to 2% in countries such as the United States and Norway, but whether Lyme disease is an important cause of stillbirths in African settings is unknown. Most large-scale serologic studies have suggested that, except in highly endemic areas, few stillbirths are associated with Lyme disease [27, 28].

Tick-borne relapsing fever, caused by *Borrelia duttonii* and transmitted to humans by the tick *Ornithodoros moubata*, is another spirochetal disease associated with adverse pregnancy outcome, which is primarily found in sub-Saharan Africa [29–32]. Studies have reported associations between *B. duttonii* and adverse pregnancy outcomes including low birthweight, preterm birth, and increased perinatal mortality risk. A study in the Democratic Republic of Congo found that as many as 6.4% of pregnant women admitted to a maternity ward were diagnosed with relapsing fever [29]. Case reports of relapsing fever during pregnancy have also been reported from the United States [33]. As with Lyme disease, in most African settings, the prevalence of tick-borne relapsing fever and its contribution to stillbirths is unknown. Finally, leptospirosis, still another spirochetal disease, has been associated with transplacental infection and stillbirth.

Other transplacental infections causing stillbirth

Listeria monocytogenes is another example of a hematogenously transmitted organism that causes fetal death [34]. The mother may acquire this infection by eating contaminated food such as unpasteurized soft cheese or undercooked meat. During bacteremia, the organisms are transmitted to the placenta causing villous necrosis and microabscesses and may also be transmitted to the fetus. Stillborns, when they occur, are attributed both to placental dysfunction and fetal infection. Transplacental infections have also been reported in association with maternal tularemia, clostridia, anthrax, typhoid fever, brucellosis, *Haemophilus influenzae*, *Pseudomonas pyocyanea*, a plant bacterium, *Agrobacterium radiobacter*, and tuberculosis [6]. With tuberculosis, in addition to the rare transplacental infection causing stillbirth, maternal cachexia also appears to be a risk factor for stillbirth [35]. Although generally still rare in pregnancy, rates of tuberculosis are increasing in many locations, especially in African countries where HIV is prevalent [36].

In summary, with the exception of syphilis, the association between bacterial transplacental infection-related stillbirths in both high- and low- and middle-income countries is largely unstudied. However, because of high maternal disease prevalence, transplacental infections with other bacteria are likely a common occurrence. In high-income countries, because of the rarity of individual infections that cause stillbirth, it is unlikely that any specific strategy for bacterial infection will substantially reduce these types of stillbirths.

Ascending bacterial infections

Organisms that ascend from the vagina into the uterus may enter the amniotic fluid either through intact choriodecidual membranes or after rupture of the membranes. The most common organ infected is the fetal lung, associated with fetal breathing of contaminated amniotic fluid. This mechanism explains why a common autopsy finding in many stillbirths is pneumonitis. Whether the fetus is stillborn with pneumonitis or is born alive with pneumonia depends on factors such as organism virulence, the fetal response, and length of time between infection and delivery. Romero et al. [37] hypothesized that a preterm infection usually elicits a fetal inflammatory response and ultimately preterm labor. However, if the fetus cannot initiate an adequate inflammatory response, the outcome is likely to be a stillbirth. Births before 28 weeks gestation appear to be strongly associated with an intrauterine bacterial infection, whereas late preterm births are less likely to have an associated intrauterine infection [5, 10]. Therefore, the apparent prevalence of this condition will depend on whether all stillbirths >20 weeks are evaluated or only later gestational age stillbirths are included. In virtually all studies, the frequency of histologic chorioamnionitis in stillbirths is at least several times greater than in controls [37–40]. In a recent study from Australia, Lahra et al. [38] found that 37% of all stillbirths were associated with histologic chorioamnionitis. The study also showed that very early preterm stillbirths as well as postterm stillbirths had substantially higher rates of histologic chorioamnionitis than other births (Figure 5.2). There are also a number of autopsy studies, predominantly from sub-Saharan Africa, where organisms such as group B *Streptococcus*, *E. coli*, and *Klebsiella* have been cultured from fetal heart blood, liver, lung, or brain [41–43]. As an example, *E. coli* was found in 25% of stillborn heart blood samples in Zimbabwe. Naeye et al. [42] studied infection-related stillbirths in Ethiopia and compared these results to findings from the U.S. Collaborative Perinatal Study. The types of organisms associated with ascending infections were similar in both locations, but the risk of stillbirth associated with infection was several times greater in Ethiopia. The authors speculated that the difference had to do with greater exposure to infectious organisms, as well as a decreased immune response, both secondary to the malnutrition which is prevalent in African populations.

Prevention of stillbirths associated with ascending bacterial infection in the presence of intact membranes has proven elusive. To date, no

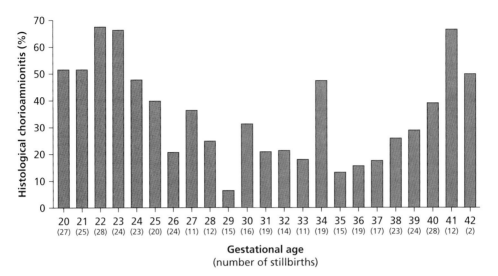

Figure 5.2 Histologic chorioamnionitis in stillborn babies by gestational age. (Data from Ref. [38].)

strategies—including antibiotic prophylaxis—appear to prevent the intrauterine infection or the associated stillbirths, although antibiotic treatment targeting bacterial vaginosis may be of value in some women [44]. In women with preterm premature membrane rupture, prophylactic antibiotics reduce histologic chorioamnionitis, but to date antibiotics have not been associated with a similar reduction in risk of stillbirth [45].

It should also be noted that both gonorrhea and chlamydia have been shown to cause stillbirth in individual case reports. To date, the extent of their relationship with stillbirth has not been evaluated in large epidemiological studies.

Viral diseases

Although it is apparent that viruses can cause stillbirths, the overall nature of the relationship between viral infection and the fetus is unknown. Many viruses are difficult to culture, a positive viral serologic result does not prove causation, and DNA or RNA viral identification, only recently widely available, is technically difficult. Few of these tests are routinely available or used in high-income countries and they are almost never available in low- or middle-income countries. For

this reason, the relative importance of maternal viral infection as a cause of stillbirth in most areas of the world is unknown.

HIV infection

Many studies show a small increase in stillbirth risk associated with maternal HIV infection, although the degree of association has been inconsistent [22, 46–50]. One meta-analysis of HIV and stillbirth suggested a threefold increase, with risk of stillbirth increasing with the severity of maternal HIV disease and with lower CD4 counts [48]. In a study conducted in four sites in southern Africa, Chi et al. found that among women who were HIV seropositive, decreasing CD4 cell counts were inversely related to stillbirth ($p < 0.0001$) suggesting that worsening maternal HIV disease may be associated with stillbirth. The authors speculated that HIV-related immunosuppression might be a contributing factor to adverse pregnancy outcomes among these women [22]. Since HIV rarely crosses the placenta or infects the fetus prior to labor, it is not likely that this increase in stillbirths was directly caused by fetal infection. Instead, the stillbirths were likely attributed to cofactors such as maternal comorbidities (such as tuberculosis) and overall poor maternal health status, both of which are of particular concern in low- and middle-income countries. In one study from western Kenya, women with both HIV and malaria had more adverse pregnancy outcomes than those with either infection alone [50]. Since the prevalence of maternal HIV infection is more than 25% in some sub-Saharan countries, the contribution of maternal HIV infection to stillbirths in those areas is likely to be high. However, at this time, it does not appear likely that *fetal* infection with HIV is causal for stillbirths, other than in those cases where the mother has a severe systemic illness resulting from the HIV.

Common childhood diseases

Maternal infections with each of the common viral childhood illnesses (rubella, measles, mumps, and chickenpox) have been implicated in stillbirths [51–56]. Maternal rubella was associated with congenital cataracts by Gregg in 1941 [54]. Subsequently, other anomalies have been documented, including major cardiac defects, some resulting in stillbirths later in pregnancy. Rubella also infects the placenta, enhancing the risk of stillbirth, and can apparently do so without fetal spread. Rubella outbreaks are routinely reported from many low- and middle-income countries; however, their contribution to stillbirths in those areas is unknown [55]. Maternal infection with both mumps and rubeola (measles) has also been implicated as a cause of stillbirth [53], and both viruses have been isolated from fetal tissues. In Guinea-Bissau, stillbirth rates were increased from four- to nine-fold if the mother was infected with measles during her pregnancy [56]. Varicella (chickenpox) infections during pregnancy may cause maternal pneumonia, placing infected women at risk for death as well as stillbirth. The virus also occasionally crosses the placenta and attacks the fetus directly [52]. These observations confirm that maternal infection with viruses that cause common childhood illnesses increase the risk of stillbirth. Because of widespread immunization in high-income countries, maternal infection with these organisms is extremely rare and few stillbirths due to these infections are reported. However, with vaccination rates less than 50% in many low- and middle-income countries, stillbirths associated with these infections likely occur.

Universal vaccination for childhood diseases should eliminate these stillbirths.

Influenza

Historically, maternal influenza infection is associated with excess maternal and fetal deaths [57]. In the recent epidemic, severe acute respiratory syndrome (SARS) was demonstrated to be associated with placental and fetal pathology, though its association with pregnancy outcome needs further research [58]. During the 2009–2010 epidemic, there were a number of reports of H1N1 influenza virus infections in pregnant women. The infection tended to be more severe in these women than in nonpregnant adults, and there were reported cases of maternal death and stillbirth associated with this infection [59]. Since influenza infections are common in low- and middle-income countries, and immunization for this virus rarely occurs in those settings, the potential for an increase in stillbirths associated with various types of influenza infections is strong. The American College of Obstetricians and Gynecologists (ACOG) has recommended immunization for all women who will be pregnant during the influenza season [60].

Parvovirus

Parvovirus (B19), which causes a common childhood exanthem known commonly as fifth disease and aplastic anemia in children with sickle cell disease, was first associated with fetal death in 1984. Subsequently, investigators have shown that parvovirus crosses the placenta and preferentially attacks erythropoietic tissue, causes fetal anemia, nonimmune hydrops, and fetal death [61–65]. The virus also attacks cardiac tissue and may cause stillbirth by this mechanism. Most stillbirths occur in the second trimester and are associated with hydrops, although parvovirus may also be an important cause of nonhydropic third-trimester fetal deaths.

Previous infection elicits an antibody response protective against subsequent maternal and fetal infection. About half of all pregnant women in the United States have had a previous infection, have circulating antibodies, and are immune. Of those not immune, with exposure, about 25% will become infected, and of these about 30% will pass the virus to their fetus. Of the infected fetuses, only about 10% will have hydrops; most of these will not die. Therefore, even with maternal infection, the risk of stillbirth is quite low. On the other hand, in a series reported from Sweden, where polymerase chain reaction (PCR) for viral DNA was used to define fetal parvovirus infection, 15% of all stillbirths were attributed to parvovirus [61] with similar results also reported from other European countries [65]. Therefore, the proportion of all stillbirths that may be attributable to parvovirus is unclear. Nevertheless, the primary mechanism leading to stillbirth involves the virus' predilection for bone marrow, resulting in fetal anemia and hydrops. The infections that result in stillbirth are generally acquired before 20 weeks gestation, and death usually occurs during the mid-trimester. Overall, in the United States, it appears that less than 1% of all stillbirths result from parvovirus infection.

Enteroviruses

The enterovirus family includes enterovirus, echovirus, Coxsackie virus, and polio. Each can cross the placenta and cause fetal death. In a detailed evaluation of unexplained perinatal deaths, Nuovo et al. [66] found Coxsackie virus present in 48% of cases. They emphasized that the histologic findings in the placenta were often nonspecific and underscored the need for molecular testing to define this relationship. Furthermore, in a case–control study from Sweden, among 21 women with stillbirth, 52% were Coxsackie virus positive, whereas among controls, only 22% were positive [67]. Echovirus and enteroviruses have also been cultured from stillborns. In most studies, unless the virus was specifically looked for at autopsy with sophisticated molecular techniques, an infectious cause of stillbirth would have been missed. Similarly, cytomegalovirus (CMV) has rarely been investigated in cases of stillbirth [68, 69]. However, in an Australian study, 9% of blood samples taken from stillbirths by cardiac puncture were positive for CMV by PCR [70]. A recent study from Greece using PCR showed significantly increased levels of CMV (16%) in the placentas of stillbirths compared to controls (3%) [71]. Since CMV is the most common cause of congenital infection in the United States, and because of its ability to infect the fetus leading to fetal growth restriction and central nervous system damage, the relationship between CMV and stillbirth should be studied in greater depth. Herpes simplex infections have also been described as a cause of fetal death.

Other viral infections and stillbirth

Viral hepatitis is caused by infection with one of the several hepatotropic viruses. Of these viruses, hepatitis E virus (HEV) infection has been associated with adverse outcomes during pregnancy, including maternal death, preterm birth, and stillbirth. HEV generally causes large-scale epidemics, usually through contaminated drinking water. Although the infection is not usually severe in men or nonpregnant women, among pregnant women' HEV often results in fulminant hepatic failure and death in up to 20% of cases. In a study from New Delhi, India, women with HEV infection were twice as likely to have a stillbirth (RR 1.8, 95% CI 1.2, 2.5) [72].

Finally, newly described viruses are being associated with stillbirth. For example, the *Ljungan virus*, a picornavirus seen in bank voles, was originally isolated in the Ljungan Valley in Sweden and since has been found in Denmark and the United States [73, 74]. A recent small study of pregnant women found the virus in 40% of stillborns but not in any tissues from normal pregnancies. The overall importance of this infection as a cause of stillbirth in any location is unknown. To be complete, the lymphocytic choriomeningitis virus has also been implicated as a cause of stillbirth.

Protozoal infections

There are a number of protozoal intrauterine infections that have been described associated with stillbirth. Among these, malaria appears to have the strongest association with stillbirth, but toxoplasmosis, Q fever, and other protozoal infections have also caused fetal death.

Malaria

Forty percent of births worldwide occur in malaria-endemic areas, and an estimated 14 million pregnant women exposed to malaria, with most of these pregnancies occurring in sub-Saharan Africa [75]. Malaria is caused by four types of intracellular parasites transmitted by several mosquito species. *Plasmodium falciparum* is the most common cause of malaria in humans and generally associated with the most adverse health effects. Women infected with *P. falciparum*, primiparas, and those previously unexposed to malaria, generally have the worst outcomes including maternal death, fetal growth restriction, preterm birth, and stillbirth [75–77]. Pregnancy outcome is also directly related to the extent of placental malaria, reported to occur in 13–63% of maternal infections [77]. Placental insufficiency results from lymphocyte and macrophage accumulation and thickening of the basement membrane, impeding blood flow through the placenta, and restricting transport of oxygen and nutrients to the fetus. Severe maternal anemia associated with malaria may also play a role in stillbirth. Malaria organisms can cross the placenta, causing congenital malaria, but the significance of these infections for stillbirth is not clear. A review of studies, mostly from endemic areas, estimated that placental malaria was associated with twice (OR 2.19) the stillbirth risk [77]. An Ethiopian population newly infected with malaria had a sevenfold increased risk [78], while a Tanzanian study showed a population attributable fraction of malaria for stillbirth of 32% [79]. Together, these findings suggest that malaria is an important cause of stillbirth. Most malaria studies have been conducted in Africa, but similar results have been found from other malaria-endemic areas [80]. Overall, because of the large number of women living in endemic areas, the high percentage of women demonstrating placental malaria, and the twofold risk of stillbirth, malaria is likely the most important preventable infectious cause of stillbirth in low- and middle-income countries. Evidence suggests that intermittent antimalarial prophylaxis and use of insecticide-impregnated bed nets may lower the risk of stillbirth and other adverse outcomes associated with malaria during pregnancy [81, 82].

Toxoplasmosis

Toxoplasma gondii is a parasite that normally spends its life cycle in animals, but may be transmitted to humans through contact with animal feces or from undercooked meat. Its human infection, toxoplasmosis, is generally asymptomatic or only causes mild disease, but has been identified in case reports as a cause of stillbirth [83]. Toxoplasmosis seropositivity in the United States is about 15%, but may be much higher in other geographic areas. For example, one study found the prevalence of toxoplasmosis antibodies to be greater than 80% among pregnant Nigerian women [84]. Prior maternal infection, indicated by the presence of specific antibodies, generally protects the pregnant woman from fetal infection.

If the mother is infected during pregnancy, toxoplasmosis, *T. gondii*, may be transmitted to the fetus via the placenta. The later in pregnancy the primary maternal infection occurs, the more likely the infection will be transmitted to the fetus. Disseminated toxoplasmosis may cause fetal death. An African study examined the role of *T. gondii* among HIV-infected women and found that HIV seropositivity was associated with a greater prevalence of *T. gondii* [85]. In a case–control study from Jordan, *T. gondii* was significantly more common in women with adverse pregnancy outcomes compared to controls (54% vs. 12%, $p < 0.02$) [83]. In Zimbabwe, serologic tests for toxoplasmosis were fourfold more common in mothers of stillbirths than in controls [86]. Thus, toxoplasmosis appears to contribute to stillbirths globally, although it appears to be less commonly found as a cause of stillbirth in the United States and other high-income countries.

Q fever

Q fever is a rickettsial infection caused by *Coxiella burnetti*. In humans this infection is generally acquired by inhalation of infected aerosols during contact with meat products, although transmission has occurred by tick bite and ingestion of infected milk. In nonpregnant adults, *C. burnetti* causes pneumonia, meningoencephalitis, hepatitis, and endocarditis. Infections may be acute or persistent, with the latter generally asymptomatic during pregnancy except when the organisms may infect the placenta, leading to abortion, stillbirth, or preterm birth. In a review of cases of acute

Q fever during pregnancy, abnormal pregnancy outcomes were found in all cases of acute maternal infection, with fetal death occurring in two-thirds [87]. Organisms were generally isolated both from placental and fetal tissue. Most of the stillbirths occurred in the second and early third trimester. The overall contribution of Q fever to stillbirths, and the actual geographic distribution of Q fever-associated stillbirths, is unknown. Rocky Mountain spotted fever, another rickettsial disease with widespread distribution in the United States, has not been associated with intrauterine infection or stillbirth.

Other protozoal infections

Two trypanosomal infections, common in tropical regions, have been associated with stillbirth. The parasite causing trypanosomiasis, *Trypanosoma brucei*, carried by the tsetse fly, has been demonstrated in placentas of stillborns [88]. Another trypanosomal illness, widespread in South America, Chagas disease, is caused by *Trypanosoma cruzi* and also infects the fetus and placenta, causing hydrops and death [89]. The extent to which maternal infection with either infection is linked to stillbirth is unknown.

Fungi

Several species of *Candida* have been reported to cause stillbirths [90, 91]. *Candida albicans* has been associated with stillbirth, and in those cases, widespread fetal dissemination involving multiple organs has been described. Interestingly, *Candida glabrata* has been reported to cause stillbirths in pregnancies originating with an in vitro fertilization (IVF) procedure. The reason for the association is not clear, but may be related to laboratory or equipment contamination at the time of the IVF.

Helminthic infections

Helminthic infections are common, especially in low-income countries where more than half of pregnant women may be infected [92]. An observational study in Sri Lanka showed significant reductions in stillbirth rates associated with antihelminthic treatment, implicating worm infestations as a possible cause of stillbirth [93]; however, a randomized controlled trial of antihelminthic treatment in Uganda where the prevalence of infection was 68% among pregnant women did not find significant reductions in stillbirth overall [94]. Cofactors including the severity of the infection, other coinfections, and maternal anemia may all be associated with the risk for stillbirth. Because of the high prevalence of this infection and its association with stillbirth, more research in this area is warranted.

Animal- and vector-borne infections

As we reviewed the infectious causes of stillbirth, it became apparent that many of these infections, whether caused by bacteria, viruses, or parasites, were animal- or vector-borne (Table 5.2). The insect vector-borne infections include malaria, Lyme disease, various tick-borne relapsing fevers, dengue fever, African sleeping sickness, Chagas disease, and tularemia. Maternal infections with a primary animal host include listeriosis, anthrax, brucellosis, leptospirosis, toxoplasmosis, Q fever, and lymphocytic choriomeningitis. Other animal-associated organisms causing stillbirth, such as the *Ljungan virus* and *Streptococcus porcinus*, have recently been identified. Because of the number of these associations, further study of the relationship between animal- and vector-borne infections and stillbirth should be undertaken.

One of the most compelling observations related to infection and stillbirths, especially in low- and middle-income countries, is the many unknowns regarding this relationship. For example, it is unknown if the high seroprevalences of Lyme disease or toxoplasmosis in African settings are associated with increased risk of stillbirth or whether African tick-borne relapsing fever is an important cause of stillbirth. Also, the risk of stillbirth associated with conditions such as worm infestations have rarely been considered. We, therefore, believe that research in a number of low- and middle-income countries settings, using both traditional and the newest molecular and culture techniques, should be conducted so that the full extent of the relationships between stillbirths and

Table 5.2 Vector-borne and animal-derived maternal infections causal for stillbirths.

Infection	Organism	Vector or animal reservoir
Malaria	*Plasmodium falciparum*	Mosquito
Lyme disease	*Borrelia burgdorferi*	Tick
Relapsing fever	*Borrelia duttonii*	Tick
Tick-borne relapsing fever	*Borrelia recurrentis*	Tick
African sleeping sickness	*Trypanosoma brucei*	Tsetse fly
Chagas disease	*Trypanosoma cruzi*	Triatomine (kissing bug)
Dengue fever	*Dengue virus*	Mosquito
Tularemia	*Francisella tularensis*	Tick or deerfly, animal carcasses, contaminated food/water
Listeriosis	*Listeria monocytogenes*	Domesticated animal products
Anthrax	*Bacillus anthracis*	Domesticated animals
Q Fever	*Coxiella burnetti*	Domesticated animals
Brucellosis	*Brucella melitensis*	Domesticated animals
Leptospirosis	*Leptospira interrogans*	Dogs, livestock, wild animals
Toxoplasmosis	*Toxoplasma gondii*	Warm-blooded animals
Lymphocytic choriomeningitis	*Lymphocytic choriomeningitis virus*	House mouse
Ljungan virus	*Ljungan virus*	Wild rodents (bank voles)
Streptococcus porcinus	*Streptococcus porcinus*	Swine

Adapted from Goldenberg et al. Ref. [2].

infection can be ascertained. Only with this type of research can we hope to define the reasons for the excessive stillbirth burden in these countries and develop strategies to reduce the stillbirth rates.

Determining infection as causal for stillbirth

Since the 1950s, more than 35 different classification systems have been developed to assign cause of stillbirth. Generally, available clinical or autopsy information about the maternal and/or fetal conditions is applied to the classification system's criteria to determine a primary or underlying cause of stillbirth. Among the systems which have been widely used are the Wigglesworth, Aberdeen, and the relevant conditions at death (ReCoDe) [95–98]. The Wigglesworth system uses a pathophysiological approach, combined with stratification by birthweight classes, to create functional groups. The first published classification system, known as the Aberdeen classification, was developed for audit and surveillance of stillbirth in 1954 by Sir Dugald Baird and colleagues. This system ascribes

the death to predisposing obstetric events or to the underlying cause. A more recent system, ReCoDe, classifies the fetal death according to the relevant maternal conditions present at the time of death in utero using a hierarchal approach. One of the challenges for all systems is the complexity of the environment in which the stillbirth occurs and, with most existing systems, an underlying cause cannot be assigned for more than half of all stillbirths [98].

Building on these existing systems, Reddy et al. [99] developed a general methodology for evaluating conditions and their causal association with stillbirth. This approach, which evaluates infectious as well as other causes of stillbirth, is based on the following principles to determine degree of the association: (1) available epidemiologic data supports the association of a specific infection with the stillbirth, (2) there is biologic plausibility that the specific infection can cause stillbirth, (3) the infection is rarely seen in live births (or significantly associated with neonatal deaths), (4) a dose–response relationship exists, (5) the infection is associated with fetal compromise, and finally (6) the stillbirth would not have occurred without that infection. Most important, in a review of the existing classification schemes, it became apparent that a rigorous method was needed to define the association between the infectious condition and the stillbirth. For example, when considering infection as a cause of stillbirth, do we consider any existing maternal infection or only those infections with certain characteristics? Using the latter approach, a group in the United States, the Stillbirth Collaborative Research Network (SCRN), has defined the criteria necessary for an infection to be considered a cause of stillbirth and also the degree of certainty of that relationship, for example, as probably causal, possibly causal, or present without sufficient evidence to implicate causation [100]. Thus, based on this work, we believe that with an appropriate evaluation and sufficient data, the degree of the relationship of an infection to the stillbirth may often be established as follows:

1. For a stillbirth to be considered caused by a maternal infection without fetal or placental involvement, we believe that the maternal infection should be severe, generally requiring hospitalization and often defined by high maternal fever, respiratory complications, and/or surgery. In addition, the stillbirth should occur in close temporal proximity to the severe maternal infection. Severe pyelonephritis, pneumonia, influenza, and a ruptured appendix are some examples.

2. Direct fetal infection as a cause of stillbirth should be demonstrated by histologic evidence of fetal organ damage plus culture, histologic or PCR evidence of the presence of a specific organism, especially in an internal fetal organ.

3. Placental infection as a cause of stillbirth should show extensive placental involvement or damage—usually in the interstitial villous area—with demonstrated presence of organisms known to cause fetal death in this manner. Placental malarial infection is the best example.

4. Infections early in pregnancy leading to congenital anomalies or other fetal conditions later associated with stillbirth are also considered an infectious cause of stillbirth. To make this diagnosis, demonstration of maternal infection at an appropriate time in pregnancy with a specific organism known to cause the fetal condition is required, as is confirmation that the fetus has that condition. First-trimester maternal rubella infection is the prime example of this type of infection; parvovirus infection with fetal hydrops is another example.

5. A number of stillbirths occur with the initiation of labor at gestational ages deemed by the provider too early (often <26 weeks) to intervene by cesarean section. The cause of the preterm labor frequently appears to be an infection of the membranes often associated with histologic chorioamnionitis. We believe that these cases should be classified as an infectious cause of stillbirth. Attributing stillbirth to this infectious pathway requires histologic chorioamnionitis plus an intrapartum death at less than 26 weeks.

As with many other conditions associated with stillbirth, it is often uncertain whether a finding related to infection should be considered causal for the stillbirth. For example, if the mother has a positive antibody test for syphilis and the fetus dies, but there is no histologic placental or autopsy evidence of lesions generally associated with syphilis, should syphilis be considered the cause of death? Similarly, if histologic chorioamnionitis is present in a fetal death at >26 weeks, and there are no other findings suggestive of an infectious etiology, should the histologic chorioamnionitis be considered the cause of death? To deal with such cases, we believe a classification system that incorporates the degree of certainty about the association between stillbirth and infection is very helpful. A stillbirth with fetal hydrops and severe anemia with a demonstrated maternal parvovirus infection was probably caused by that parvovirus infection. It is less certain that a stillbirth with only histologic chorioamnionitis was actually caused by that condition. Therefore, we believe that in a classification system that includes infection as a potential cause of death, a measure of the certainty of the association should be presented. If signs of infection are present but do not meet carefully defined criteria, those infections should simply be noted as present, but not described as the cause of death.

Evaluation

Once a stillbirth occurs, the question often arises about which tests to review or order to confirm or rule out an infectious cause of death. Various authors and the ACOG have evaluated the utility of available diagnostic tests [100, 101]. From the routine prenatal laboratory tests, the results for syphilis, HIV, hepatitis B virus, rubella, chlamydia, and gonorrhea should be reviewed. In cases of stillbirth, a repeat evaluation for syphilis is usually recommended. TORCH titers (toxoplasmosis, rubella, CMV, herpes, and "other") are also often recommended, but Silver et al. [102] noted that although these have traditionally been advised in the evaluation of stillbirth, these titers are rarely clinically useful. Maternal serology for parvovirus may be informative in select cases. Most useful is a careful placental histological examination and autopsy with specific bacterial cultures and specimens for viral culture and PCR drawn and evaluated based on the pregnancy history and findings at autopsy. Because of contamination following membrane rupture or vaginal contamination during delivery, routine bacterial culture of the placenta is usually not useful. Culture of fetal heart blood or fluid from uncontaminated fetal sites during autopsy, however, occasionally provides surprising and useful information to determine an infectious etiology.

Reducing infection-related stillbirth

The stillbirth ratio in the United States is approximately 6–7 per 1,000 births. With infections accounting for 10–24% of all stillbirths, this means that in about 1 in 1,000 births there will be a stillbirth caused by infection. With the relative rarity of this condition, the many varieties of bacteria, viruses, fungi, and protozoa that may cause an infection-related stillbirth, and the different strategies necessary to prevent these infections, it is unlikely that further substantial reductions in U.S. infection-related stillbirths will be achieved in the foreseeable future. That said, a number of strategies

implemented fully should reduce the risk of stillbirth associated with infection. Prenatal screening for infections such as syphilis is important because women identified early and appropriately treated have a stillbirth risk not much higher than the general population. The U.S. Public Health Task Force recently recommended routine screening of all pregnant women for syphilis to allow for prompt treatment to reduce stillbirths associated with this infection. Further, in high incidence areas, repeat testing in the third trimester may help to prevent stillbirths later in pregnancy. In addition, screening and treatment of other sexually transmitted infections, including chlamydia and gonorrhea, should minimize stillbirths associated with these infections. Screening for group B streptococcus (GBS) and treatment with antibiotics in labor may reduce the stillbirths associated with that infection. Some stillbirths have been associated with ascending bacterial infection after premature rupture of membranes (PROM).The current recommended antibiotic treatment strategies certainly reduce chorioamnionitis and improve several other newborn outcomes, and may reduce stillbirth as well. Although many of the viral infections related to stillbirth are not preventable by vaccines, continued high rates of routine immunizations for childhood illness (e.g., measles, mumps, rubella, varicella) should prevent stillbirth associated with those infections. Timely immunization of all pregnant women against influenza as recommended by ACOG should eliminate the stillbirths associated with that infection. Reducing exposure to cat litter boxes and to soft cheeses should reduce the few stillbirths associated with toxoplasmosis and listeriosis. From a research perspective—since ascending bacterial infection prior to membrane rupture seems to be the most important infectious cause of stillbirths—developing a better understanding of this infection as well as methods to reduce its occurrence is crucial to reducing the infection-related stillbirths in the United States.

In many low- and middle-income countries, the infectious disease burden during pregnancy is extremely high, and it is likely that the stillbirth rate is also high as a result of these infections. Therefore, in some countries, programs that screen for and treat syphilis should have a major impact on the number of stillbirths. Antibiotic treatment for syphilis-infected women appears to be effective in reducing the stillbirth risk almost to that of noninfected women. Reducing maternal malaria infections in endemic areas should also reduce the stillbirth rate. Antimalarial strategies have been evaluated specifically for implementation during pregnancy. These include malaria prophylaxis—and particularly intermittent therapy—as well as use of bed nets impregnated with insecticides. To date, while these strategies have clearly reduced malaria and outcomes such as severe anemia, most studies have not been powered to show improvements in rarer outcomes such as stillbirth. In low- and middle-income countries, it is also likely that a reduction in bacterial intrauterine infections, if achievable, will have a substantial impact on stillbirth rates. Achieving high antiviral vaccination rates (rubella, rubeola, varicella, polio) should reduce the stillbirths associated with these infections.

Overall, it is clear that a high-quality evaluation is crucial to determine causality of infection for any particular stillbirth. The best evidence of an infectious etiology for a stillbirth is obtained from a carefully performed autopsy and placental examination with appropriate serologic studies, cultures, and DNA specimens taken for the organisms discussed in this report. New organisms associated with stillbirth should be sought. However, even if an autopsy is not performed, a histologic study of the placenta, membranes, and umbilical cord, with appropriate bacterial, viral, and protozoan serologic studies, culture, and DNA isolation techniques, will often provide evidence for an infectious etiology.

References

1. Stanton C, Lawn JE, Rahman H, et al. Stillbirth rates: delivering estimates in 190 countries. Lancet 2006;367(9521):1487–94.
2. Goldenberg RL, McClure EM, Saleem S, Reddy U. Infection-related stillbirth. Lancet 2010;375(9724):1482–90.
3. Di Mario S, Say L, Lincetto O. Risk factors for stillbirth in developing countries: a systematic review of the literature. Sex Transm Dis 2007;34(7):S11–21.
4. Rawlinson WD, Hall B, Jones CA, et al. Viruses and other infections in stillbirth: what is the evidence and what should we be doing? Pathology 2008;40(2):149–60.
5. Gibbs RS. The origins of stillbirth: infectious diseases. Semin Perinatol 2002;26:75–8.
6. Goldenberg RL, Thompson C. The infectious origin of stillbirth. Am J Obstet Gynecol 2003;189:861–73.
7. Copper RL, Goldenberg RL, DuBard MB, Davis RO. Risk factors for fetal death in white, black, and Hispanic women. Obstet Gynecol 1994;84:490–5.
8. Korteweg FJ, Gordijn SJ, Timmer A, et al. A placental cause of intra-uterine fetal death depends on the perinatal mortality classification system used. Placenta 2008;29:71–80.
9. McClure EM, Phiri M, Goldenberg RL. Stillbirth in developing countries: a review of the literature. Int J Gynaecol Obstet 2006;94(2):82–90.
10. Lumbiganon P, Piaggio G, Villar J, et al. The epidemiology of syphilis in pregnancy. Int J STD AIDS 2002;13:486–94.
11. Genc M, Ledger WJ. Syphilis in pregnancy. Sex Transm Infect 2000;76:73–9.
12. CDC. Congenital syphilis—United States, 2000. MMWR Morb Mortal Wkly Rep 2001;50:573–7.
13. Folgosa E, Osman NB, Gonzalez C, et al. Syphilis seroprevalence among pregnant women and its role as a risk factor for stillbirth in Maputo, Mozambique. Genitourin Med 1996;72:339–42.
14. Potter D, Goldenberg RL, Read JS, et al. Correlates of syphilis seroreactivity among pregnant women: the HIVNET 024 trial in Malawi, Tanzania and Zambia. Sex Transm Dis 2006;33:604–9.
15. Schmid GP, Stoner BP, Hawkes S, Broutet N. The need and plan for global elimination of congenital syphilis. Sex Transm Dis 2007;34:S5–10.
16. Sheffield JS, Sanchez PJ, Wendel GD, et al. Placental histopathology of congenital syphilis. Obstet Gynecol 2002;100:126–33.
17. Watson-Jones D, Changalucha J, Gumadoka B, et al. Syphilis in pregnancy in Tanzania. I. Impact of maternal syphilis on outcome of pregnancy. J Infect Dis 2002;186:940–7.
18. Salakhov E, Tikhonova L, Southwick K, et al. Congenital syphilis in Russia: the value of counting epidemiologic cases and clinical cases. Sex Transm Dis 2004;31:127–32.
19. Sethi S, Sharma K, Dhaliwal LK, et al. Declining trends in syphilis prevalence among antenatal women in northern India: a 10-year analysis from a tertiary healthcare centre. Sex Transm Infect 2007;83:592.

20. Vásquez-Manzanilla O, Dickson-Gonzalez SM, Salas JG, et al. Congenital syphilis in Valera, Venezuela. J Trop Pediatr 2007;53:274–7.

21. Watson-Jones D, Weiss HA, Changalucha JM, et al. Adverse birth outcomes in United Republic of Tanzania—impact and prevention of maternal risk factors. Bull World Health Organ 2007;85:9–17.

22. Chi BH, Wang L, Read JS, et al. Predictors of stillbirth in sub-Saharan Africa. Obstet Gynecol 2007; 110:989–97.

23. Rydzak CE, Goldie SJ. Cost-effectiveness of rapid point-of-care prenatal syphilis screening in sub-Saharan Africa. Sex Transm Dis 2008;35:775–84.

24. Schmid GP. Economic and programmatic aspects of congenital syphilis elimination. Bull World Health Organ 2004;82:402–9.

25. Hossain M, Broutet N, Hawkes S. The elimination of congenital syphilis: a comparison of the proposed World Health Organization Action Plan for the elimination of congenital syphilis with existing national maternal and congenital syphilis policies. Sex Transm Dis 2007;34:S22–30.

26. MacDonald A, Benach J, Burgdorfer W. Stillbirth following maternal Lyme disease. N Y State J Med 1987;87:615–16.

27. Strobino BA, Williams CL, Abid S, et al. Lyme disease and pregnancy outcome: a prospective study of two thousand prenatal patients. Am J Obstet Gynecol 1993;169:367–74.

28. Mhalu FS, Matre R. Serological evidence of lyme borreliosis in Africa: results from studies in Dar Es Salaam, Tanzania. East Afr Med J 1996;73:583–5.

29. Dupont HT, La Scola B, Williams R, Raoult D. A focus of tick-borne relapsing fever in southern Zaire. Clin Infect Dis 1997;25:139–44.

30. McConnell J. Tick-borne relapsing fever under-reported. Lancet Infect Dis 2003;3:604.

31. Jongen VH, van Roosmalen J, Tiems J, et al. Tick-borne relapsing fever and pregnancy outcome in rural Tanzania. Acta Obstet Gynecol Scand 1997;76:834–8.

32. Melkert PW. Relapsing fever in pregnancy: analysis of high-risk factors. Br J Obstet Gynaecol 1988; 95:1070–2.

33. Guggenheim JN, Haverkamp AD. Tick-borne fever during pregnancy: a case report. J Reprod Med 2005;50(9):727.

34. Smith B, Kemp M, Ethelberg S, et al. *Listeria monocytogenes*: maternal-foetal infections in Denmark 1994–2005. Scand J Infect Dis 2009;41:21–5.

35. Jana N, Vasishta K, Jindal SK, et al. Perinatal outcome in pregnancies complicated by pulmonary tuberculosis. Int J Gynaecol Obstet 1994;44:119–24.

36. Pillay T, Sturm AW, Khan M, et al. Vertical transmission of *Mycobacterium tuberculosis* in KwaZulu Natal: impact of HIV-1 co-infection. Int J Tuberc Lung Dis 2004;8:59–69.

37. Romero R, Gomez R, Ghezzi F, et al. A fetal systemic inflammatory response is followed by the spontaneous onset of preterm parturition. Am J Obstet Gynecol 1998;179:186–93.

38. Lahra MM, Gordon A, Jeffery HE. Chorioamnionitis and fetal response in stillbirth. Am J Obstet Gynecol 2007;196:e1–4.

39. Madan E, Meyer MP, Amortegui A. Chorioamnionitis: a study of organisms isolated in perinatal autopsies. Ann Clin Lab Sci 1988;18:39–45.

40. Blackwell S, Romero R, Chaiworapongsa T, et al. Maternal and fetal inflammatory responses in unexplained fetal death. J Matern Fetal Neonatal Med 2003;14:151–7.

41. Axemo P, Ching C, Machungo F, et al. Intrauterine infections and their association with stillbirth and preterm birth in Maputo, Mozambique. Gynecol Obstet Invest 1993;35:108–13.

42. Naeye RL, Tafari N, Judge D, et al. Amniotic fluid infections in an African city. J Pediatr 1977; 90:965–70.

43. Goldenberg RL, Mudenda V, Read JS, et al., for the HPTN 024 Study Team. HPTN 024: histologic chorioamnionitis, antibiotics and adverse infant outcomes in a predominantly HIV-1-infected African population. Am J Obstet Gynecol 2006;195: 1065–74.

44. Lamont R. Infection in the prediction and antibiotics in the prevention of spontaneous preterm labour and preterm birth. BJOG 2003;110(20):71–5.

45. Kenyon S, Boulvain M, Neilson JP. Antibiotics for preterm rupture of membranes. Cochrane Database Syst Rev 2003;Issue 2:Art. No.: CD001058.

46. Tuomala RE, Shapiro DE, Mofenson LM, et al. Antiretroviral therapy during pregnancy and the risk of an adverse outcome. N Engl J Med 2002; 346:1863–70.

47. Olagbuji BN, Ezeanochie MC, Ande AB, Oboro VO. Obstetric and perinatal outcome in HIV positive women receiving HAART in urban Nigeria. Arch Gynecol Obstet 2010;281(6):991–4.

48. Brocklehurst P, French R. The association between maternal HIV infection and perinatal outcome: a systematic review of the literature and meta-analysis. Br J Obstet Gynaecol 1998;105:836–48.

49. Cotter AM, Garcia AG, Duthely ML, et al. Is antiretroviral therapy during pregnancy associated with an increased risk of preterm delivery, low birth weight, or stillbirth? J Infect Dis 2006;193:1195–201.

50. Ayisia JG, van Eijka AM, ter Kuilea FO, et al. The effect of dual infection with HIV and malaria on pregnancy outcome in western Kenya. AIDS 2003; 17:585–94.

51. Cutts FT, Robertson SE, Diaz-Ortega JL, Samuel R. Control of rubella and congenital rubella syndrome (CRS) in developing countries, Part 1: burden of disease from CRS. Bull World Health Organ 1997; 75:55–68.

52. Gershon AA. Chickenpox, measles and mumps. In: Remington JS, Klein JO (eds), Infectious diseases of fetus and newborn infant. Philadelphia, PA: WB Saunders; 2006, pp. 693–738.

53. Ornoy A, Tenenbaum A. Pregnancy outcome following infections by coxsackie, echo, measles, mumps, hepatitis, polio and encephalitis viruses. Reprod Toxicol 2006;21:446–57.

54. Gregg NM. Congenital cataract following German measles in the mother. Trans Ophthalmol Soc Aust 1941;3:35–46.

55. Dayan GH, Zimmerman L, Shteinke L, et al. Investigation of a rubella outbreak in Kyrgyzstan in 2001: implications for an integrated approach to measles elimination and prevention of congenital rubella syndrome. J Infect Dis 2003;187:S235–40.

56. Aaby P, Bukh J, Lisse IM, et al. Increased perinatal mortality among children of mothers exposed to measles during pregnancy. Lancet 1988;1:516–19.

57. Stanwell-Smith R, Parker AM, Chakraverty P, et al. Possible association of influenza A with fetal loss: investigation of a cluster of spontaneous abortions and stillbirths. Commun Dis Rep CDR Rev 1994;3: R28–32.

58. Ng WF, Wong SF, Lam A, et al. The placentas of patients with severe acute respiratory syndrome: a pathophysiological evaluation. Pathology 2006; 38:210–18.

59. Jamieson DJ, Honein MA, Rasmussen SA, et al., Novel Influenza A (H1N1) Pregnancy Working Group. H1N1 2009 influenza virus infection during pregnancy in the USA. Lancet 2009;374:451–8.

60. ACOG Committee on Obstetric Practice. ACOG committee opinion number 305, November 2004. Influenza vaccination and treatment during pregnancy. Obstet Gynecol 2004;104(5 Pt 1):1125–6.

61. Enders M, Weidner A, Zoellner I, et al. Fetal morbidity and mortality after acute human parvovirus B19 infection in pregnancy: a prospective evaluation of 1018 cases. Prenat Diagn 2004; 24(7):513–18.

62. Riipinen A, Väisänen E, Nuutila M, et al. Parvovirus b19 infection in fetal deaths. Clin Infect Dis 2008; 47:1519–25.

63. [No authors listed]. Prospective study of human parvovirus (B19) infection in pregnancy. Public health laboratory service working party on fifth disease: BMJ 1990;300:1166–70.

64. Tolfvenstam T, Papadogiannakis N, Norbeck O, et al. Frequency of human parvovirus B19 infection in intrauterine fetal death. Lancet 2001;357: 1494–7.

65. Silingardi E, Santunione AL, Rivasi F, et al. Unexpected intrauterine fetal death in parvovirus B19 fetal infection. Am J Forensic Med Pathol 2009;30(4):394.

66. Nuovo GJ, Cooper LD, Bartholomew D. Histologic, infectious, and molecular correlates of idiopathic spontaneous abortion and perinatal mortality. Diagn Mol Pathol 2005;14(3):152–8.

67. Frisk G, Diderholm H. Increased frequency of Coxsackie B virus IgM in women with spontaneous abortion. J Infect 1992;24:141–5.

68. Maruyama Y, Sameshima H, Kamitomo M, et al. Fetal manifestations and poor outcomes of congenital cytomegalovirus infections: possible candidates for intrauterine antiviral treatments. J Obstet Gynaecol Res 2007;33:619–23.

69. Tongsong T, Sukpan K, Wanapirak C, Phadungkiatwattna P. Fetal cytomegalovirus infection associated with cerebral hemorrhage, hydrops fetalis, and echogenic bowel: case report. Fetal Diagn Ther 2008;23:169–72.

70. Howard J, Hall B, Brennan LE, et al. Utility of newborn screening cards for detecting CMV infection in cases of stillbirth. J Clin Virol 2009;44:215–18.

71. Syridou G, Spanakis N, Konstantinidou A, et al. Detection of cytomegalovirus, parvovirus B19 and herpes simplex viruses in cases of intrauterine fetal death: association with pathological findings. J Med Virol 2008;80:1776–82.

72. Patra S, Kumar A, Trivedi SS, et al. Maternal and fetal outcomes in pregnant women with acute hepatitis E virus infection. Ann Intern Med 2007;147(1):28–33.

73. Samsioe A, Papadogiannakis N, Hultman T, et al. *Ljungan virus* present in intrauterine fetal death diagnosed by both immunohistochemistry and PCR. Birth Defects Res A Clin Mol Teratol 2009;85(3):227–9.

74. Niklasson B, Samsioe A, Papadogiannakis N, et al. Association of zoonotic *Ljungan virus* with intrauterine fetal deaths. Birth Defects Res A Clin Mol Teratol 2007;79:488–93.

75. Desai M, Oter Kuile F, Nosten F, et al. Epidemiology and burden of malaria in pregnancy. Lancet Infect Dis 2007;7:93–104.

76. McGregor IA, Wilson ME, Billewicz WZ. Malaria infection of the placenta in The Gambia, West Africa: its incidence and relationship to stillbirth, birth weight, and placenta weight. Trans R Soc Trop Med Hyg 1983;77:232–44.

77. Dorman EK, Shulman CE, Kingdom J, et al. Impaired uteroplacental blood flow in pregnancies complicated by falciparum malaria. Ultrasound Obstet Gynecol 2002;19:165–70.

78. Van Geertruyden JP, Thomas F, Erhart A, D'Alessandro U. The contribution of malaria in pregnancy to perinatal mortality. Am J Trop Med Hyg 2004;71 (Suppl.):35–40.

79. Newman RD, Hailemariam A, Jimma D, et al. Burden of malaria during pregnancy in areas of stable and unstable transmission in Ethiopia during a non-epidemic year. J Infect Dis 2003;187:1765–72.

80. Kumar A, Valecha N, Jain T, Dash AP. Burden of malaria in India: retrospective and prospective view. Am J Trop Med Hyg 2007;77:69–78.

81. Coll O, Menedez C, Botet F, Dayal R, WAPM Perinatal Infections Working Group. Treatment and prevention of malaria in pregnancy and newborn. J Perinat Med 2008;36:15–29.

82. Okie S. A new attack on malaria. N Engl J Med 2008;358:2425–8.

83. Jones JL, Lopez A, Wilson M, et al. Congenital toxoplasmosis: a review. Obstet Gynecol Surv 2001; 56:296–305.

84. Onadeko MO, Joynson DH, Payne RA, Francis J. The prevalence of toxoplasma antibodies in pregnant Nigerian women and the occurrence of stillbirth and congenital malformation. Afr J Med Med Sci 1996;25:331–4.

85. Nimri L, Pelloux H, Elkhatib L. Detection of *Toxoplasma gondii* DNA and specific antibodies in high-risk pregnant women. Am J Trop Med Hyg 2004; 71:831–5.

86. Demar M, Ajzenberg D, Maubon D, et al. Fatal outbreak of human toxoplasmosis along the Maroni River: epidemiological, clinical, and parasitological aspects. Clin Infect Dis 2007;45(7):e88–95.

87. Carcopino X, Raoult D, Bretelle F, et al. Q Fever during pregnancy: a cause of poor fetal and maternal outcome. Ann N Y Acad Sci 2009;1166:79–89.

88. Lingam S, Marshall WC, Wilson J, et al. Congenital trypanosomiasis in a child born in London. Dev Med Child Neurol 1985;27:664–74.

89. Buekens P, Almendares O, Carlier Y, et al. Mother-to-child transmission of Chagas' disease in North America: why don't we do more? Matern Child Health J 2008;12(3):283–6.

90. Gürgan T, Diker KS, Haziroglu R, et al. In vitro infection of human fetal membranes with *Candida* species. Gynecol Obstet Invest 1994;37(3):164–7.

91. Sfameni S, Talbot JM, Chow S, et al. *Candida glabrata* chorioamnionitis following in vitro fertilization and embryo transfer. Aust N Z J Obstet Gynaecol 1997;37(1):88.

92. Haider BA, Humayun Q, Bhutta ZA. Effect of administration of antihelminthics for soil transmitted helminths during pregnancy. Cochrane Database Syst Rev 2009;2:CD005547.

93. De Silva N, Sirisena J, Gunasekera D, et al. Effect of mebendazole therapy during pregnancy on birth outcomes. Lancet 1999;353:145–9.

94. Ndibazza J, Muhangi L, Akishule D, et al. Effects of deworming during pregnancy on maternal and perinatal outcomes in Entebbe, Uganda: a randomized controlled trial. Clin Infect Dis 2010;50(4):531–40.

95. Wigglesworth J. Classification of perinatal deaths. Soc Prev Med 1994;39:11–14.

96. Pattinson RC, De Jong G, Theron GB. Primary causes of total perinatally related wastage at Tygerberg Hospital. S Afr Med J 1989;75:50–3.

97. Gardosi J, Kady SM, McGeown P, et al. Classification of stillbirth by relevant condition at death (ReCoDe): population based cohort study. BMJ 2005;331(7525): 1113–17.

98. Flenady V, Frøen JF, Pinar H, et al. An evaluation of classification systems for stillbirth. BMC Pregnancy Childbirth 2009;9:24.

99. Reddy UM, Goldenberg RL, Silver R, et al. Stillbirth classification—developing an international consensus for research. Obstet Gynecol 2009;114(4):901–14.

100. Dudley DJ, Goldenberg RL, Conway D, et al. For the Stillbirth Collaborative Research Network: A New System for Determining the Causes of Stillbirth. Obstet Gynecol 2010;116:254–60.

101. ACOG Practice Bulletin No. 102: management of stillbirth. Obstet Gynecol 2009;113(3):748–61.

102. Silver RM, Varner MW, Reddy U, et al. Work-up of stillbirth: a review of the evidence. Am J Obstet Gynecol 2007;196(5):433–44.

CHAPTER 6
Genetics

Ronald Wapner, MD
Division of Maternal Fetal Medicine, Department of Obstetrics and Gynecology, Columbia University, College of
Physicians and Surgeons, New York, NY, USA

Of the over 4 million births that occur in the United States per year, approximately 26,000 will end in a stillborn infant. The exact percentage of these that are due to a "genetic" cause is uncertain and depends on how specific one is in defining a "genetic" etiology. If any stillborn infant with a fetal structural anomaly is considered to be due to a "genetic etiology," then approximately a quarter of stillbirths will be included. Forty percent will have single malformations, 40% multiple anomalies, and the other 20% disruption or dysplasia syndromes [1]. Among these, there is heterogeneity of diagnoses with more than 90 potential disorders with no single diagnosis accounting for more than 1.5%. However, if one requires laboratory confirmation that the in utero death was caused by an alteration of the fetal, maternal, or placental genome, then a much smaller proportion will qualify as genetic. Even among stillborns with multiple malformations, a specific diagnosis of a genetic syndrome is unlikely and can be accomplished in only about one quarter of cases.

When a stillbirth is associated with a fetal structural anomaly or has a confirmed genetic diagnosis, it is still not certain that this was the cause of death. In general, a stillbirth should be considered due to a fetal malformation or genetic etiology when (1) there is epidemiologic data demonstrating an excess of intrauterine mortality associated with the disorder, (2) the process is only rarely seen in liveborns and when a live birth occurs it frequently results in neonatal death, and (3) there

is biologic plausibility that the anomalies contributed to the death. If multiple criteria are met, then the likelihood that the process caused death is increased [2].

Cytogenetic causes of stillbirth

Chromosomal abnormalities of either the fetus or the placenta is a frequently described cause of stillbirth, but the exact mechanisms by which this occurs is often unknown. Factors that appear to have an impact on lethality include the specific chromosome error involved, the associated fetal structural anomalies that occur, and the distribution of the abnormal cell line within the fetus and/ or the placenta.

Cytogenetic abnormalities of the fetus

Overall, fetal cytogenetic abnormalities are associated with approximately 6–17% of all stillbirths with the proportion being higher for macerated or malformed fetuses [1, 3–8]. In a large study of 750 stillbirths, 38% of those with morphologic abnormalities were aneuploid when compared to 4.6% of those that were structurally normal [6]. The distribution of abnormal karyotypes in stillborns is similar to that seen in liveborns, that is, 23% 45X, 23% trisomy 21, 21% trisomy 18, 8% trisomy 13, with mosaics, autosomal monosomies, deletions, unbalanced translocations, and marker chromosomes making up the rest [1, 3, 9].

As alluded to above, a cytogenetic imbalance occurring in a stillbirth does not completely account for the fetal death since many of the same chromosomal abnormalities associated with stillbirths also result in live-born infants. For example, of trisomy 21 pregnancies surviving into the second trimester only 9.5% will result in a stillbirth after 20 weeks and 6.8% after 24 weeks [10]. Among trisomy 18 fetuses, only about a third surviving to 20 weeks will result in a fetal death so that factors other than the karyotype must contribute to the outcome. The most significant contributing factor to fetal death in trisomy 21 appears to be the presence of specific structural anomalies. For example, Won et al. [10] have shown that slightly more than half of surviving Down syndrome pregnancies have no major structural anomalies, whereas all of those resulting in stillbirth had significant malformations such as hydrops or severe cardiac malformations which were the likely cause of the fetal death.

The karyotype of the placenta may also play a role in determining survival of an aneuploid fetus. For example, of the 30–40% of trisomy 18 and 60% of trisomy 13 gestations that survive to term [11–13], most have a coexisting normal cell line in the cytotrophoblast cells within the placenta despite having 100% aneuploid cells in the fetus and other extraembryonic tissues. In their series of placentas from aneuploid pregnancies, Kalousek et al. [14] found that all trisomy 13 and 18 fetuses surviving the intrauterine period had a euploid cell line present within the cytotrophoblast demonstrating the role confined placental mosaicism (CPM, described in detail later in this chapter) plays in placental function. Interestingly, this effect appears to be chromosome specific since most surviving trisomy 21 fetuses have only aneuploid cytotrophoblast cells.

It is likely that cytogenetic abnormalities contribute to a greater proportion of stillbirths than is presently recognized, since the macerated tissue available from stillborn fetuses is difficult to culture and karyotype. In most series, karyotyping is unsuccessful in almost half of the cases [1, 3, 15]. In addition, many series investigating the karyotype of stillborn infants were performed more than 20 years ago so that only whole chromosome aneuploidy or other relatively large abnormalities were detectable.

Recently, technologies that directly analyze fetal DNA and do not require tissue culture have been used to investigate pregnancy loss. Florescent in situ hybridization (FISH) can be used to confirm suspected abnormalities, but is limited by the need to prospectively anticipate which chromosomes may be involved. More recently, comparative genomic hybridization (CGH) has been utilized. With this approach (Figure 6.1), the entire genome can be simultaneously evaluated and small microdeletions and duplications that are 1 Mb or smaller can be identified. This resolution is superior to standard karyotyping, in which abnormalities of 5 Mb or smaller are usually not detected. Analysis of stillbirths using CGH has recently been investigated by members of the Wisconsin Stillbirth Service Program (WISP) [16]. In 15 cases tested, two chromosomal abnormalities not seen with standard karyotyping were identified. In this pilot evaluation, only cases with multiple structural anomalies were evaluated so that the rate of subtle chromosome errors in the overall evaluation of stillbirths still needs further investigation. However, if additional series confirm this success, then CGH may supplant karyotyping for evaluation of stillborn fetuses since tissue culture is not required and it has higher resolution identifying small imbalances. Of equal importance is the potential that identification of small deletions associated with fetal death will provide clues useful to the identification of genes underlying many of these defects.

Placental cytogenetics

The karyotype of the placenta can differ from that of the fetus and in certain cases this difference may alter the anticipated outcome of the pregnancy. In approximately 1–2% of pregnancies, the placenta will be mosaic (i.e., contain two distinct cell lines) despite an entirely euploid fetal karyotype [17–19].

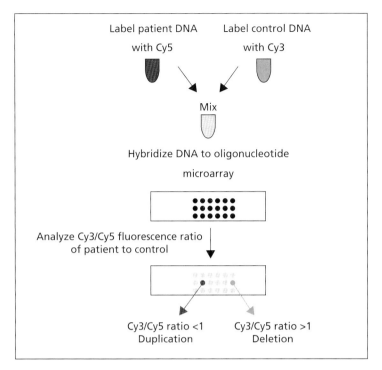

Figure 6.1 The potential use of array CGH to diagnose structural genomic changes in stillbirth. This figure illustrates the general principal underlying CGH that is used to identify DNA deletions or duplications. In this technique, fluorescently labeled DNA from a normal control sample is mixed with a test sample that is labeled with a different colored dye. The mixture is then hybridized to an array containing hundreds of thousands of small, well-defined DNA probes. Regional differences in the fluorescence ratio can be detected and used for identifying abnormal regions in the genome. Courtesy of Dr. Ronald Wapner (modified from Ref. [2]).

This is referred to as CPM and as described later may have significant clinical sequelae, including stillbirth.

There are two mechanisms leading to CPM (Figure 6.2). In one, postzygotic (mitotic) nondisjunction occurring during early development of the zygote will lead to a trisomic population of cells along with the population of normal euploid cells. At the time of blastula development and differentiation, cells from the trisomic population may segregate along with the euploid cells into the inner cell mass and become incorporated into the embryo, migrate exclusively into extrafetal tissues such as the placenta or be incorporated into both. True fetal mosaicism results when both euploid and aneuploidy cells are present in the fetus, whereas CPM implies that the trisomic cells are only found in extrafetal tissues such as the placenta. In a second mechanism, a meiotic error occurs during gametogenesis resulting in a trisomic zygote which frequently will result in a miscarriage. However, if a second error (e.g., anaphase lag) involving the trisomic chromosomes occurs during early mitotic divisions, a disomic cell line will result rescuing the potentially lethal embryo. The morula then will contain both euploid and aneuploid cells and again, by chance, the aneuploid cells may segregate entirely into the trophoblast [20, 21]. Since meiotic errors occur more frequently with advancing maternal age, it is not surprising that CPM resulting from "trisomy rescue" occurs more frequently in older mothers.

CPM has significant clinical implications and results in an altered perinatal outcome in up to 20% of cases. It is associated not only with stillbirth, but also has been shown to increase the risk of first- and second-trimester fetal losses and intrauterine growth retardation [22, 23]. The significance of CPM in any particular pregnancy is determined by a number of factors including the specific chromosome involved, persistence of the aneuploid cell line to term, the percentage of abnormal cells, and the presence of uniparental disomy which may occur when the cell line rescued from a meiotic error contains a pair of chromosomes both of which emanate from the same parent (Figure 6.3) [5, 21–25].

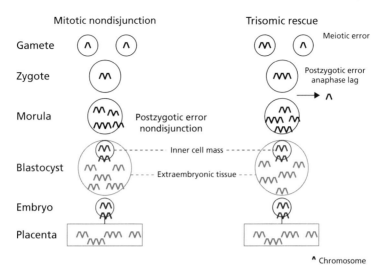

Figure 6.2 Mechanisms leading to CPM. This figure demonstrates two mechanisms capable of causing CPM. Mitotic nondisjunction early in embryo development may lead to a mosaic morula containing a normal and an aneuploid cell line. Alternatively, a meiotic error can lead to a trisomic embryo; many of which will result in a spontaneous miscarriage. However, a second error (anaphase lag) may occur converting a trisomic cell to disomy. In both mechanisms the morula is mosaic. Subsequently, cells are then randomly distributed to various compartments. Aneuploid cells distributed to the inner cell mass will result in true fetal mosaicism. If the aneuploid cells are distributed exclusively to the extra fetal lineage, CPM will occur. Courtesy of Dr. Ronald Wapner.

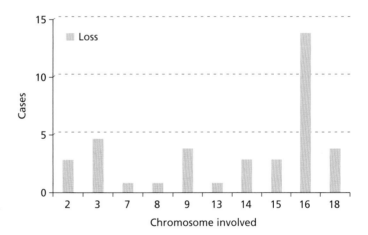

Figure 6.3 CPM: fetal loss by chromosome involved. (Data from Ref. [5].)

CPM involving cell lines containing chromosomes 2, 3, 9, 14, 15, 16, and 18 are associated with a particularly high risk of a poor perinatal outcome [14, 22, 26, 27]. Although it is tempting to propose that genes on these chromosomes are particularly important in placental function, these are also the chromosomes that are frequently involved in trisomic rescue producing a relatively higher proportion of trisomic cells in the placenta. Persistence of the abnormal cell line is also important in determining its clinical impact. Kalousek et al. [28] have shown that in cases where CPM is identified during a first-trimester chorionic villus sampling (CVS) procedure and the cell line persists to term, approximately 29% of fetuses will be growth retarded. In normally grown fetuses, it is unusual to find the cell line at term.

CPM involving chromosome 16 is particularly illustrative of the impact of an aneuploid cell line within the placenta and is the abnormality most likely to result in stillbirth. Benn [22] has shown that, despite the presence of a chromosomally normal fetus, approximately 1 in 5 pregnancies with CPM for chromosome 16 diagnosed at the time of a first-trimester CVS will result in a stillbirth. In addition, preterm birth, early pregnancy loss, and intrauterine growth retardation occur relatively more frequently, suggesting a continuum of effect based on the degree of placental involvement. The exact pathophysiology by which CPM leads to stillbirth and the incremental impact of uniparental disomy which occurs in up to one-third of cases of CPM resulting from meiotic rescue are still poorly understood and deserving of additional study.

Single-gene disorders

For some of single-gene disorders associated with stillbirth (Table 6.1), the genetic defect and the resulting pathophysiology leading to fetal death is fairly well understood. For example, alpha thalassemia leading to lethal hydrops occurs secondary to deletion of the four genes on chromosome 16 involved in alpha chain production. This results in the utilization of hemoglobin Barts ($\gamma4$) as the predominant hemoglobin. The inability of hemoglobin Barts to appropriately transfer oxygen to tissues as well as severe hemolysis of red cells containing this abnormal hemoglobin results in fetal anemia, excessive extramedullary hematopoiesis resulting in obstructive umbilical venous return and subsequent in utero death. Similarly, lysosomal storage diseases may also result in hydrops causing fetal death, but the mechanisms are less well defined and depending on the specific primary defect may include some mechanisms similar to those seen with the hemoglobinopathies such as obstruction of umbilical venous return and anemia. However, rather than being secondary to abnormal hemoglobin production, the hepatic venous obstruction and anemia are a result of organomegaly (frequently liver and spleen) from replacement of erythropoietic stem cells with storage cells. In addition, depending on

Table 6.1 Single-gene disorders associated with stillbirth.

Category	Disorders
Lysosomal storage disease	Pompe disease
	Gaucher: perinatal lethal type
	I-cell disease
	Sialidosis type II
	Galactosialidosis
	Fabry disease
	Sandhoff disease
	GM1 Gangliosidosis
	Schindler disease
	Niemann-Pick type A and C
	MPS IV and VII
Fetal energy production	Mitochondrial respiratory chain diseases
	Pyruvate dehydrogenase complex deficiency
Skeletal dysplasia	Achondrogenesis type 1B, IA
	Osteogenesis imperfecta type II
	Chondrodysplasia punctata lethal neonatal (Conradi Hunermann)
	Thanatophoric dysplasia
	Melnick-Needles syndrome (Otopalatal digital type II)
CNS	X-linked hydrocephalus
	Fetal akinesia hypokinesia (Pena Shokier type I)
	Rett syndrome
Skin	Incontinentia pigmenti
Hemoglobinopathy	Alpha thalassemia
Others	Meckel syndrome
	Fryns syndrome

the disorder, excess lysosomal storage may involve other systems including the placenta, the fetal brain and brain stem, the fetal heart (cardiomyopathy) and conduction system (lethal arrhythmia), or liver (hypoproteinemia).

For some disorders, stillbirth may occur as a direct result of the fetal metabolic alteration. Smith-Lemli-Opitz syndrome is an autosomal recessive multiple congenital anomaly (MCA)/mental retardation syndrome caused by a defect in cholesterol synthesis. Affected individuals usually have low to absent plasma cholesterol levels and elevated levels of cholesterol precursors, including 7-dehydrocholesterol. Severely affected individuals (those with the condition formerly referred to as Smith-Lemli-Opitz syndrome type II) in addition to multiple congenital malformations are often stillborn. In these cases, fetal malformations and death may occur from either the accumulated toxic cholesterol precursors or from the absence of cholesterol which has a significant role in fetal development. Other disorders, in which the metabolic defect is likely to be the direct cause of death, include those involving fetal energy production.

Since many of the metabolic disorders that result in fetal death also result in live births with varying degrees of neonatal and infant impairment, stillbirth should be thought of as one end of a continuum with the phenotype dependent on the specific gene defect. Gaucher disease (GD), an autosomal recessive lysosomal storage disease caused by a deficiency or absence of glucosylceramidase, is an excellent example of the phenotypic spectrum of these disorders. Type I is a relatively common disorder with mild phenotypic consequences including hepatosplenomegaly, bone alterations, mild anemia, and thrombocytopenia. Type 2, caused by different mutations of the same gene is an acute neuronopathic disorder, presenting in infancy and having a devastating neurologic course. There is a subset of type 2 disease that manifests in utero, with severe neurologic signs including strabismus, trismus, retroflexion of the head, and opisthotonos [29]. Another rare severe variant of GD is associated with hydrocephalus, corneal opacities, deformed toes, gastroesophageal reflux, and fibrous thickening of the splenic and hepatic capsules [13].

Finally, there is a perinatal lethal form manifesting as nonimmune hydrops fetalis and in utero demise [30]. Arthrogryposis and distinctive facial features are seen in 35–43% [31]. The perinatal lethal form can also be associated with hepatosplenomegaly, pancytopenia, and skin changes presenting clinically as ichthyosiform or collodion skin abnormalities (Figure 6.4) [32]. While in general, most patients with Gaucher disease have some residual enzyme activity, the majority of the perinatal lethal cases are caused by null alleles, leading to absent or severely deficient glucosylceramidase activity [29, 31–44].

In evaluating stillborn infants, the diagnosis of Mendelian disorders such as Gaucher disease is often missed due to the early lethality and the failure to recognize the association between lysosomal disorders, hydrops fetalis, and the other clinical findings not usually seen in the more common milder forms of the diseases. The incidence of severe perinatal lethal Gaucher disease as well as other Mendelian causes of stillbirth may prove more common than currently appreciated with greater physician awareness of the disorders and increasing use of molecular diagnostic techniques.

Some Mendelian disorders resulting in stillbirth have autosomal dominant inheritance. Since the lethal forms of these disorders are not consistent with reproduction, most of these stillbirths result from spontaneous mutations leading to lethal structural anomalies (e.g., skeletal dysplasias). However, on rare occasions, fetal death may occur secondary

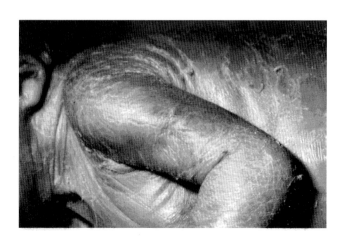

Figure 6.4 Skin lesions associated with the perinatal lethal form of Gaucher disease. (Reproduced from Ref. [32], with permission from Informa Healthcare.)

to inheritance of a parental mutation with lethal potential that is expressed in utero. For example, the long QT syndrome (LQTS) is a rare congenital heart condition in which delayed repolarization of the heart increases the risk of arrhythmias originating in the ventricles. In adults, these episodes may present as palpitations or fainting, but sudden death due to ventricular fibrillation can occur. In rare cases, stillbirth from an arrhythmia has occurred in a fetus inheriting the underlying genetic predisposition from a parent [45, 46].

There are a number of X-linked dominant disorders that are lethal in male fetuses (e.g., incontinentia pigmenti, X-linked hydrocephalus, Melnick-Needles syndrome, Rett syndrome) and result in stillbirth. In many of these cases the fetal demise occurs early in gestation, but near-term deaths can also occur depending on the disorder. A thorough examination of the mother may reveal characteristics of the disorder but because of possible skewed X inactivation the maternal phenotype may be normal. Accordingly, when repetitive losses of male fetuses occur, a clinically normal mother does not preclude an X-linked disorder as a cause of recurrent stillbirth. If an X-linked etiology of recurrent loss is suspected, evaluation for skewed X inactivation in the mother may help in evaluating this possibility. As with most Mendelian disorders associated with stillbirth, a spectrum of phenotypes is possible with X-linked dominant inheritance so that a pedigree including early male miscarriages, stillbirths, neonatal deaths, and severely effected infants may occur in the same family [47, 48].

As with cytogenetic disorders, the frequency of single-gene disorders contributing to stillbirth is underappreciated for a number of reasons. First, even though the live-born phenotype associated with a Mendelian disorder may be well described, when the same genetic disorder leads to stillbirth the phenotype may be significantly different and may not be recognized by clinical dysmorphologists nor well described in the literature. This is compounded by the fact that there is not a detailed registry of recognizable stillbirth syndromes. In most series of fetal deaths, those with structural anomalies and normal karyotypes are lumped together as "MCA syndromes" preventing further characterization. Finally, only recently have molecular tools been developed in which a panel of potential gene defects can be evaluated simultaneously. As this technology expands, it is anticipated that additional Mendelian causes of stillbirths will be identified.

Evaluation of stillborn pregnancies to identify genetic causes

Identifying a genetic etiology of a stillbirth is not only of academic interest but has serious implication for future pregnancies. In most cases in which a cytogenetic abnormality is determined, the couple can be counseled with increased precision about the risk of recurrence. When a 45X karyotype is identified, there is no increased risk of recurrence. For other trisomies including trisomy 21, the recurrence risk is based on the age of the mother at the time of delivery and her age at the next conception [49]. If she was 30 years old or older at the time of a trisomic stillbirth, she can be counseled that her risk of recurrence in a future pregnancy is only slightly greater than her age-related risk in that pregnancy. However, if the trisomic stillbirth occurred in a younger woman, the recurrence risk is usually quoted as 1%. It should also be remembered that women with a previous trisomic stillbirth have a recurrence risk for a trisomy other than the one seen in the initial stillbirth. Cytogenetic abnormalities other than trisomy (e.g., unbalanced translocation, marker chromosome) may require evaluation of the parents' karyotype with the outlook for future pregnancies based on the results.

The recurrence risk for autosomal recessive, X-linked, and familial and de novo autosomal dominant disorders are well defined. However, it is important to make sure that parents are aware that even when a well-defined autosomal dominant disorder is identified (e.g., a lethal form of osteogenis imperfect) and the parents are unaffected, there remains a small recurrence risk because of the possibility of parental germ cell mosaicism.

Confirming a genetic etiology of a stillbirth requires a comprehensive evaluation which is best initiated when the stillbirth is still in utero rather than waiting until after delivery. Analysis by amniocentesis or transabdominal placental biopsy will provide a successful karyotype more consistently than fetal skin or tissue sampling collected after delivery [6, 50–52]. Postdelivery tissue culture is complicated by contamination and maceration and fails from 30% to 60% of the time [6]. Alternatively, predelivery invasive procedures will be successful in almost all cases. In utero sampling should be strongly considered when fetal structural anomalies are identified since the probability of a cytogenetic abnormality is highest in these cases [7]. However, on occasion, phenotypic findings suggestive of aneuploidy are subtle and may not be seen prenatally, suggesting that sampling all prenatal demises seem justified.

After delivery, the stillborn infant should ideally be examined and autopsied by a pathologist or pediatric dysmorphologist with expertise in the evaluation of stillborn infants. If this is not possible, then detailed photographs should be obtained, which provide an overview of the fetus and close ups of anomalies. If a skeletal dysplasia is present, whole body X-rays should be obtained so that a specific diagnosis can be attempted. Even if in utero sampling was performed, fetal tissue should be obtained and a portion saved and stored for future DNA analysis. Tissue samples for karyotype should be taken from the placenta to exclude CPM. While it is likely that over the next few years molecular cytogenetic techniques (such as array CGH) which do not require tissue culture and can identify small genomic alterations will replace karyotypes, this transition awaits further evaluation. However, even when molecular techniques are used, karyotype is still advised since low-level mosaicism, particularly of the placenta, is not routinely identified by array CGH. In addition, some cases of triploidy may be missed by microarray analysis.

The clinician can help facilitate postmortem evaluation by providing the pathologist with the results of prenatal ultrasound or fetal magnetic resonance imaging (MRI) examinations since fetal tissue, particularly the brain, will be distorted from maceration and delivery. In addition, some in utero findings such as an abnormal amniotic fluid volume will not be evident at autopsy. For example, knowing that fetal ascites was present may suggest a lysosomal storage disorder which will require additional stains to diagnose [53]. Similarly, the absence of amniotic fluid may explain some deformations that otherwise might be considered to be malformations. In addition, providing the pathologist or geneticist with results of any prenatal testing will be beneficial as certain patterns of maternal serum analytes may suggest a particular cause of fetal death. For example, CPM for trisomy 16 is known to have alpha feto protein (AFP) and human chorionic gonadotropin (HCG) levels 7–10 times those of a normal pregnancy [22] and Smith-Lemli-Opitz syndrome will have extremely low maternal estriol levels [54].

Evaluation of whether a genetic factor was responsible for the fetal death requires a detailed pedigree through third-degree relatives. Stillborn infants and recurrent pregnancy losses should be identified, as should the presence of live-born individuals with developmental delay or structural anomalies since these may be clues to single-gene disorders. Consanguinity should be identified because of the increased possibility of severe autosomal recessive disorders. A detailed history for arrhythmias and sudden death (including sudden infant dealth syndrome [SIDS]) should be obtained since prolonged QT syndrome may be more prevalent in these cases than initially thought. If the stillborn was a male, the mother should be examined looking for subtle characteristics of an X-linked disorder that could be lethal in males.

Conclusion

Understanding the role that genetic abnormalities play in causing fetal death is evolving. Previous tools used to evaluate stillborn infants such as karyotyping and autopsy are being replaced by improved imaging techniques such as MRI and more detailed fetal DNA analysis. As data from these evaluations accrues, it is likely that an increasing understanding of the role of genetic disorders in stillbirths will occur.

References

1. Pauli, R.M. and C.A. Reiser. Wisconsin Stillbirth Service Program: II. Analysis of diagnoses and

diagnostic categories in the first 1,000 referrals. Am J Med Genet 1994;50(2): 35–53.

2. Reddy, U.M., R. Goldenberg, R. Silver, et al. Stillbirth classification--developing an international consensus for research: executive summary of a National Institute of Child Health and Human Development workshop. Obstet Gynecol 2009;114(4):901–14.

3. Pauli, R.M., C.A. Reiser, R.M. Lebovitz, et al. Wisconsin Stillbirth Service Program: I. Establishment and assessment of a community-based program for etiologic investigation of intrauterine deaths. Am J Med Genet 1994;50(2):116–34.

4. ACOG Committee Opinion. Committee on Genetics. Genetic evaluation of stillbirths and neonatal deaths. Obstet Gynecol, 2001;97(5 Pt 1):suppl 1–3.

5. Kalousek, D.K. and I. Barrett. Confined placental mosaicism and stillbirth. Pediatr Pathol, 1994;14(1):151–9.

6. Korteweg, F.J., K. Bouman, J.J. Erwich, et al. Cytogenetic analysis after evaluation of 750 fetal deaths: proposal for diagnostic workup. Obstet Gynecol 2008;111(4):865–74.

7. Pinar, H., M. Carpenter, B.J. Martin, et al. Utility of fetal karyotype in the evaluation of phenotypically abnormal stillbirths. Pediatr Dev Pathol 2009;12(3):217–21.

8. Wapner, R.J. and D. Lewis. Genetics and metabolic causes of stillbirth. Semin Perinatol 2002;26(1):70–4.

9. Tyson, R.W., Kalousek, D.K. Chromosomal abnormalities in stillbirth and neonatal death, in Developmental Pathology of the Embyro and Fetus, J.E. Dimmick, Kalousek, D.K. (eds), Editor. 1992, Lippincott: Philadelphia, PA. 83–110.

10. Won, R.H., R.J. Currier, F. Lorey, et al. The timing of demise in fetuses with trisomy 21 and trisomy 18. Prenat Diagn, 2005;25(7):608–11.

11. Hook, E.B. Chromosome abnormalities and spontaneous fetal death following amniocentesis: further data and associations with maternal age. Am J Hum Genet 1983;35(1):110–6.

12. Hook, E.B., B.B. Topol, and P.K. Cross. The natural history of cytogenetically abnormal fetuses detected at midtrimester amniocentesis which are not terminated electively: new data and estimates of the excess and relative risk of late fetal death associated with 47,+21 and some other abnormal karyotypes. Am J Hum Genet 1989;45(6):855–61.

13. Hook, E.B., D.E. Mutton, R. Ide, et al. The natural history of Down syndrome conceptuses diagnosed prenatally that are not electively terminated. Am J Hum Genet 1995;57(4):875–81.

14. Kalousek, D.K., I.J. Barrett, and B.C. McGillivray, Placental mosaicism and intrauterine survival of trisomies 13 and 18. Am J Hum Genet 1989; 44(3):338–43.

15. Christiaens, G.C., J. Vissers, P.J. Poddighe, et al. Comparative genomic hybridization for cytogenetic evaluation of stillbirth. Obstet Gynecol, 2000. 96(2): 281–6.

16. Raca, G., A. Artzer, L. Thorson, et al., Array-based comparative genomic hybridization (aCGH) in the genetic evaluation of stillbirth. Am J Med Genet A 2009;149A(11):2437–43.

17. Hahnemann, J.M. and L.O. Vejerslev, European collaborative research on mosaicism in CVS (EUCROMIC)–fetal and extrafetal cell lineages in 192 gestations with CVS mosaicism involving single autosomal trisomy. Am J Med Genet 1997;70(2):179–87.

18. Ledbetter, D.H., J.M. Zachary, J.L. Simpson, et al. Cytogenetic results from the U.S. Collaborative Study on CVS. Prenat Diagn, 1992;12(5):317–45.

19. Kalousek, D.K. and F.J. Dill, Chromosomal mosaicism confined to the placenta in human conceptions. Science, 1983;221(4611):665–7.

20. Johnson, A. and R.J. Wapner, Mosaicism: implications for postnatal outcome. Curr Opin Obstet Gynecol, 1997;9(2):p. 126-35.

21. Kalousek, D.K. and M. Vekemans. Confined placental mosaicism. J Med Genet 1996;33(7):529–33.

22. Benn, P., Trisomy 16 and trisomy 16 Mosaicism: a review. Am J Med Genet 1998;79(2):121–33.

23. Lestou, V.S. and D.K. Kalousek, Confined placental mosaicism and intrauterine fetal growth. Arch Dis Child Fetal Neonatal Ed, 1998;79(3):F223–6.

24. Kalousek, D.K. Pathogenesis of chromosomal mosaicism and its effect on early human development. Am J Med Genet 2000;91(1):39–45.

25. Kotzot, D. Abnormal phenotypes in uniparental disomy (UPD): fundamental aspects and a critical review with bibliography of UPD other than 15. Am J Med Genet 1999;82(3):265–74.

26. Kalousek, D.K., S. Langlois, W.P. Robinson, et al. Trisomy 7 CVS mosaicism: pregnancy outcome, placental and DNA analysis in 14 cases. Am J Med Genet 1996;65(4):348–2.

27. Wolstenholme, J., D.E. Rooney, and E.V. Davison. Confined placental mosaicism, IUGR, and adverse pregnancy outcome: a controlled retrospective U.K. collaborative survey. Prenat Diagn 1994;14(5): 345–61.

28. Kalousek, D.K., P.N. Howard-Peebles, S.B. Olson, et al. Confirmation of CVS mosaicism in term placentae and high frequency of intrauterine growth retardation

association with confined placental mosaicism. Prenat Diagn 1991;11(10):743–50.

29. Staretz-Chacham, O., T.C. Lang, M.E. LaMarca, et al. Lysosomal storage disorders in the newborn. Pediatrics, 2009;123(4):1191–207.

30. Mignot, C., D. Doummar, I. Maire, et al. Type 2 Gaucher disease: 15 new cases and review of the literature. Brain Dev, 2006;28(1):39–48.

31. Mignot, C., A. Gelot, B. Bessieres, et al. Perinatal-lethal Gaucher disease. Am J Med Genet A 2003; 120A(3):338–44.

32. Eblan, M.J., O. Goker-Alpan, and E. Sidransky. Perinatal lethal Gaucher disease: a distinct phenotype along the neuronopathic continuum. Fetal Pediatr Pathol 2005;24(4–5):205–22.

33. Finn, L.S., M. Zhang, S.H. Chen, et al. Severe type II Gaucher disease with ichthyosis, arthrogryposis and neuronal apoptosis: molecular and pathological analyses. Am J Med Genet 2000;91(3):222–6.

34. Strasberg, P.M., M.A. Skomorowski, I.B. Warren, et al. Homozygous presence of the crossover (fusion gene) mutation identified in a type II Gaucher disease fetus: is this analogous to the Gaucher knockout mouse model? Biochem Med Metab Biol 1994;53(1):16–21.

35. Sherer, D.M., L.A. Metlay, R.A. Sinkin, et al. Congenital ichthyosis with restrictive dermopathy and Gaucher disease: a new syndrome with associated prenatal diagnostic and pathology findings. Obstet Gynecol, 1993;81(5 (Pt 2)):842–4.

36. Sidransky, E., D.M. Sherer, and E.I. Ginns. Gaucher disease in the neonate: a distinct Gaucher phenotype is analogous to a mouse model created by targeted disruption of the glucocerebrosidase gene. Pediatr Res 1992;32(4):494–8.

37. Sun, C.C., S. Panny, J. Combs, et al. Hydrops fetalis associated with Gaucher disease. Pathol Res Pract 1984;179(1):101–4.

38. Ginsburg, S.J. and M. Groll, Hydrops fetalis due to infantile Gaucher's disease. J Pediatr, 1973; 82(6):1046–8.

39. Girgensohn, H., H. Kellner, and H. Sudhof. [Congenital Gaucher's disease in erythroblastosis and vascular sclerosis.]. Klin Wochenschr 1954; 32(3–4):57–64.

40. Sidransky, E., M. Fartasch, R.E. Lee, et al. Epidermal abnormalities may distinguish type 2 from type 1 and type 3 of Gaucher disease. Pediatr Res 1996; 39(1):134–41.

41. Sidransky, E., N. Tayebi, B.K. Stubblefield, et al. The clinical, molecular, and pathological characterisation of a family with two cases of lethal perinatal type 2 Gaucher disease. J Med Genet 1996;33(2):132–6.

42. Tayebi, N., S.R. Cushner, W. Kleijer, et al. Prenatal lethality of a homozygous null mutation in the human glucocerebrosidase gene. Am J Med Genet 1997;73(1):41–7.

43. Stone, D.L., N. Tayebi, E. Orvisky, et al. Glucocerebrosidase gene mutations in patients with type 2 Gaucher disease. Hum Mutat 2000;15(2):181–8.

44. Church, H.J., A. Cooper, F. Stewart, et al. Homozygous loss of a cysteine residue in the glucocerebrosidase gene results in Gaucher's disease with a hydropic phenotype. Eur J Hum Genet 2004;12(11):975–8.

45. Bhuiyan, Z.A., T.S. Momenah, Q. Gong, et al. Recurrent intrauterine fetal loss due to near absence of HERG: clinical and functional characterization of a homozygous nonsense HERG Q1070X mutation. Heart Rhythm 2008;5(4):553–61.

46. Schwartz, P.J., Stillbirths, sudden infant deaths, and long-QT syndrome: puzzle or mosaic, the pieces of the Jigsaw are being fitted together. Circulation 2004;109(24):2930–2.

47. Villard, L., A. Kpebe, C. Cardoso, et al. Two affected boys in a Rett syndrome family: clinical and molecular findings. Neurology 2000;55(8):1188–93.

48. Fyfe, S., H. Leonard, D. Dye, et al. Patterns of pregnancy loss, perinatal mortality, and postneonatal childhood deaths in families of girls with Rett syndrome. J Child Neurol 1999;14(7):440–5.

49. Warburton, D., L. Dallaire, M. Thangavelu, et al. Trisomy recurrence: a reconsideration based on North American data. Am J Hum Genet 2004;75(3):376–85.

50. Brady, K., P. Duff, F.E. Harlass, et al. Role of amniotic fluid cytogenetic analysis in the evaluation of recent fetal death. Am J Perinatol 1991;8(1):68–70.

51. Khare, M., E. Howarth, J. Sadler, et al. A comparison of prenatal versus postnatal karyotyping for the investigation of intrauterine fetal death after the first trimester of pregnancy. Prenat Diagn 2005;25(13):1192–5.

52. Neiger, R. and C.S. Croom. Cytogenetic study of amniotic fluid in the evaluation of fetal death. J Perinatol 1990;10(1):32–4.

53. Konstantinidou, A.E., H. Anninos, S. Dertinger, et al. Placental involvement in glycogen storage disease type IV. Placenta, 2008;29(4):378–81.

54. Schoen, E., C. Norem, J. O'Keefe, et al. Maternal serum unconjugated estriol as a predictor for Smith-Lemli-Opitz syndrome and other fetal conditions. Obstet Gynecol, 2003;102(1):167–72.

CHAPTER 7

Fetal Growth Restriction

Jason Gardosi, MD, FRCOG
West Midlands Perinatal Institute, Birmingham, UK

Unexplained stillbirths

Many causes and factors associated with stillbirth are known and have been detailed in other chapters. They include congenital anomalies (chromosomal and structural defects) (Chapters 6 and 11); maternal medical conditions such as hypertension and preeclampsia; diabetes and other endocrinological disorders; systemic lupus erythematosus, thrombophilias, cholestasis; transplacental and ascending infections, intrapartum-related deaths and multiple pregnancy-related conditions such as twin–twin transfusion syndrome (see Chapters 5, 8, 9 and 10).

However, according to the commonly used Wigglesworth pathophysiological classification and the Aberdeen "Obstetric" classifications applied in national reviews such as those by CESDI [1] (Chapter 3), the majority of stillbirth is designated as "unspecified" or "unexplained." Such a preponderance of cases being "unexplained" is a good prompt for further research, but not useful in everyday care, as often such terms are taken as being synonymous with "unavoidable." This has connotations for all parties concerned: the parents who are seeking explanations and are trying to come to terms with the loss; the clinicians who want to advise the mother on the implications and plans for management of future pregnancies; the health care institutions which need to review the service they are providing; and the health service planners and commissioners who wish to improve the service.

Fetal growth restriction: the hidden factor

Until recently, there has been little consideration of fetal growth restriction and its underlying causes as factors which can lead to stillbirth. This has been mostly due to the prevalent failure to recognize growth restriction both ante- and postnatally.

During *antenatal* care, audits have repeatedly shown that most cases of intrauterine growth restriction (IUGR) are not detected [2] and the detection rate is even lower in pregnancies considered low risk [3], probably because of a lower level of suspicion. Yet most stillbirths occur in pregnancies considered "low risk." There is furthermore a treatment paradox in operation: when IUGR *is* suspected and diagnosed antenatally, for example by ultrasound and Doppler, it is more likely that those most at risk are delivered iatrogenically, and stillbirth is avoided.

In *postnatal*, that is, retrospective assessment of birthweight, the lack of good birthweight standards may hinder the recognition of IUGR. For example, a standard for preterm deliveries, which is based on neonatal weights, hides the fact that many preterm live births are IUGR [4, 5] (Figure 7.1). Amongst stillbirths, the most severe IUGR cases occur in the preterm period [7].

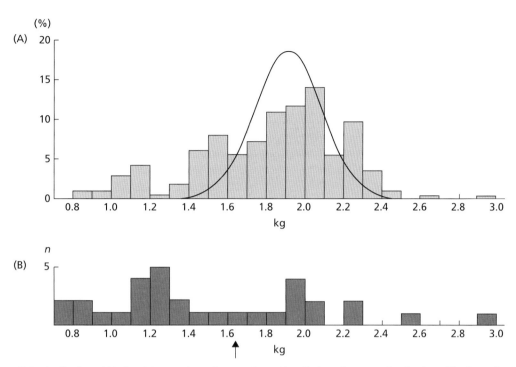

Figure 7.1 Distribution of birthweights at 32 weeks gestation. (A) Bell-shaped curve—distribution of fetal weights in pregnancies destined for normal-term delivery, and histogram of preterm birthweights showing negative skewness; (B) Stillbirths weights at 32 weeks, showing left shift. Most cases are below the 10th fetal weight centile (here 1,621 g, indicated by the arrow). (Reproduced from Ref. [6], with permission from Blackwell Publishing.)

Pathological examination and IUGR

A histopathological assessment can provide definitive means to diagnose pathological processes such as growth failure. However, postmortem rates vary substantially between countries and over time. Pathological examination is often either not available as a service, especially in developing countries where most stillbirths occur; or it is not affordable, in countries where it is available but not provided as a free service. In some communities, postmortems are not accepted on cultural or religious grounds.

A cursory examination will easily miss the presence of IUGR. A full postmortem by trained perinatal pathologists will include fetal organs and weight ratios, such as that between brain and liver. Failing that, there should at least be an assessment of whether the weight of the stillborn baby was adequate or small for gestational age (SGA).

However, until not long ago, pathologists used weight standards that were based on *other* stillbirths [8]. For organ weights, this is unavoidable, but unless birthweight standards are based on normal-term deliveries, they will mask the fact that many stillbirths are significantly smaller than their live-born counterparts [6].

Placental examination is also often not undertaken, but increasingly recognized as an essential component of the postmortem (see also Chapter 10). Recent work has highlighted the frequent presence of placental pathology associated with IUGR [9]. Two main distinctive patterns have been described—placental bed pathology which is associated with stillbirths in the early preterm period, mostly between 24 and 32 weeks; and "developmental" placental pathology manifesting as placental hypoplasia which occurs more frequently after 32 weeks. Placental villus immaturity was also observed, occurring typically later in the third trimester.

Assessing stillbirth by the fetal growth potential

While a fetal weight-based standard can give an overall indication of the preponderance of still-births with a low weight-for-gestation, it cannot define which babies were smaller than the weight which they individually should have achieved. A full appreciation of the link between stillbirth and IUGR is made possible with the development of the concept of the growth potential, where the weight actually achieved is measured against an optimum predicted for a normal pregnancy. The standard excludes pathological factors such as smoking, hypertension, and preterm birth, and is adjusted for maternal characteristics including height, weight, parity, and ethnic origin as well as sex and gestational age [10]. Receiver operator curves found the 10th customized centile to be an appropriate cutoff for predicting perinatal morbidity [11]. A customized

standard based on fetal growth potential has been found to be a better predictor of adverse outcome in databases from the United Kingdom, France, Sweden, Australia, New Zealand, and the United States [7, 12, 13]. Importantly, the new individual standard identifies additional cases at risk which are not identified by the population standard, while reclassifying as normal those cases which are only constitutionally small (Figure 7.2).

For the assessment of weight-for-gestational age centiles in the study of databases with stillbirths, the appropriate gestational age at fetal death needs to be estimated. Although the clinical scenario of an intrauterine death occurring with spontaneous onset of labor delayed by days or even weeks is well known, it is relatively rare. Most pregnancies with stillbirth deliver within 48h, either after spontaneous onset of labor or iatrogenically, after the mother presents with no fetal movements. This is supported by histopathological studies [14],

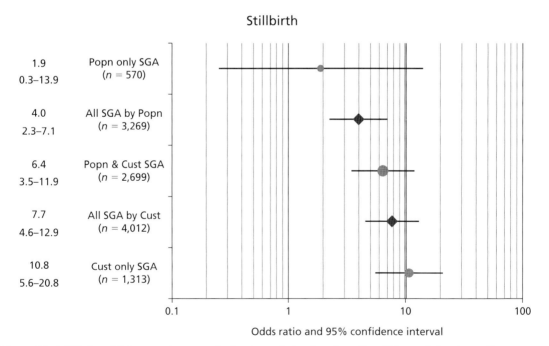

Figure 7.2 Stillbirth and SGA status by customized and population-based centiles. SGA was defined according to population-based centiles (All SGA by Popn) and SGA by customized centiles (All SGA by Cust) (diamond markers). Subgroups are shown that are SGA by both methods (Popn & Cust SGA), by the population method only (Popn only SGA), or by the customized method only (Cust only SGA) (round markers). Odds ratios and 95% confidence intervals are shown. (Reproduced from Ref. [7], with permission from Mosby.)

which show that the average third-trimester delay between intrauterine demise and delivery is 48 h, with an estimated 85% of cases delivering within 72 h. Therefore, in practice, 2 days are deducted from gestational age at delivery in the study of weight-for-gestation of stillbirths, and <10th customized centile is used to denote "IUGR" [6].

It is sometimes claimed that the fetus loses weight after death in utero, but there is little evidence for this, and no ready pathological explanation how this would come about. To the contrary, the weight recorded for a stillborn baby at delivery may be artificially high due to third space fluid. Often, such fluid can be observed on the sheets at the time of the postmortem a day or two later. Postmortem weights were found on average to be 28 g less than the weight recorded at delivery, regardless of the degree of maceration [6].

Prevalence of IUGR amongst stillbirths

The concept of growth potential allows examination of the prevalence of IUGR in stillbirths, and include IUGR as its own category when classifying stillbirths.

Conventional stillbirth classification systems, such as Wigglesworth and Obstetric/Aberdeen, have consistently reported most cases to be "unexplained" [1]. Many systems claim to establish "causes" but in fact describe conditions which relate to the demise. For example, diabetes and multiple pregnancy are not in themselves a cause for stillbirth, and most pregnancies with these conditions have a normal outcome. However, they are known to represent increased risk. Similarly, IUGR is not a cause, but usually the clinical manifestation of underlying placental dysfunction.

In a study of 2,625 consecutive stillbirths from 24 weeks gestation recorded on the West Midlands perinatal mortality register, IUGR was the single largest category or "relevant clinical condition," accounting for over 40% of deaths [15]. After excluding congenital anomalies, over half of all normally formed stillbirths were below the 10th centile of each individual fetuses own growth potential.

In an additional, unknown number of fetuses, the growth has slowed substantially before demise but the birthweight was still within normal limits. As a result of the inclusion of IUGR as a category, the proportion of "unexplained" or "unclassified" deaths dropped to 16% [15].

Such reductions in the proportion of unexplained stillbirths through the use of customized centiles to define IUGR have been confirmed in other studies [16, 17]. In one Norwegian cohort of stillbirths, which were considered "unexplained" even after undergoing comprehensive investigations including postmortems, over half of cases were found to have had fetal growth restriction [17].

IUGR in epidemiological research

The ability to define IUGR retrospectively on the basis of the individual growth potential provides a useful tool for further research, which in turn can point to clinical strategies aiming to reduce adverse outcome.

This is illustrated by the recent progress in understanding the well-known association between maternal obesity and perinatal mortality. Until recently, fetal growth was not considered a potential cause, and obesity was in fact claimed to be a protective factor for SGA [18]. But such a finding is in fact an artifact caused by the use of nonspecific population standards for birthweight, which fail to recognize that large mothers should expect to have larger babies, and an average birthweight in the pregnancy of a high body mass index (BMI) mother may in fact be relatively small and indicate the presence of IUGR.

Application of the concept of fetal growth potential is able to identify firstly that high BMI mothers have an increased risk of IUGR, and secondly that this BMI-associated risk mirrors the increased risk of perinatal mortality in a dose-dependent relationship [19], as illustrated in Figure 7.3. Combined with emerging findings that the detection of IUGR is substantially poorer in obese mothers, this points to the need of increased surveillance of fetal growth in these pregnancies by serial ultrasound biometry.

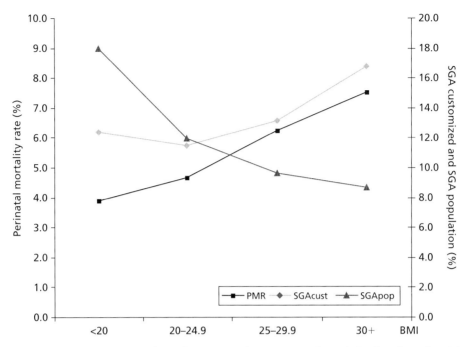

Figure 7.3 Perinatal mortality rate (PMR) and SGA by customized (SGAcust) and population-based centiles (SGApop), according to maternal BMI. Comparison test for difference of slopes: PMR versus SGAcust: $p = 0.753$; PMR versus SGApop: $p = 0.007$. (Reproduced from Ref. [19], with permission from Blackwell Publishing Ltd.)

IUGR and clinical strategies for stillbirth prevention

Good antenatal care requires awareness of the contribution of medical and social risk to pregnancy outcome and implementation of the appropriate protocols for maternity care. IUGR risk is associated with poor obstetric history, smoking, drug abuse, social deprivation, high maternal age, diabetes, and pregnancy complications such as antepartum hemorrhage, hypertension, lupus and antiphospholipid syndromes, thrombophilias, and multiple pregnancy. A detailed discussion of all risk factors and their interactions is beyond the scope of this chapter, but any factor that increases the risk of IUGR requires more intensive surveillance of fetal growth during pregnancy.

There is currently no direct evidence that antenatal detection of IUGR prevents stillbirth, and it would require considerably large multicenter trials to demonstrate a significant effect on such a relatively rare outcome. However, circumstantial evidence is fairly strong. Detection of SGA improves outcome [20] and systematic reviews [21] show that appropriate identification and further evaluation including umbilical artery Doppler studies reduce stillbirths. Interestingly, while detection increases iatrogenic prematurity, such intervention does not appear to result in increased neonatal morbidity and mortality [21], suggesting that babies are delivered in better condition as a result. This often requires a fine balance between the risks of prematurity and intrauterine demise to determine the optimal time for delivery.

While appropriate investigation and management of high-risk pregnancy is an essential element of maternity care, most pregnancies are low risk, and most stillbirths occur in low-risk pregnancies. Further research is needed to identify and predict risk when it develops in "low-risk" pregnancy.

The placental changes that lead to preeclampsia, growth failure, and related complications are often unpredicted. They occur early in pregnancy, and serum markers such as pregnancy associated plasma protein A, alfpa fetoprotein and estriol are being investigated as potentially useful indicators. Similarly, second-trimester assessment of Doppler, looking for notching of the uterine arteries, has been proposed as markers of pregnancies at increased risk of subsequent preeclampsia and growth restriction. It is likely that a combination of serum markers and ultrasound/Doppler will identify pregnancies that require increased surveillance.

Until such evidence emerges, it is essential that all pregnancies receive an appropriate standard of surveillance of fetal well-being in the form of serial assessment of growth. In high-risk pregnancies, this consists of serial biometry at regular, 2–3 weekly intervals throughout the third trimester. In pregnancies without known risk factors, serial scans have not been shown to result in increased detection of IUGR, and are hardly affordable. In these cases, serial assessment by regular fundal height measurement and plotting on customized growth charts are recommended [22], and have been shown to significantly improve detection [23].

Clinical practice points

- Many stillbirths currently categorized as "unexplained" have evidence of fetal growth restriction.
- Postnatal and postmortem diagnosis of IUGR requires as standard which is based on fetal growth potential.
- Antenatal detection, investigation, and management of fetal growth restriction can lead to stillbirth prevention.

References

1. Gardosi J. Clinical implications of "unexplained" stillbirths (Commentary). Maternal and Child Health Consortium. CESDI 8th Annual Report: Confidential Enquiry of Stillbirths and Deaths in Infancy, London, 2001:40–7.

2. Hepburn M, Rosenberg K. An audit of the detection and management of small-for-gestational age babies. Br J Obstet Gynaecol 1986;93:212–16.

3. Kean LH, Liu DT. Antenatal care as a screening tool for the detection of small for gestational age babies in the low risk population. J Obstet Gynaecol 1996;16:77–82.

4. Tamura RK, Sabbagha RE, Depp R, et al. Diminished growth in fetuses born preterm after spontaneous labor or rupture of membranes. Am J Obstet Gynecol 1984;148:1105–10.

5. Gardosi JO. Prematurity and fetal growth restriction. Early Hum Dev 2005;81:43–9.

6. Gardosi J, Mul T, Mongelli M, Fagan D. Analysis of birthweight and gestational age in antepartum stillbirths. BJOG 1998;105:524–30.

7. Gardosi J, Francis A. Adverse pregnancy outcome and association with smallness for gestational age by customised and population based birthweight percentiles. Am J Obstet Gynecol 2009;201(28):e1–8.

8. Singer DB, Sung CJ, Wigglesworth JS. Fetal growth and maturation: with standards for body and organ development. In: Wigglesworth JS, Singer DB (eds), Textbook of fetal and perinatal pathology. Oxford: Blackwell Science; 1991, pp. 11–47.

9. Korteweg FJ, Erwich JJ, Holm JP, et al. Diverse placental pathologies as the main causes of fetal death. Obstet Gynecol 2009;114(4):809–17.

10. Gardosi J, Mongelli M, Wilcox M, et al. An adjustable fetal weight standard. Ultrasound Obstet Gynecol 1995;6:168–74.

11. De Jong CL, Francis A, Van Geijn HP, et al. Customized fetal weight limits for antenatal detection of fetal growth restriction. Ultrasound Obstet Gynecol 2000;15:36–40.

12. Clausson B, Gardosi J, Francis A, et al. Perinatal outcome in SGA births defined by customised versus population-based birthweight standards. BJOG 2001;108:830–4.

13. McCowan L, Harding JE, Stewart AW. Customised birthweight centiles predict SGA pregnancies with perinatal morbidity. BJOG 2005;112:1026–33.

14. Genest DR, Williams MA, Greene MF. Estimating the time of death in stillborn fetuses: I. Histologic evaluation of fetal organs; an autopsy study of 150 stillborns. Obstet Gynecol 1992;80(4):575–84.

15. Gardosi J, Kady SM, McGeown P, et al. Classification of stillbirth by relevant condition at death (ReCoDe): population based cohort study. BMJ 2005;331:1113–17.

16. Vergani P, Cozzolino S, Pozzi E, et al. Identifying the causes of stillbirth: a comparison of four classification systems. Am J Obstet Gynecol 2008;199(3):319e1–4.

17. Froen JF, Gardosi J, Thurmann A, et al. Restricted fetal growth in sudden intrauterine unexplained death. Acta Obstet Gynecol Scand 2004;83:81–7.

18. Cnattingius S, Bergstrom R, Lipworth L, et al. Prepregnancy weight and the risk of adverse pregnancy outcomes. N Engl J Med 1998;338:147–52.

19. Gardosi J, Clausson B, Francis A. The value of customised centiles in assessing perinatal mortality risk associated with parity and maternal size. BJOG 2009;116:1356–63.

20. Lindqvist PG, Molin J. Does antenatal identification of small-for-gestational age fetuses significantly improve their outcome? Ultrasound Obstet Gynecol 2005;25(3):258–64.

21. Alfirevic Z, Neilson JP. Doppler ultrasonography in high-risk pregnancies: systematic review with meta-analysis. Am J Obstet Gynecol 1995;172(5):1379–87.

22. Royal College of Obstetrics and Gynaecology Green-Top Guidelines. The investigation and management of the small-for-gestational-age fetus. London, England: Royal College of Obstetrics and Gynaecology; 2002.

23. Morse K, Williams A, Gardosi J. Fetal growth screening by fundal height measurement. Best Pract Res Clin Obstet Gynaecol 2009;23(6):809–18.

CHAPTER 8
Maternal Medical Conditions

Deborah L. Conway, MD

Department of Obstetrics and Gynecology, Division of Maternal–Fetal Medicine, University of Texas School of Medicine at San Antonio, San Antonio, TX, USA

The risk of stillbirth is increased among pregnant women with certain medical disorders compared to women without comorbid conditions [1]. The reasons for this increased risk vary according to underlying condition. Disease processes in the mother impact fetal well-being via many avenues, including compromised placental circulation, inadequate oxygenation or removal of waste products, inflammatory processes, and congenital anomalies (see also Chapter 11). For many conditions, we have a fairly clear understanding of the pathophysiologic derangements that lead to fetal demise. For other conditions, the clinical link between disease and stillbirth is well established, but the causative mechanism is poorly understood. In such instances, prediction and prevention of fetal loss are particularly challenging.

In order to prevent the devastating outcome of stillbirth in women at risk by virtue of their medical comorbidities, it is imperative that obstetric care providers are armed with knowledge and skill regarding:
- which maternal medical conditions carry an increased risk for fetal loss;
- the magnitude of that risk, and factors that mitigate or heighten that risk, including preconception factors;
- the mechanism or pathway that leads to stillbirth in a given condition;
- critical periods during gestation when risk is the highest;

- ways to identify a compromised fetus;
- prudent interventions to optimize outcomes.

In this chapter, we will discuss several maternal diseases and conditions that are associated with an increased stillbirth risk, following the template in this list for each disease entity or condition. It must be noted that, in many cases, the epidemiologic link between a condition and fetal loss is strong, but the causative pathway is unclear. In such circumstances, recommendations for clinical care, including fetal surveillance and timing of delivery, may be extrapolated from similar conditions where more evidence exists.

Type 1 and type 2 diabetes mellitus

Stillbirth rate

The perinatal loss rate in pregnancies complicated by type 1 and type 2 diabetes mellitus (DM) has been steadily declining over the last century. Before the advent of therapeutic insulin, pregnancy in women with type 1 DM resulted in a maternal mortality rate of 30% and a perinatal mortality rate (PMR) of 65% [2]. Once insulin administration became the norm, this rate was reduced dramatically, in part, due to improved maternal survival. Further reductions in perinatal loss resulted from improved attention to lowering maternal glucose levels, incorporation of fetal surveillance tests into the therapeutic regimen, and advances in neonatal care.

Despite these advances, however, the modern-day stillbirth rate in women with preexisting DM remains elevated above that of the nondiabetic population. Most modern series that compare stillbirth rates between diabetic women and normal controls report a two- to six-fold increased risk [2]. For example, a population-based study from the United Kingdom used 2002 data from the Confidential Enquiry into Maternal and Child Health to report a stillbirth rate of 26.8/1,000 in women with preexisting DM, compared to 5.7/1,000 in the general population, with a relative risk of 4.7 (95% CI 3.7–6.0) [3].

Although type 1 DM is assumed by many to be the greater risk, several recent reports suggest that type 2 DM carries at least as high, if not higher, a chance for stillbirth as type 1 DM [3–5]. Several explanations for this are possible. First, both types of DM have some components of pathophysiology and metabolic derangement in common, and thus might be expected to result in similar outcomes for the fetus. In addition, women with type 2 DM are more likely than those with type 1 DM to be socioeconomically disadvantaged and/or obese, two additional risk factors for fetal death [3, 5]. Type 1 DM is more likely to result in congenital anomaly than type 2 DM [3, 5], while type 2 DM is more likely to result in stillbirth later in gestation [5]. A systematic review and meta-analysis found no significant difference in stillbirth rate or neonatal death between type 1 and type 2 DM, although when the two were combined to calculate the PMR, women with type 2 DM were at significantly higher risk (OR 1.50, 95% CI 1.15–1.96) [6].

Mechanism of fetal death

Preexisting maternal diabetes threatens the well-being of the fetus by multiple mechanisms. First, an increased risk of congenital anomalies contributes to the fetal death rate. Second, fetal mortality is high during episodes of diabetic ketoacidosis (DKA). This is, in part, due to the risk of maternal death, which had historically been as high as 5–15%. More modern series put the maternal mortality rate in DKA at approximately 1%, which is substantially higher

than the background rate [7]. With maternal survival, the risk of fetal death remains high because of the severe metabolic derangements involved. Acidemia, hyperglycemia, severe dehydration, and profound electrolyte disturbances are the hallmarks of the maternal disease, and they combine to place the fetus at risk (Figure 8.1). Stillbirth rate in relation to an episode of DKA (occurring either during the acute episode or within a short time afterward) has been reported to be as high as 35%, though the authors of this series note that no fetal deaths occurred once maternal treatment was underway [8]. Another series reported a fetal loss in one patient out of a series of 11 diagnosed with DKA, occurring in a mother with severe acidemia at 27 weeks gestation [9].

Once anomalous fetuses and DKA-related fetal deaths are removed from the total stillbirths in diabetic women, a substantial portion remain "unexplained." However, many are thought to be due to a metabolic cascade that begins with maternal hyperglycemia and ends with fetal metabolic acidosis and death. The link between maternal hyperglycemia and fetal acidosis appears to be fetal hyperinsulinemia, produced in response to the increased glucose load crossing from mother to fetus. Insulin drives growth in the fetus, and this anabolic state may outstrip the capability of the placenta to supply sufficient oxygen for aerobic metabolic processes. In animal models, the integrated effects of chronic hyperglycemia, hyperinsulinemia, and fetal oxygen consumption have been demonstrated, supporting this theoretical mechanism of fetal death in humans [10, 11].

It must be noted that excessive, disproportionate fetal growth due to fetal hyperinsulinemia may result in intrapartum stillbirth as a result of obstructed labor, or severe, unresolved shoulder dystocia in isolated cases. The contribution of such cases to the overall burden of stillbirth among diabetic gravidas is small in developed countries.

Finally, when a stillbirth occurs, it is crucial that the simple presence of maternal diabetes is not uniformly assumed to be the direct cause of fetal death, to the exclusion of considering other causative or contributing factors. There are certainly extreme circumstances, such as fetal death in the

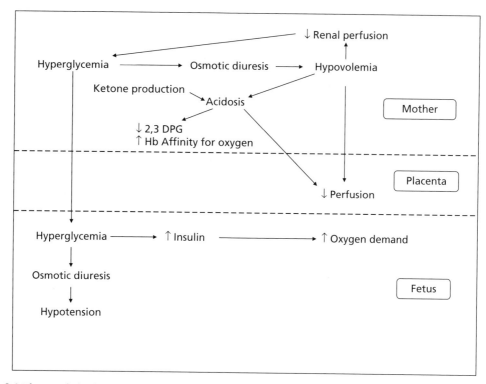

Figure 8.1 The metabolic derangements in DKA and their contribution to risk of fetal death.

course of an episode of maternal DKA, when it is clear that the fetus would be alive but for the presence of diabetes. As a general rule, however, all women with DM who suffer a stillbirth should be offered a full work-up, including laboratory tests, placental and fetal pathology, and a detailed assessment of other sociodemographic and medical risk factors [12, 13].

Risk factors

In addition to the direct impact of the metabolic derangements of diabetes on fetal health, women with diabetes often have additional risk factors for stillbirth [14]. These include hypertensive disease, obesity, Black race, prior cesarean delivery, poverty/health-related disparities, and advanced maternal age (see also Chapter 4). Evidence for diabetes-related end-organ damage, such as retinopathy or nephropathy, also increases the stillbirth risk (50/1,000 in a recent report on diabetic nephropathy [15]). Current theories to explain the added

risk of fetal death with vasculopathy include dysfunctional or abnormal placental vasculature, and excessive oxidative stress associated with advanced disease [16] (See also Chapters 9 and 10).

Identifying the compromised fetus and management options to reduce risk

Strategies for reducing fetal death in pregnancies complicated by diabetes should target the underlying mechanism for stillbirth whenever possible. For this reason, intervention is best initiated prior to pregnancy, with attention to glucose control and folic acid supplementation to reduce the rate of major fetal anomalies. Multidimensional, multidisciplinary programs that were developed to achieve optimal preconception preparation in women with type 1 DM report successful reduction in not only fetal anomalies, but also fetal death [17]. Routing women to appropriate providers of preconception counseling and care can be a significant challenge, however. In one successful program [17], glycemic targets in the preconception and early pregnancy periods were: premeal <100 mg/dl and 90-min postmeal <140 mg/dl. Using hemoglobin A1C values as a proxy for frequent self-monitored blood glucose levels, a target of 6.3% or lower results in rates of anomalies similar to a nondiabetic population [18]. Once pregnancy is achieved, continued scrupulous attention to glucose levels is warranted. Attempts to normalize blood glucose levels should be made, getting as close to nondiabetic values as possible, balanced with the goal of avoiding hypoglycemia. No specific insulin regimen or route of insulin delivery (intermittent injections vs. subcutaneous continuous infusion by pump) has been shown to have an impact on stillbirth rate.

Pregnancies complicated by preexisting diabetes warrant fetal surveillance beginning in the third trimester. The proposed mechanism of fetal death at this point in gestation is accelerated fetal metabolism and resultant fetal hypoxia, as described earlier. This is typically thought to be a chronic process, and thus is amenable to weekly or twice weekly routine tests of fetal well-being, such as the nonstress test (NST) or the biophysical profile (BPP). No single surveillance regimen has been sufficiently tested in a prospective manner to prove its superiority over other regimens to identify the compromised fetus with high sensitivity and specificity, much less lead to fewer stillbirths. The key, then, appears to be applying a modality that an individual provider can interpret accurately, and ensuring patient compliance with the testing regimen.

The ideal timing of initiation of a fetal surveillance regimen also has not been identified, and likely varies with the presence of other comorbid conditions that increase stillbirth risk (Table 8.1). In women with preexisting DM and one or more of the conditions noted in Table 8.1, consideration should be given to start the testing regimen at 28–30 weeks gestation. In women without additional risk factors, surveillance should begin by 32–34 weeks gestation.

Delivery of the fetus can certainly be considered among the strategies used to prevent stillbirth. It is impossible to predict with certainty which

Table 8.1 Comorbid conditions that increase stillbirth risk in diabetes.

Fetal growth restriction
Hypertensive disorders
Evidence of fetal hyperinsulinemia, excessive growth
Other vascular complications, e.g., nephropathy
Poor patient cooperation with care regimen
Stillbirth in prior pregnancy

pregnancies will benefit from such intervention, and which can safely be managed expectantly until 39–40 weeks gestation without delivery [19]. Once again, knowledge of the risk factors for stillbirth in this setting is essential, followed by a careful search for these factors in each patient as term approaches. Absent frank evidence for fetal hypoxia or a condition mandating delivery (e.g., severe preeclampsia), it is rare that a patient would warrant delivery prior to 37 weeks gestation. In the setting of an episode of DKA, intervention on fetal behalf due to abnormal tests of fetal well-being must be carefully weighed against the mother's ability at that point in time to withstand the insult of cesarean delivery.

Gestational diabetes mellitus

The current definition of gestational diabetes mellitus (GDM) refers to carbohydrate intolerance with onset or first recognition during pregnancy [20]. By virtue of this definition, some proportion of women labeled "GDM" actually enter pregnancy with undiagnosed preexisting DM (almost always type 2 DM and rarely type 1 DM). Indeed, approximately 8% of women met criteria for DM shortly after delivery in one series of socioeconomically disadvantaged Mexican-American women [21]. This is important to consider when assessing the impact of GDM on stillbirth risk, both within the literature and for individual patient management.

Studies exist to support the concept that efforts to identify and treat GDM can reduce perinatal mortality [22, 23]. In Australia, as thresholds for diagnosis of GDM were lowered and monitoring and treatment were intensified over time, corresponding

Table 8.2 Stillbirth rates in studies of mild gestational diabetes.

Reference	Study type	Sample size	SB rate
Casey et al. (1997) [24]	Retrospective cohort	874 GDM (FPG < 105 mg/dl)	5/1,000
		61,209 normal glucose testing	4/1,000
HAPO Study (2008) [25]	Prospective cohort; blinded 2-h, 75 g OGTT	25,505 (FPG ≤ 105 mg/dl and 2-h glucose ≤ 200 mg/dl)	5.6/1,000*
MFMU GDM Trial (2009) [26]	RCT of treatment versus no treatment of GDM when FPG on OGTT is <95 mg/dl	485 unblinded, treated as GDM	0/1,000
		473 blinded, untreated	0/1,000

GDM, gestational diabetes mellitus; FPG, fasting plasma glucose; HAPO, Hyperglycemia and Adverse Pregnancy Outcome; OGTT, oral glucose tolerance test; MFMU, Maternal–Fetal Medicine Units Network; RCT, randomized clinical trial.

*Perinatal mortality rate; the rate of stillbirth alone was not reported.

decreases in perinatal mortality and stillbirths were noted [22]. In a more recent randomized clinical trial (RCT) [23], women were randomized to treatment or no treatment of GDM following a 75 g, 2-h oral glucose tolerance test (OGTT). Women who were randomized to "no treatment" were informed that they did not have GDM, in accordance with predetermined study plans. While the "treated GDM" group of 490 women experienced no fetal or neonatal losses, the untreated group of 512 women contained five perinatal deaths, including three stillbirths. This difference approached statistical significance ($p = 0.07$) in this relatively small group, in a study not powered to detect a difference in PMR as an isolated outcome. It is important to note, however, that OGTT thresholds for eligibility for this RCT included fasting plasma glucose (FPG) values up to 140 mg/dl and 2-h values up to 198 mg/dl, making the inclusion of some women with undiagnosed type 2 DM a possibility.

It is difficult, on the other hand, to implicate mild forms of GDM as a cause for stillbirth. Studies that limit their population to women with OGTT results well below established cutoffs for frank DM report PMR and stillbirth rates comparable to normal pregnancies, with or without treatment [24–26] (Table 8.2). The presence of mild GDM [24, 26] or increasing degrees of glycemia [25]

result in increased rates of large-for-gestational age (LGA) and macrosomic infants, as well as increased adiposity in the neonate [27]. This indicates the presence of fetal hyperinsulinemia in utero. Despite this, there is little indication that risk of fetal death is increased over nondiabetic pregnancies. This is demonstrated best in the Hyperglycemia and Adverse Pregnancy Outcomes study [25], where all OGTT results were blinded and the low PMR cannot be attributed to heightened fetal surveillance or intervention by delivery.

Thus, clinical management strategies to avoid stillbirth in pregnancies with GDM can be targeted to women with OGTT values or self-monitored blood glucose readings indicative of frank DM or prediabetes, or when there is substantial evidence for diabetic fetopathy (Table 8.3). Fetal surveillance algorithms and timing of delivery in such women can mimic recommendations for preexisting DM, as described earlier. By the same token, women with GDM who do not have fasting hyperglycemia, who are well controlled (not just treated) on diet alone, who have no other comorbidities that add to risk of stillbirth, and who show no evidence of abnormal fetal growth likely do not benefit from enhanced fetal surveillance because it is unlikely that they carry a higher risk of stillbirth than the general population.

Table 8.3 Clinical criteria suggesting increased risk for stillbirth in women with GDM.

FPG on OGTT > 105 mg/dl
Need for medication to achieve glycemic targets
Comorbid conditions that increase stillbirth risk
(e.g., hypertension)
Evidence for diabetic fetopathy—EFW > 90th percentile for gestational age and any of the following:
Hydramnios
Sonographic evidence of disproportionate fetal growth/ adiposity, e.g.:
Low HC/AC ratio
Humeral soft tissue thickness > 12 mm
Fetal growth restriction

GDM, gestational diabetes mellitus; FPG, fasting plasma glucose; OGTT, oral glucose tolerance test; EFW, estimated fetal weight; HC/AC, head circumference/abdominal circumference.

Chronic hypertension and hypertensive disorders of pregnancy

Stillbirth rate by type of hypertension

The risk of fetal death is increased when hypertension complicates pregnancy. The magnitude of the risk varies with the nature and severity of the hypertensive disorder, as well as the presence of additional risk factors, such as diabetes, or warning signs of fetal compromise, such as growth restriction. In a population-based study [28] with a stillbirth rate of 4/1,000 among normotensive women, women with hypertension had a stillbirth rate of 5.2/1,000, a significant increase in risk (RR 1.4, 95% CI 1.1–1.8). With nearly 14,000 hypertensive women in this cohort, distinctions could be drawn between various hypertensive disorders in terms of their stillbirth risk. Thus, the highest risk of stillbirth occurred in women with pregnancy-induced hypertension (PIH) superimposed on preexisting chronic hypertension (stillbirth rate 17/1,000, RR 4.4, 95% CI 2.2–8.8), and risk was significantly increased in all women with preexisting chronic hypertension. Conversely, no significant increase in risk was detected in women with gestational-onset hypertension, including HELLP syndrome (hemolysis, elevated liver enzymes, low platelets). There were 32 women with eclampsia, and no stillbirths were

encountered in this group. However, given the small number in this subset and the severity of this clinical entity, it would be unwise to assume absence of fetal risk in the setting of eclampsia.

Data from the Calcium for Preeclampsia Prevention Trial also suggest that gestational-onset hypertensive disorders (preeclampsia, pregnancy-associated/gestational hypertension) do not increase the risk of fetal death [29]. In fact, women with mild hypertensive disease had a significantly lower risk of stillbirth than the normotensive population in this study, possibly due to the enhanced fetal and maternal surveillance that accompanied the diagnosis of hypertension.

Nonetheless, when dealing with a patient with apparent gestational-onset hypertension, it is incumbent upon obstetric care providers to obtain a careful, thorough history, backed up and corroborated by medical records whenever possible in order to answer the following question: how sure are you that the hypertension is truly "gestational onset"? Like preexisting DM that is recognized only as gestational diabetes, stillbirth risk is increased for women with undiagnosed chronic hypertension. The fetus and placenta are affected by the pathophysiology of the underlying disease, whether or not its presence is conveyed by the mother, or discerned by the care provider.

Mechanism of fetal death

Like preexisting DM, hypertension in pregnancy threatens fetal well-being in a number of ways. In a small subset of cases, the mother may be in a critically ill state, such as eclampsia, hypertensive crisis, or congestive heart failure, and uteroplacental blood flow is acutely and critically diminished. Far more common is a chronic picture of uteroplacental vasoconstriction. Diminished intervillous blood flow leads to fetal hypoxia, which in turn can result in fetal growth restriction and oligohydramnios. In such cases, fetal death can result from chronic hypoxia and acidosis, or from acute anoxia due to umbilical cord compression when amniotic fluid volume is low [30].

Identifying the compromised fetus and management options to reduce risk

Interventions aimed at preventing the occurrence of PIH/preeclampsia, or at mitigating its severity, might also hold promise in reducing the increased rate of stillbirth associated with the disease. While a Cochrane review of calcium supplementation to prevent hypertensive disorders in pregnancy found a reduced risk of hypertension, preeclampsia, maternal death, and serious morbidity in women who received calcium compared to those receiving placebo, no impact on stillbirth rate was seen (RR = 0.90, 95% CI 0.74–1.09) [31]. Individual trials and meta-analyses of antioxidant treatment (vitamins C and E) suggest no benefit in well-nourished study populations in preventing PIH/preeclampsia, or stillbirth associated with the disease [32, 33]. Conversely, low-dose antiplatelet agents, such as aspirin or dipyridamole, not only reduced the risk of PIH (particularly in women at high-risk for the disease), but resulted in significantly lower combined fetal, neonatal, and infant death when compared to no treatment or placebo (RR 0.86, 95% CI 0.76–0.98) [34]. However, this meta-analysis could not detect differences between antiplatelet treatment and no treatment/placebo in any single category of baby death, suggesting that the effects on stillbirth alone are very small or nonexistent. In women with a diagnosis of PIH/preeclampsia, we lack sufficient data to conclude whether limiting physical activity (at home or in hospital) affects the fetal loss rate. Small trials that have included this outcome have shown no benefit, however [35].

In women with chronic hypertension, a Cochrane review of randomized trials of antihypertensive medication versus placebo showed no impact on death of the baby (RR = 0.73, 95% CI 0.50–1.08); the only subgroup in which the impact appeared to reach significance was for reduction of early miscarriage [36]. The same review also examined comparative trials of various antihypertensive medications, and no drug was superior to another in rates of fetal or neonatal loss.

Fetal surveillance in women with preexisting or pregnancy-associated hypertension should consist of serial ultrasound studies to monitor fetal growth. If growth restriction is suspected, serial amniotic fluid measurements and possibly Doppler studies can be added. The utility of antepartum fetal heart rate testing in all patients with chronic hypertension is controversial [30]. The American College of Obstetricians and Gynecologists, following the National High Blood Pressure Working Group on High Blood Pressure in Pregnancy recommendations, states that fetal surveillance is not indicated in pregnancies in which fetal growth restriction and superimposed preeclampsia have been ruled out [37].

Obesity

As the worldwide obesity epidemic has taken root, data have been emerging over the past decade that maternal obesity is an independent risk factor for stillbirth. In a bellwether report from Sweden in 1998 [38], the odds ratio for late-pregnancy stillbirth rose with increasing prepregnancy body mass index (BMI), reaching an adjusted OR of 2.7 (95% CI 1.8–4.1) for women with prepregnancy BMI ≥ 30. Numerous similar reports followed examining various populations, and a meta-analysis of nine studies was published in 2007 [39]. The nine studies selected for inclusion were ones that had good data on maternal prepregnancy or early pregnancy weight, included a comparison group of normal-weight women, reported stillbirths separate from neonatal deaths, and reported all stillbirths (not just a subset, e.g., unexplained stillbirths). Stillbirth risk was significantly increased in overweight (OR 1.47, 95% CI 1.08–1.94) and obese women (OR 2.07, 95% CI 1.59–2.74). Thus, there is a dose-dependent impact of maternal BMI on stillbirth risk, independent of other risk factors, such as diabetes and hypertension.

Among obese women, additional risk factors have been identified that heighten the stillbirth risk still further. In a study using Missouri state birth data [40], Black race conferred an approximately 50% increased risk for stillbirth compared to White race among obese women, who overall had a higher stillbirth rate than normal-weight women, similar to other studies. Advancing gestational age, particularly after 40 weeks, also appears to add to stillbirth risk in obese women more so than in normal-weight women. In the Danish National Birth Cohort between 1998 and 2001, the stillbirth

Table 8.4 Stillbirth risk increases with gestational age in obese women.

Gestational period (weeks)	Crude SB rate* in obese[†]	Crude SB rate in normal[‡]	Adjusted HR (95% CI)
20–27	0.5	0.3	1.9 (1.1–3.3)
28–36	0.2	0.1	2.1 (1.0–4.4)
37–40	1.3	0.4	3.5 (1.9–6.4)
>40	1.8	0.4	4.6 (1.6–13.4)

Adapted from Ref. [41].
SB, stillbirth; HR, hazard ratio.
*Expected number of fetal deaths when 1,000 women are followed for 1 week.
†BMI ⩾ 30.
‡BMI, 18.5–24.9.

rate was again higher in obese women compared to lean women, but the magnitude of the heightened risk increased with increasing gestational age [41] (Table 8.4).

Mechanism of fetal death

In pregnancies where obesity, hypertension, and DM coexist, any one or a combination of these factors can initiate events that culminate in stillbirth. However, obesity is a risk factor for stillbirth by itself, and the mechanism underlying this risk is still a matter of speculation and investigation as of this writing. One proposed mechanism linking maternal obesity to fetal death relates to the chronic inflammatory characteristics of the obese state [39]. Others have focused their concern on the occurrence of maternal hypoxia in obese women with obstructive sleep apnea (OSA). The answer is unlikely to be a simple one, and, like diabetes and hypertension, obesity may have numerous causal pathways for fetal death. In some cases, of course, undiagnosed diabetes, hypertension, or other condition may be the cause of stillbirth in an obese woman, though obesity is her only clinically recognized risk factor. That possibility notwithstanding, obesity is a common finding in otherwise unexplained stillbirths. This was described in a series from Canada, where increased prepregnancy weight (>68 kg) was the strongest independent risk factor among 196 unexplained fetal deaths [42].

Identifying the compromised fetus and management options to reduce risk

Interventions that reduce the risk of stillbirth in obese women are not well described. This is in part due to the relatively recent increase in obesity rates, the lack of a clear understanding of the mechanism leading to fetal death in obesity, as well as the daunting prospect of enrolling large numbers of women in a prospective study to show an impact on a relatively rare, though devastating, outcome. Thus, most recommendations for clinical care to reduce stillbirth in obese women are extrapolated from management of other high-risk pregnancies, and targeted to what appear to be risk factors for stillbirth among obese women.

Beginning prior to pregnancy, whenever possible, overweight and obese women should be encouraged and supported in efforts to normalize, or at least reduce their BMI. This is ideal, but rarely achieved. Failing this, obese women who are pregnant should be educated about and monitored for appropriate gestational weight gain, according to recent Institute of Medicine guidelines: 11–20 lb across the entire pregnancy. The potential benefit in achieving this goal, in terms of stillbirth risk, is the associated reduction in rates of hypertensive disorders and LGA babies that occurs when women gain within the recommended range [43]. There is no evidence that performing antenatal surveillance with NST or BPP for the sole indication of obesity is warranted, and it is not currently recommended by the American College of Obstetricians and Gynecologists [44]. As in all pregnancies, fetal movement counts, with immediate notification of care providers if abnormal, should be regularly and repeatedly encouraged.

Renal disease

Maternal renal disease comprises a range of disease entities, degrees of severity, and comorbid conditions, all of which have different implications for the chance of fetal death. For example, regardless of underlying mechanism of renal failure, the need for dialysis in pregnancy is associated with an extremely high fetal loss rate. The specific entities of diabetic nephropathy and lupus nephritis are discussed elsewhere in this chapter in greater detail.

It is difficult to distinguish the stillbirth rate in pregnancies complicated by maternal renal disease, as many reports combine all antenatal losses, or report PMR without breaking out stillbirths. Because of the association between maternal renal disease and iatrogenic prematurity due to severe growth restriction, early-onset severe preeclampsia, or deterioration of the maternal condition, neonatal death is significantly increased. Some series report "fetal loss" rates that include neonatal deaths. Nonetheless, live birth rates are consistently reported to be 75–95% in various series since the 1980s [45]. Successful pregnancy outcome is more likely with mild-to-moderate renal impairment (serum creatinine below 2.4–2.8 mg/dl), with a four- to five-fold increase in PMR with creatinine above these levels [46]. Presence of hypertension at the time of conception is another predictor of poor pregnancy outcome, including perinatal death. This is true regardless of the underlying source of the renal dysfunction: primary glomerular processes, such as IgA nephropathy, chronic reflux disease, or DM and systemic lupus erythematosus (SLE) [45].

Fetal death in maternal renal disease is likely caused by one or a combination of placental dysfunction/fetal growth restriction, direct effects of the underlying cause of renal damage (e.g., diabetes or lupus), or other comorbid conditions. Underlying disease management, including blood glucose control in DM and blood pressure control in hypertension, can have a beneficial impact on fetal survival [47]. Fetal surveillance algorithms, to include serial assessment of fetal growth, should be rigorously followed. Difficult decisions surrounding iatrogenic premature delivery will arise, but delivery is warranted if maternal or fetal condition is deteriorating.

Worthy of separate consideration are patients undergoing renal dialysis during pregnancy. The stillbirth rate is among the highest of any maternal condition. Case series comprising the past three decades report live birth rates of 25–50% [45], partly due to a high neonatal death rate because of premature delivery. Stillbirth rate has been reported as approximately 60–80/1,000, even in a very recent series of cases between 1988 and 2008 [48]. The development of preeclampsia was highly associated with fetal death in this report, while the presence of hydramnios (common in dialyzed pregnant patients) carried a good prognosis for the fetus, with a 95% survival.

Systemic lupus erythematosus

Women with SLE carry an increased risk for stillbirth, approximately 36–71/1,000 [49, 50]. Fetal death can result from fetal atrioventricular block due to antibody destruction of the conduction fibers by maternal SSA and SSB autoantibodies that cross the placenta [51]. Development of fetal hydrops in these cases presages fetal death in one-third of cases [52]. Controversy exists regarding whether treatment of heart block with steroids administered to the mother is beneficial. Some investigators have also proposed prophylactic steroids for women with SLE who have SSA and SSB antibodies to prevent heart block. A review of studies in this arena suggested that complete heart block could not be reversed with steroids, and prophylactic treatment did not appear beneficial either [51].

The presence of antiphospholipid antibodies also increases the risk of stillbirth in women with SLE. Although traditionally thought to result from vascular thrombotic events in placental vasculature, more recent data point to placental dysfunction due to autoimmune inflammation and oxidant-mediated damage, as well as antibody-mediated faulty trophoblast invasion, as the more likely mechanisms for fetal compromise leading to fetal death [53].

The highest risk of fetal loss in women with SLE is found in patients with lupus nephritis, who have reported live birth rates/neonatal survival of 58–84% after exclusion of pregnancy terminations [54]. Fetal death between 23 and 36 weeks gestation occurred in 7.8% (5/64 women, stillbirth rate 78/1,000) of cases in one large series at an experienced center [55]. Independent predictors of fetal loss in women with lupus nephritis include hypertension (OR 6.4,

95% CI 1.4–28.9), presence of antiphospholipid antibodies (OR 17.8, 95% CI 3.8–81.4), and proteinuria (OR 13.3, 95% CI 2.6–66.6) [55].

Few data exist to link any particular intervention in women with SLE directly to improved fetal survival. Beginning pregnancy when the disease is in a quiescent state improves overall outcomes, even in women with a history of lupus nephritis [45]. Monitoring for fetal growth restriction is essential, accompanied by tests of fetal well-being beginning early in the third trimester. Particularly when fetal growth is compromised, the addition of Doppler velocimetry to the testing algorithm may provide additional information about fetal status.

Thyroid disorders

The nature of the relationship between thyroid disorders and stillbirth is not entirely clear. Stillbirth is not a frequent outcome in women with overt hypo- and hyperthyroidism (stillbirth rate 12–20/1,000), but is associated with an increased risk compared to the general population (OR 2.2–3.0) [1]. Whether stillbirth is a direct result of the metabolic derangements or autoantibodies associated with thyroid dysfunction, or rather results from the comorbid conditions in women with thyroid disease, is not known. From the standpoint of clinical management and stillbirth prevention, it is not necessary to determine the presence or absence of antithyroid antibodies. Achieving a euthyroid state with appropriate medications is more important, and standard fetal surveillance techniques can be employed in women with suboptimal control of their thyroid disease.

Much attention and controversy has surrounded the detection and treatment of subclinical hypothyroidism in recent years. In this condition, thyroid stimulating hormone (TSH) levels are elevated, but thyroid hormone levels are normal. Associations of subclinical hypothyroidism with multiple adverse pregnancy outcomes have been reported, including stillbirth. In a retrospective study, TSH levels were analyzed from stored serum samples drawn in mid-pregnancy for routine prenatal tests. When TSH was ≥ 6 mU/l, the stillbirth rate was 3.8%, an OR of 4.4 (95% CI 1.9–9.5) compared to pregnancies with lower TSH levels [56]. No difference in stillbirth rate was noted in a large prospective study designed to further investigate the pregnancy implications of subclinical hypothyroidism, which these investigators defined as >97.5th percentile for gestational age [57]. At this time, screening asymptomatic women for subclinical hypothyroidism is not warranted in an effort to prevent stillbirth.

Intrahepatic cholestasis of pregnancy

Intrahepatic cholestasis of pregnancy (ICP) is the most common liver disorder unique to pregnancy. It is characterized by pruritis and abnormal liver tests, specifically increased serum levels of bile acids, aminotransferases, and bilirubin. The onset is typically in the second or third trimester of pregnancy, and it can recur in subsequent pregnancies in 40–60% of cases [58]. While carrying little implication for the mother other than intense discomfort from pruritis, ICP is clearly associated with an increased risk of stillbirth compared to an unaffected population. Reported stillbirth rates in ICP range from 12 to 35/1,000 [1, 59], roughly 2–4 times the rate in the general population. The etiology of ICP is multifactorial and not completely understood, but is influenced by genetic, environmental, and hormonal factors [60].

Mechanism of fetal death in ICP
To date, the mechanism leading to fetal death in women with ICP is incompletely understood. We do know that bile acids cross the placenta from mother to fetus along a concentration gradient, so that increased amounts of these potentially toxic substances are presented to the fetus in ICP [61]. Bile acids have been shown to affect transport and hormone production in the placenta, and cause chorionic vessel constriction [60]. How these changes impact upon the fetus to result in death is not clear, though some sort of placental dysfunction is hypothesized. Fetal hypoxia is suggested in the

frequently reported increase in meconium-stained amniotic fluid in all pregnancies with ICP [58, 62], and particularly in women with ICP and stillbirth, where meconium staining is found in 86% of cases [63]. However, the hypoxia does not appear to be chronic in nature. Support for acute anoxia as the lethal event in ICP is found in postmortem examinations of stillbirths, where petechial bleeding in adrenals, pleura, and pericardium are described in the absence of signs of chronic hypoxia [64]. Indirect evidence for an acute anoxic event, rather than chronic hypoxia, as the cause of fetal death includes normal rates of fetal growth restriction in affected pregnancies [65], normal umbilical artery Doppler velocimetry [66], and the inability of routine tests of fetal well-being to eliminate stillbirth in women with ICP [67].

The increased incidence of meconium-stained amniotic fluid in pregnancies complicated by ICP may be both an effect of the pathophysiology (fetal hypoxia resulting in meconium passage in utero) as well as a contributor to stillbirth risk. There is evidence that meconium causes umbilical cord and placental vasoconstriction [68], possibly compounding the vasoconstriction produced by increased bile acid levels in the amniotic fluid.

Identifying the compromised fetus and management options to reduce risk

Because the mechanism leading to fetal death is not completely understood, we cannot target our prevention of ICP-related fetal death to the specific cause. Total serum bile acid levels (TBA), the laboratory hallmark of the disease, have been correlated to risk of adverse events in pregnancy [69], with higher TBA levels associated with more complications, including "asphyxial events." These authors found no increase in adverse outcomes when TBA levels were <40 μmol/l, and suggested that women with ICP and TBA levels below this threshold could be treated as normal, without additional surveillance or intervention. Others report isolated cases of fetal death despite relatively low TBA levels and favorable maternal responses to medication [70].

Pharmacologic treatment of women with ICP with ursodeoxycholic acid (UDCA) has been reported to reduce pruritus, maternal serum TBA and aminotransferase levels, and transfer of TBA to the fetus [71–73]. UDCA is a normal minor fraction of TBA and is a Pregnancy Category B drug that does not cross the placenta [74]. Although there are apparent benefits to treatment with UDCA in terms of maternal symptoms and improved laboratory values, attributing improved fetal outcomes, particularly avoidance of stillbirth, to UDCA treatment is difficult because of the relatively small number of reported cases currently available. It is possible that a properly designed and adequately powered study could shed light on the impact of UDCA treatment on the stillbirth rate in ICP some time in the future. For now, reassuring safety data are accumulating for UDCA use in the second and third trimesters of pregnancy for women with ICP. Recommended doses range from 10–15 mg/kg/day up to 1.5–2.0 g/day [71, 73].

Increased fetal surveillance and timely intervention by delivery are the current mainstays of avoiding stillbirth in ICP. By instituting such programs, several centers have been able to achieve fetal loss rates comparable to an unaffected population [62, 63]. Others report that routine means of fetal surveillance, such as NST weekly or twice-weekly, are not sufficient to prevent all deaths [67, 70]. Because of the association between ICP, meconium passage, and fetal death, some clinical algorithms incorporate transcervical amnioscopy or amniocentesis, with delivery upon detection of meconium in the amniotic fluid [63]. In this series of 206 women with ICP, approximately 20% of all indicated preterm deliveries were performed due to detection of meconium. A summary of this surveillance and intervention algorithm is shown in Figure 8.2. Using this algorithm, no stillbirths occurred in 218 fetuses of 206 women with ICP.

Once a diagnosis of ICP is made, it is generally accepted that delivery should be effected no later than 37–38 weeks gestation, or at 36 weeks gestation if amniocentesis suggests low risk of fetal lung immaturity [75]. Prolonging pregnancy beyond 38 weeks gestation should be approached with extreme caution and vigilance.

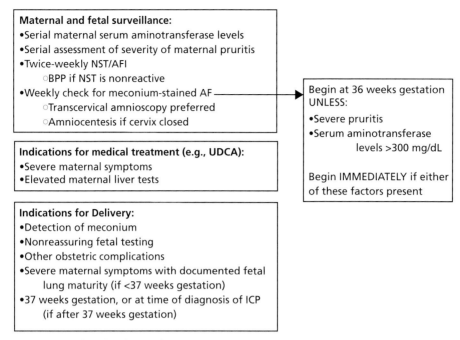

Maternal and fetal surveillance:
- Serial maternal serum aminotransferase levels
- Serial assessment of severity of maternal pruritis
- Twice-weekly NST/AFI
  - BPP if NST is nonreactive
- Weekly check for meconium-stained AF
  - Transcervical amnioscopy preferred
  - Amniocentesis if cervix closed

Begin at 36 weeks gestation UNLESS:
- Severe pruritis
- Serum aminotransferase levels >300 mg/dL

Begin IMMEDIATELY if either of these factors present

Indications for medical treatment (e.g., UDCA):
- Severe maternal symptoms
- Elevated maternal liver tests

Indications for Delivery:
- Detection of meconium
- Nonreassuring fetal testing
- Other obstetric complications
- Severe maternal symptoms with documented fetal lung maturity (if <37 weeks gestation)
- 37 weeks gestation, or at time of diagnosis of ICP (if after 37 weeks gestation)

Figure 8.2 Management algorithm for intrahepatic cholestasis of pregnancy. (Adapted from Ref. [62].)

Conclusion/summary

Finally, it is important to remember that the potential impact of the clinical recommendations in this chapter rely on at-risk patients being identified and treated as "at-risk." This requires not only clinical expertise on the part of obstetric care providers, but also unrestricted patient access to antenatal care programs that focus on effective interventions, as well as availability of high-level emergency obstetric services and neonatal intensive care.

References

1. Fretts RC. Etiology and prevention of stillbirth. Obstet Gynecol 2005;193(6):1923–35.
2. Dudley DJ. Diabetic-associated stillbirth: incidence, pathophysiology, and prevention. Obstet Gynecol Clin North Am 2007;34(2):293–307.
3. Macintosh MC, Fleming KM, Bailey JA, et al. Perinatal mortality and congenital anomalies in babies of women with type 1 or type 2 diabetes in England, Wales, and Northern Ireland: population based study. BMJ 2006;333(7560):177.
4. Cundy T, Gamble G, Townend K, et al. Perinatal mortality in Type 2 diabetes mellitus. Diabet Med 2000;17(1):33–9.
5. Cundy T, Gamble G, Neale L, et al. Differing causes of pregnancy loss in type 1 and type 2 diabetes. Diabetes Care 2007;30(10):2603–7.
6. Balsells M, Garcia-Patterson A, Gich I, Corcoy R. Maternal and fetal outcome in women with type 2 versus type 1 diabetes mellitus: a systematic review and metaanalysis. J Clin Endocrinol Metab 2009; 94(11):4284–91.
7. Parker JA, Conway DL. Diabetic ketoacidosis in pregnancy. Obstet Gynecol Clin North Am 2007; 34(3):533–43.
8. Montoro MN, Myers VP, Mestman JH, et al. Outcome of pregnancy in diabetic ketoacidosis. Am J Perinatol 1993;10(1):17–20.
9. Cullen MT, Reece EA, Homko CJ, Sivan E. The changing presentations of diabetic ketoacidosis during pregnancy. Am J Perinatol 1996;13(7):449–51.
10. Philipps AF, Porte PJ, Stabinsky S, et al. Effects of chronic fetal hyperglycemia upon oxygen consumption in the ovine uterus and conceptus. J Clin Invest 1984;74(1):279–86.
11. Philips AF, Dubin JW, Matty PJ, Raye JR. Arterial hypoxemia and hyperinsulinemia in the chronically

hyperglycemic fetal lamb. Pediatr Res 1982;16(8): 653–8.

12. Silver RM, Varner MW, Reddy U, et al. Work-up of stillbirth: a review of the evidence. Obstet Gynecol 2007;196(5):433–44.

13. Dudley DJ, Goldenberg R, Conway D, et al. A new system for determining the causes of stillbirth. Obstet Gynecol 2010;116(2):254–60.

14. Gonzalez-Gonzalez N, Ramirez O, Mozas J, et al. Factors influencing pregnancy outcome in women with type 2 versus type 1 diabetes mellitus. Acta Obstet Gynecol Scand 2008;87(1):43–9.

15. Reece EA, Leguizamon G, Homko C. Pregnancy performance and outcomes associated with diabetic nephropathy. Am J Perinatol 1998;15(7):413–21.

16. Giugliano D, Ceriello A, Paolisso G. Oxidative stress and diabetic vascular complications. Diabetes Care 1996;19(3):257–67.

17. McElvy SS, Miodovnik M, Rosenn B, et al. A focused preconceptional and early pregnancy program in women with type 1 diabetes reduces perinatal mortality and malformation rates to general population levels. J Matern Fetal Med 2000;9(1):14–20.

18. Kitzmiller JL, Jovanovic L, Brown F, et al. (eds). Managing preexisting diabetes and pregnancy: technical reviews and consensus recommendations for care. Alexandria, VA: American Diabetes Association; 2008.

19. ACOG Practice Bulletin. Pregestational diabetes mellitus. Obstet Gynecol 2005;105(3):675–85.

20. ACOG Practice Bulletin. Gestational diabetes. Obstet Gynecol 2001;98(3):525–38.

21. Conway DL, Langer O. Effects of new criteria for type 2 diabetes on the rate of postpartum glucose intolerance in women with gestational diabetes. Obstet Gynecol 1999;181(3):610–14.

22. Beischer NA, Wein P, Sheedy MT, Steffen B. Identification and treatment of women with hyperglycaemia diagnosed during pregnancy can significantly reduce perinatal mortality rates. Aust N Z J Obstet Gynaecol 1996;36(3):239–47.

23. Crowther CA, Hiller JE, Moss JR, et al. Australian Carbohydrate Intolerance Study in Pregnant Women (ACHOIS) Trial Group. Effect of treatment of gestational diabetes mellitus on pregnancy outcomes. N Engl J Med 2005;352(24):2477–86.

24. Casey BM, Lucas MJ, Mcintire DD, Leveno KJ. Pregnancy outcomes in women with gestational diabetes compared with the general obstetric population. Obstet Gynecol 1997;90(6):869–73.

25. HAPO Study Cooperative Research Group. Hyperglycemia and adverse pregnancy outcomes. N Engl J Med 2008;358(19):1991–2002.

26. Landon MB, Spong CY, Thom E, et al. A multicenter, randomized trial of treatment for mild gestational diabetes. N Engl J Med 2009;361(14):1339–48.

27. HAPO Study Cooperative Research Group. Hyperglycemia and Adverse Pregnancy Outcome (HAPO) Study: associations with neonatal anthropometrics. Diabetes 2009;58(2):453–9.

28. Allen VM, Joseph K, Murphy KE, et al. The effect of hypertensive disorders in pregnancy on small for gestational age and stillbirth: a population based study. BMC Pregnancy Childbirth 2004;4(1):17.

29. Hauth JC, Ewell MG, Levine RJ, et al. Pregnancy outcomes in healthy nulliparas who developed hypertension. Calcium for Preeclampsia Prevention Study Group. Obstet Gynecol 2000;95(1):24–8.

30. Freeman RK. Antepartum testing in patients with hypertensive disorders in pregnancy. Semin Perinatol 2008;32(4):271–3.

31. Hofmeyr GJ, Lawrie TA, Atallah AN, et al. Calcium supplementation during pregnancy for preventing hypertensive disorders and related problems. Cochrane Database Syst Rev 2010;8:CD001059; DOI: 10.1002/14651858.CD001059.pub3.

32. Roberts JM, Myatt L, Spong CY, et al. Vitamins C and E to prevent complications of pregnancy-associated hypertension. N Engl J Med 2010;362(14):1282–91.

33. Rumbold A, Duley L, Crowther CA, et al. Antioxidants for preventing pre-eclampsia. Cochrane Database Syst Rev 2008;1:CD004227; DOI: 10.1002/14651858.CD004227.pub3.

34. Duley L, Henderson-Smart DJ, Meher S, et al. Antiplatelet agents for preventing pre-eclampsia and its complications. Cochrane Database Syst Rev 2007;2: CD004659; DOI: 10.1002/14651858.CD004659.pub2.

35. Meher S, Abalos E, Carroli G. Bed rest with or without hospitalisation for hypertension during pregnancy. Cochrane Database Syst Rev 2005;4: CD004659; DOI: 10.1002/14651858.CD004659.pub2.

36. Abalos E, Duley L, Steyn DW, et al. Antihypertensive drug therapy for mild to moderate hypertension during pregnancy. Cochrane Database Syst Rev 2007;1: CD002252; DOI: 10.1002/14651858.CD002252.pub2.

37. ACOG Practice Bulletin. Chronic hypertension in pregnancy. Obstet Gynecol 2001;98(1):suppl. 77–85.

38. Cnattingius S, Bergstrom R, Lipworth L, Kramer MS. Prepregnancy weight and the risk of adverse pregnancy outcomes. N Engl J Med 1998;338(3):147–52.

39. Chu SY, Kim SY, Lau J, et al. Maternal obesity and risk of stillbirth: a metaanalysis. Obstet Gynecol 2007;197(3):223–8.

40. Salihu HM, Dunlop AL, Hedayatzadeh M, et al. Extreme obesity and risk of stillbirth among black

and white gravidas. Obstet Gynecol 2007;110(3): 552–7.

41. Nohr EA, Bodil HB, Michael JD, et al. Prepregnancy obesity and fetal death: a study within the Danish National Birth Cohort. Obstet Gynecol 2005;106(2): 250–9.

42. Huang DY, Usher RH, Kramer MS, et al. Determinants of unexplained antepartum fetal deaths. Obstet Gynecol 2000;95(2):215–21.

43. Kiel DW, Dodson EA, Artal R, et al. Gestational weight gain and pregnancy outcomes in obese women: how much is enough? Obstet Gynecol 2007;110(4): 752–8.

44. ACOG Committee Opinion. Obesity in pregnancy. Obstet Gynecol 2005;106(3):671–5.

45. Jungers P, Chauveau D. Pregnancy in renal disease. Kidney Int 1997;52(4):871–85.

46. Vidaeff AC, Yeomans ER, Ramin SM. Pregnancy in women with renal disease. Part I: general principles. Am J Perinatol 2008;25(7):385–97.

47. Packham DK, North RA, Fairley KF, et al. Primary glomerulonephritis and pregnancy. Q J Med 1989;71(266):537–53.

48. Luders C, Castro MC, Titan SM, et al. Obstetric outcome in pregnant women on long-term dialysis: a case series. Am J Kidney Dis 2010;56(1):77–85.

49. Smyth A, Oliveira GH, Lahr BD, et al. A systematic review and meta-analysis of pregnancy outcomes in patients with systemic lupus erythematosus and lupus nephritis. Clin J Am Soc Nephrol 2010;5(11), 2060–8.

50. Madazli R, Bulut B, Erenel H, et al. Systemic lupus erythematosus and pregnancy. J Obstet Gynaecol 2010;30(1):17–20.

51. Breur JM, Visser GH, Kruize AA, et al. Treatment of fetal heart block with maternal steroid therapy: case report and review of the literature. Ultrasound Obstet Gynecol 2004;24(4):467–72.

52. Coletta J, Simpson LL. Maternal medical disease and stillbirth. Clin Obstet Gynecol 2010;53(3): 607–16.

53. Branch DW. Antiphospholipid antibodies and fetal compromise. Thromb Res 2004;114(5–6):415–18.

54. Vidaeff AC, Yeomans ER, Ramin SM. Pregnancy in women with renal disease. Part II: specific underlying renal conditions. Am J Perinatol 2008;25(7): 399–405.

55. Moroni G, Quaglini S, Banfi G, et al. Pregnancy in lupus nephritis. Am J Kidney Dis 2002;40(4): 713–20.

56. Allan WC, Haddow JE, Palomaki GE, et al. Maternal thyroid deficiency and pregnancy complications: implications for population screening. J Med Screen 2000;7(3):127–30.

57. Casey BM, Dashe JS, Wells CE, et al. Subclinical hypothyroidism and pregnancy outcomes. Obstet Gynecol 2005;105(2):239–45.

58. Reyes H. Review: intrahepatic cholestasis. A puzzling disorder of pregnancy. J Gastroenterol Hepatol 1997;12(3):211–16.

59. Fisk NM, Storey GN. Fetal outcome in obstetric cholestasis. Br J Obstet Gynaecol 1988;95(11): 1137–43.

60. Kondrackiene J, Kupcinskas L. Intrahepatic cholestasis of pregnancy—current achievements and unsolved problems. World J Gastroenterol 2008;14(38): 781–8.

61. Rodrigues CM, Marin JJ, Brites D. Bile acid patterns in meconium are influenced by cholestasis of pregnancy and not altered by ursodeoxycholic acid treatment. Gut 1999;45(3):446–52.

62. Rioseco AJ, Ivankovic MB, Manzur A, et al. Intrahepatic cholestasis of pregnancy: a retrospective case-control study of perinatal outcome. Obstet Gynecol 1994;170(3):890–5.

63. Roncaglia N, Arreghini A, Locatelli A, et al. Obstetric cholestasis: outcome with active management. Eur J Obstet Gynecol Reprod Biol 2002;100(2):167–70.

64. Reid R, Ivey KJ, Rencoret RH, Storey B. Fetal complications of obstetric cholestasis. Br Med J 1976;1(6014):870–2.

65. Heinonen S, Kirkinen P. Pregnancy outcome with intrahepatic cholestasis. Obstet Gynecol 1999;94(2): 189–93.

66. Zimmermann P, Koskinen J, Vaalamo P, Ranta T. Doppler umbilical artery velocimetry in pregnancies complicated by intrahepatic cholestasis. J Perinat Med 1991;19(5):351–5.

67. Alsulyman OM, Ouzounian JG, Ames-Castro M, Goodwin TM. Intrahepatic cholestasis of pregnancy: perinatal outcome associated with expectant management. Obstet Gynecol 1996;175(4):957–60.

68. Altshuler G, Hyde S. Meconium-induced vasocontraction: a potential cause of cerebral and other fetal hypoperfusion and of poor pregnancy outcome. J Child Neurol 1989;4(2):137–42.

69. Glantz A, Marschall HU, Mattsson LA. Intrahepatic cholestasis of pregnancy: relationships between bile acid levels and fetal complication rates. Hepatology 2004;40(2):467–74.

70. Sentilhes L, Verspyck E, Pia P, Marpeau L. Fetal death in a patient with intrahepatic cholestasis of pregnancy. Obstet Gynecol 2006;107(2):458–60.

71. Palma J, Reyes H, Ribalta J, et al. Ursodeoxycholic acid in the treatment of cholestasis of pregnancy: a randomized, double-blind study controlled with placebo. J Hepatol 1997;27(6):1022–8.

72. Brites D, Rodrigues DM, Oliveira N, et al. Correction of maternal serum bile acid profile during ursode-oxycholic acid therapy in cholestasis of pregnancy. J Hepatol 1998;28(1):91–8.

73. Mazzella G, Rizzo N, Azzaroli F, et al. Ursodeoxycholic acid administration in patients with cholestasis of pregnancy: effects on primary bile acids in babies and mothers. Hepatology 2001;33(3):504–8.

74. PDR® Electronic Library™ (n.d.). Retrieved on August 19, 2010, from http://www.thomsonhc.com.libproxy.uthscsa.edu. Greenwood Village, CO: Thomson Reuters (Healthcare) Inc.

75. Parvin CA, Kaplan LA, Chapman JF, et al. Predicting respiratory distress syndrome using gestational age and fetal lung maturity by fluorescent polarization. Obstet Gynecol 2005;192(1):199–207.

CHAPTER 9
Vascular/Thrombotic

Fabio Facchinetti and Francesca Monari
Mother-Infant Department, Unit of Obstetrics and Gynecology, University of Modena and Reggio Emilia, Modena, Italy

Thrombosis-related phenomena came to the attention of obstetricians after the milestone paper of Michael Kuperminc et al. [1] reported an association of some thrombophilic traits and adverse pregnancy outcomes. Despite subsequent research and significant debate on the relationship, many physicians have overinterpreted the association and frequently order numerous laboratory tests to evaluate for thrombophilia. Indeed, in many countries there is widespread (ab)use of heparin administration throughout pregnancy for "prophylaxis."

This chapter will review thrombophilia and stillbirth, other vascular risk factors, and the management of these conditions.

Thrombophilia and stillbirth

Stillbirth, as well as preeclampsia, fetal growth restriction (FGR), and placental abruption (PA) are serious pregnancy complications that represent important contributors to both perinatal and maternal morbidity and mortality, and the precise causes of these conditions are largely idiopathic. A common finding among patients experiencing such complications is the presence of areas of thrombosis at histologic examination of the placenta [2, 3] (also see Chapter 10). This suggests that disturbances in coagulation may contribute to the etiology (Figure 9.1).

A large number of case–control studies have reported associations between adverse pregnancy outcomes and thrombophilias, but the results have been heterogeneous. The most troubling issue is the definition of "unexplained stillbirth" which largely depends on the extension of diagnostic work-up performed in each one of the primary studies.

To date, the data are conflicting regarding the association between inherited thrombophilias and adverse reproductive outcomes, including stillbirth. Some show a positive relationship between thrombophilias and adverse outcomes, whereas others report no association. Thrombophilia is a condition quite common in normal individuals, especially of Caucasian ethnicity.

Lockwood [4] found that heritable thrombophilias increased the risk of stillbirth by 3.6-fold in a general population. In a meta-analysis of 31 studies, factor V Leiden mutation (OR 3.26, 95%CI 1.82–5.83), prothrombin G20210A gene mutation (OR 2.30, 95%CI 1.09–4.87), and protein S deficiency (OR 7.39, 95%CI 1.28–42.63) were associated with late nonrecurrent fetal loss. However, such definition varied among studies and ranged from 14 to 22 weeks of gestational age [5]. A systematic review, which analyzed the association between adverse obstetric outcomes and inherited and acquired thrombophilias, found that unexplained stillbirth, when compared with controls, was more often associated with heterozygous factor V Leiden mutation, protein S deficiency, activated protein C (APC) resistance, anticardiolipin IgG antibodies, or lupus anticoagulant, but not

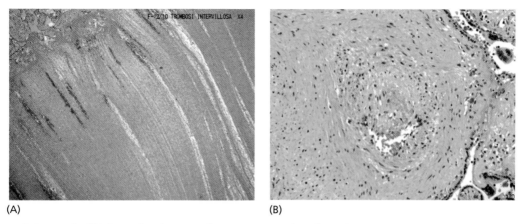

Figure 9.1 Case of stillbirth: (A) female, 32 weeks, 950 g. Recent thrombosis showing a laminar pattern, with few fibrin inserts. The villi are pushed toward vessel extremity. (B) Male, 34+5 weeks, 2,300 g. Thrombosis of a vessel of chorionic plaque partially occluding lumen. Fibroblasts proliferation is evident. Both (A) and (B) are reprinted by courtesy of Prof. G. Rivasi, Pathologist of the University of Modena and Reggio Emilia, Italy.

with protein C deficiency [6]. Several prospective studies [7, 8] failed to demonstrate an association between factor V Leiden mutation and fetal death. Gonen et al. [9] did not find an association between unexplained third-trimester intrauterine fetal death and inherited thrombophilia. Thrombophilia is more likely to contribute to a fetal death if there is objective evidence of placental insufficiency (FGR, abnormal blood flow, placental infarction, or PA).

Antithrombin, protein C, and protein S deficiency

Deficiency of antithrombin (AT) is inherited in autosomal dominant pattern. The prevalence of the heterozygous state in the general population is estimated at 1:2,000 to 1:5,000. The gene for AT is at 1q23-25 and a database of mutations is associated with AT deficiency. Venous thrombo-embolism (VTE) tends to occur at early age in individuals heterozygous for AT deficiency with a median age of presentation of 24 (with 67% first presenting between 10 and 35 years). AT deficiency is considered to carry a higher risk for thrombosis than any other thrombophilia. In family studies, the incidence of VTE in individuals with AT deficiency was 1.1–1.6% per year. The incidence of VTE increased

to 20% in individuals exposed to risk factors such as pregnancy or surgery [10].

A descriptive retrospective study showed that inherited AT deficiency is associated with a high risk of VTE during pregnancy and the puerperium and a high incidence of poor pregnancy outcome. Eighteen pregnancies were registered among nine AT-deficient women during 1991–2005. This cohort included women without antithrombotic treatment because AT deficiency was not known at the time of their pregnancies. In 12 pregnancies (66.7%) anticoagulant therapy with low-molecular-weight heparin (LMWH) was given, and three episodes of VTE were recorded (16.7%). Among all pregnancies, 10 suffered an adverse outcome (55.6%), including miscarriage (11.1%), stillbirth (11.1%), intrauterine growth restriction (33.3%), PA (6.7%), preeclampsia (6.7%), and intrapartum fetal distress (23.1%). A lower incidence of pregnancy complications was observed among women with antithrombotic treatment [11].

Protein C deficiency has a prevalence in heterozygous form in the general population ranging from 2.7% to 4.6%, but in young people with recurrent VTE this may be as high as 8.6%. The structure for protein C has been determined and the gene maps to chromosome 2q13-q14. Missense

Table 9.1 Prevalence of heterozygous Factor V Leiden (FV) in unexplained stillbirth group versus controls.

FV heterozygous	GA (weeks)	Stillbirth group	Controls	OR (95%CI)
Gris et al. (1999) [13]	>22	15/232 (6.5)	7/464 (1.5)	4.5 (1.7–12.4)
Martinelli et al. [14]	>20	5/67 (7)	6/232 (3)	3.2 (1.0–10.9)
Many et al. [20]	>27	3/40 (7.5)	3/80 (3.8)	1.5 (0.7–3.6)
Alonso et al. [22]	>23	0/8	1/75 (1)	/
Facchinetti et al. (2009) [58]	>23	7/132 (5.3)	8/310 (2.6)	2.0 (0.6–6.4)
Said JM et al. (2010) [8]	>20	?/663	?/1379	1.9 (1.1–3.3)

We included only those studies where the diagnostic work-up has been described. Data are reported as N and % in brackets. OR is reported with 95%CI.

mutation accounts for the majority of protein C deficiency cases. Clinical presentation with thrombotic disease in protein C deficiency tends to occur early in life. Homozygosity is associated with severe thrombosis and neonatal purpura fulminans. Among heterozygous individuals, the median age of the first thrombotic event is 29 years. Pregnancy does not modify protein C levels, which remain constant through all three trimesters. It is controversial whether protein C deficiency is associated with stillbirth [6].

Protein S is a cofactor for protein C, thereby acting as a natural inhibitor of the coagulation cascade. Protein S circulates in plasma in two forms, about 40% in the free active form and 60% bound to C4b-binding protein, a regulator of the complement system. Levels of C4b-binding protein are increased in pregnancy, with the combined oral contraceptive pill and in inflammation. An increase in the level of C4b-binding protein leads to a reduction in the level of free active protein S, possibly contributing to a thrombophilic state [10].

The prevalence of *protein S deficiency* is less than 1% in general population. Fifty percent of individuals with protein S deficiency experienced their first VTE by 26 years of age. Free protein S levels fall to 40–60% of normal levels in the first trimester of pregnancy and remain low throughout pregnancy and into the puerperium. A diagnosis of protein S deficiency is therefore not possible during pregnancy and requires confirmation at least 3 months postdelivery. Protein S deficiency has been associated with unexplained stillbirth.

Factor V Leiden

The prevalence of the factor V Leiden mutation in European populations is approximately 5%. The mutation renders factor V refractory to proteolysis by APC, therefore increasing the risk for VTE. The most recent meta-analysis found that a heterozygous factor V Leiden mutation is associated with twofold increased risk for a late unexplained fetal loss and a fourfold higher risk for loss in second trimester compared to the first trimester [12]. Table 9.1 summarizes the available data in studies where the diagnostic work-up was described. One explanation is that the late-pregnancy losses reflect thrombosis of the placental vessels, in contrast to first-trimester losses, which are more commonly attributable to other causes. In several studies, the majority of placentas from women heterozygous for factor V Leiden and fetal loss had evidence of thrombotic vasculopathy or infarction, supporting this hypothesis [13, 14]. However, specific studies have not found a correlation between placental finding and thrombophilia [15].

Although other adverse pregnancy outcomes, such as preeclampsia, intrauterine growth restriction, and PA, may also involve impaired placental perfusion, their association with thrombophilia remains controversial. The conflicting results reported in different studies may reflect the varying diagnostic and selection criteria, different ethnic groups, and small number of cases included. Many trials are retrospective and underpowered to detect a significant association with any of the thrombophilias [16, 17].

Table 9.2 Prevalence of factor II mutation heterozygous in stillbirth group versus controls.

FII heterozygous	GA (weeks)	Stillbirth group	Controls	OR
Gris et al. (1999) [13]	>22	2/232 (0.9)	5/464 (1)	0.8 (2.9–4.7)
Martinelli et al. [14]	>20	6/67 (9)	7/232 (3)	3.3 (1.1–10.3)
Many et al. [20]	>27	5/40 (12.5)	2/80 (3.8)	1.5 (0.7–3.6)
Alonso et al. [22]	>23	1/8 (12)	2/75 (3)	5 (0.4–64)
Facchinetti et al. (2009) [58]	>23	12/124 (9.7)	9/310 (2.9)	3.3 (1.3–8.8)
Said JM et al. (2010) [8]	>20			No association

We included only those studies where diagnostic work-up has been described. Data are reported as N and % in brackets. OR is reported with 95%CI.

Prothrombin gene mutation (factor II)

Prothrombin G20210A mutation is a point mutation that results in elevated circulating prothrombin levels and is characterized by VTE which manifest most commonly in adults as deep venous thrombosis (DVT) in the legs or pulmonary embolism. It is present in approximately 3% of European and in 2.4% of Australian antenatal population [18], and it has been reported to account for 17% of cases of VTE in pregnancy.

Heterozygous G20210A mutation was found in 4–9% of women with recurrent pregnancy loss (the majority in the first trimester), compared with 1–2% of those with uncomplicated pregnancies, with OR ranging from 2 to 9 [19]. Two other studies found heterozygous G20210A in 9–13% of women with a first unexplained third-trimester loss, compared with 2–3% of controls, suggesting a two- to three-fold increase in the risk [14, 20]. However, other studies found no significant association with fetal loss [13, 21]. A large meta-analysis concluded that heterozygous G20210A was associated with a two- to three-fold increase in risk of all recurrent, early first-trimester recurrent, and late nonrecurrent fetal loss [5, 22]. Moreover, in the recent prospective study by Said et al. [8], the prothrombin gene mutation was significantly associated with stillbirth (OR 3.58, 95%CI 1.20–10.61) although the number of events was very low. However, in the most recent study involving a geographically based population of women with stillbirth and matched controls, the stillbirth collaborative research network found no association between the prothrombin gene mutation and stillbirth. The data from studies where diagnostic work-up was described are summarized in Table 9.2.

The data about association between prothrombin gene mutation (heterozygous G20210A) and other adverse pregnancy outcomes are also controversial. In one study, heterozygous G20210A did not increase the risk of severe preeclampsia; however, women heterozygous for G20210A had a significantly earlier onset of preeclampsia [23]. The inconsistent results may reflect varying definitions of these complications, different ethnic groups and selection criteria, and the small number of individuals studied. The majority of published studies are too small to yield statistically significant results.

Other inherited thrombophilias

Methylentetrahydrofolate reductase (MTHFR). In their meta-analysis, Rey et al. [5] showed that individuals homozygous for the MTHFR mutation are not at increased risk of fetal loss. A subsequent meta-analysis by Nelen et al. [24] showed an association between recurrent early loss and separately hyperhomocysteinemia and MTHFR mutation. Homozygous MTHFR mutation is a very frequent finding in Caucasian population ranging 20–40%, and unless it is associated with hyperhomocysteinemia, it is not considered a risk factor for thrombosis. On the other hand, hyperhomocysteinemia per se could be dependent on several other factors such as reduced intake of folic acid or vitamin B12. For all these reasons the relationship between stillbirth and such a mutation has not been considered to be relevant. Moreover, the recent guidelines released from the Royal College of Obstetricians and Gynaecologists on thrombosis and pregnancy state that the thermolabile variant of the gene for MTHFR (in homozygous form) is sometimes included in thrombophilia testing, but there is no evidence of its association with a clinically relevant increase of VTE in pregnancy [25].

Plasminogen activator inhibitor (PAI-1). Such mutation could be related to adverse pregnancy outcomes. To assess the hypofibrinolytic 4G/4G mutation of the PAI-1 gene as a possible factor contributing to severe preeclampsia, abruption of the placenta, FGR, and stillbirth, Glueck et al. [26] compared 94 patients to 95 controls with normal pregnancies, matched for ethnic background and age. Women having had obstetric complications (30 of 94, 32%) were more likely to be homozygous for 4G/4G mutation (OR = 2.0; 95%CI 1.02–3.90) than controls (18 of 95, 19%). In such women who had increased incidence of the hypofibrinolytic 4G/4G mutation of the PAI-1 gene, there is a frequent association with the thrombophilic factor V Leiden mutation, further predisposing them to thrombosis [26]. However, no other data are available and the possible relationship between PAI-1 mutation and stillbirth need to be further investigated.

Acquired thrombophilia

Antiphospholipid syndrome (APLAS) is an autoimmune disorder defined by the presence of an adverse pregnancy outcome and a laboratory test positive for circulating antiphospholipid antibodies (aPL). They are a diverse group of antibodies with specificity for protein binding negatively charged phospholipids on cell surfaces. The aPL antibodies that are best characterized are lupus anticoagulant and anticardiolipin antibodies. The most common

and serious complications associated with APLAS are thromboses in both venous and arterial sides, most thrombotic events being venous (65–70%). Although the most frequent site of VTE is at lower extremities, thrombosis can occur in almost any blood vessel in the body, and occlusions in unusual locations should prompt clinicians to consider the diagnosis of APLAS.

The risk of thrombosis is significantly increased during pregnancy in patients with APLAS. Arterial thrombosis is also associated with aPL antibodies and can occur in atypical sites, such as retinal, subclavian, digital, or brachial arteries. Stroke is the most common arterial event, and the most frequently involved vessel is the middle cerebral artery. A variety of other diseases have been associated with aPL antibodies, including transient ischemic attacks and *amaurosis fugax*, stroke in young women (<50 years), coronary occlusions, and autoimmune thrombocytopenia.

Pregnancy losses related to aPL antibodies are typically second- or third-trimester fetal deaths. APLAS is also associated with an increased risk of preeclampsia, FGR, uteroplacental insufficiency, and preterm delivery [27]. A plausible explanation for fetal losses in APLAS is thrombosis of the uteroplacental vasculature and placental infarction. The prothrombotic nature of aPL is supported by the finding that the antibodies can bind and activate platelets and endothelial cells, inhibit fibrinolysis, and may interfere with the protein C pathway [27].

Few data are available on APLAS prevalence in unexplained stillbirth. Three studies with a total of 549 investigated patients are available, just one reporting a statistical significant association. However, summarizing the findings reported in Table 9.3, it could be concluded that APLAS

Table 9.3 Prevalence of acquired thrombophilia in stillbirth group versus controls.

Acquired thrombophilia	GA (weeks)	Stillbirth group	Controls	OR
Gris et al. (2001)	>22	18/232 (7.7)	6/464 (1.3)	6.4 (2.4–18.3)
Alonso et al. [22]	>23	6/75 (8)	0/75 (0)	0
Facchinetti et al. (2009)	>23	10/142 (7)	11/326 (3.4)	2.2 (0.8–5.6)
Total		34/549	17/865	3.39 (1.76–6.21)

We included only those studies where diagnostic work-up has been explicated. Data are reported as *N* and % in brackets. OR is reported with 95%CI.

represents a risk factor for stillbirth (OR = 3.29; 95%CI 1.76–6.21).

Other vascular risk factors

Maternal hemorrhage

Maternal hemorrhage can jeopardize the fetus at any time in pregnancy. Apart from incidental cases due to vessel trauma, the majority are due to PA or abnormal placentation such as placenta previa or accreta.

In a retrospective cohort study performed in the United States, the rates of PA were 6.2, 12.2, and 15.6 per 1,000 pregnancies, in single, twins, and triplets, respectively. In singletons, the stillbirth rate was 8.3% as compared to 0.42% in pregnancies not complicated by abruption, with an adjusted OR of 18. 9 (95%CI 16.9–20.8) [28]. Several etiologic determinants of PA have been reported, and most of them have been independently associated with stillbirth, such as severe FGR, chorioamnionitis, and hypertension [29]. The picture is further complicated by the strong association existing between PA and inherited thrombophilia [30]. Despite the knowledge of several risk factors, neither prediction nor prevention of PA is possible. PA is one of the most important causes of stillbirth.

Another risk factor for maternal bleeding is when the placenta covers the internal os (complete previa) or, to a lesser extent, is just around it (marginal previa), with bleeding occurring in 48–57% of cases, especially in the setting of uterine contractility. In the setting of placenta previa or accreta, the risk for stillbirth is not increased [31].

Vasa previa is a rare condition (0.2–0.3%) where umbilical vessels course in between placenta lobes or have a velamentous insertion, beyond the internal os. The lack of Warthon jelly around these vessels allows for the potential of massive hemorrhage when the membranes rupture. Perinatal mortality is up to 36%, with stillbirth accounting for around 20%. Antenatal diagnosis through Doppler evaluation and subsequent planned cesarean delivery may substantially reduce mortality to 3% as compared to 44% in cases lacking a prenatal diagnosis [32].

Feto–maternal hemorrhage

The passage of small amounts of fetal blood into the maternal compartment during pregnancy is a relatively common phenomenon. There is no known level of fetal blood in the maternal circulation that is known to cause fetal death. The incidence of fetal–maternal hemorrhage (FMH) is in the range of 1–3 per 1,000 pregnancies according to the blood exchange which has been defined to be 80 or 30 ml [33]. Silver and colleagues reported that a massive FMH is found in 5–14% of fetal deaths [34].

Despite the intermingling of fetal and maternal blood in the placental intervillar spaces, a physiological barrier separates the two compartments. The rupture of this functional barrier may occur in the setting of abdominal trauma, placental disorders (placenta previa, chorioangioma), invasive diagnostic procedures (i.e., villocentesis), and traumatic procedures (including external cephalic version). Fetal anemia whether directly related to blood loss or indirectly caused by Rh-immunization is the final cause resulting in stillbirth. A Kleihauer–Betke or flow cytometry testing should be performed as a routine for every case of stillbirth, preferably prior to delivery [35].

Multiple gestation

As compared to singletons, multiple gestations carry an increased risk of stillbirth, occurring in 1.2% in twins and 3.4% in triplets [36]. In monochorionic diamniotic twins, the vascular complications related to twin to twin transfusion syndrome (TTTS) account for 50% of deaths. In dichorionic diamniotic twins, FGR is the major cause of stillbirth [37]. In triplets, tri-chorionicity is the rule with less than 20% being mono- or dichorionic. However, in the latter, stillbirth rates are very high, predominately due to vascular disorders such as TTTS and twin reversed arterial perfusion sequence (TRAP) [38]. In addition to the fetal loss in monochorionic pregnancy, the prognosis of the co-twin is poor with a 12% risk of death and 18% risk of neurological sequelae [39].

Laser therapy may be successful in these cases [40], thus the timely diagnosis of vascular disorders is important. Due to other reasons including congenital anomalies, the rate of stillbirth in multiple gestations remains elevated.

Management

Inherited thrombophilia

Clinicians are often faced with the difficult situation of what to do with a woman with a previous adverse pregnancy outcome, such as stillbirth, who tested positive for thrombophilia (see also Chapter 15). Gris et al. [41] performed a small multicenter randomized controlled trial in 160 thrombophilic women (factor V Leiden, prothrombin mutation, or protein S deficiency) with one prior pregnancy loss at $\geq$10 weeks. All women preconceptionally received 5 mg folic acid daily. At eighth week of pregnancy, they were randomized to low dose of aspirin (100 mg/day) or enoxaparin (40 mg/day). The addition of enoxaparin, an LMWH, was associated with a significant improvement of live birth which occurred in 86% compared to 29% in low dose of aspirin only group (OR = 15.5; 95%CI 7–34). The improvement in live birth rates with enoxaparin was similar for each one of the thrombophilias. Moreover, low birthweight occurred less (10%) in women treated with LMWH with respect to those treated with low-dose aspirin (30%). In another study, Brenner et al. reported that the percentage of live births in women with inherited thrombophilia and recurrent early pregnancy loss increased from 20% without therapy to 75% following treatment with LMWH [42].

Bloomenthal et al. [43] wrote a summary of published documents outlining expert opinion on possible management strategies in these women, that is, treatment with LMWH (either Enoxaparin 40 mg or Deltaparin 5,000 UI sc once/day or twice/day) during pregnancy followed by warfarin for 6–12 weeks in the postpartum period. Similarly, the "Consensus Report and recommendations for prevention and treatment of venous thromboembolism

and adverse pregnancy outcomes" made from the Pregnancy and Thrombosis Working Group stated that women with a moderate risk assessment (i.e., a history of adverse obstetric outcome such as severe preeclampsia, FGR <fifth percentile or fetal loss at $\geq$20 weeks) should receive antepartum therapy with Enoxaparin 4,000 UI sc or Deltaparin 5,000 UI sc once/day to prevent the recurrence of adverse obstetric outcome.

Despite these experts opinions, there is no substantial data supporting their recommendations since the trials we quoted included only very few cases of correctly defined stillbirth whereas they mostly refer to earlier pregnancy losses [44]. To remove uncertainties, there are several ongoing international trials about efficacy (or not) of LMWH prophylaxis of asymptomatic carriers with a previous adverse obstetric outcome which may provide evidence in the near future.

Acquired thrombophilia

Current recommendations are that women with APLAS and without a history of thrombosis should receive low-dose aspirin (0.1 g/day) and prophylactic doses of LMWH (5,000 UI twice/day) during pregnancy. This management strategy is documented by small well-controlled prospective studies and it is recommended by the American College of Chest Physicians (ACCP) (grade 1A recommendation). The treatment is stepwise: starts with aspirin before conception or at positive pregnancy test and adds heparin either with a positive pregnancy test or when fetal heart activity was demonstrated. The treatment should continue until 6 weeks after delivery, considering that these women are at high risk of VTE [45].

A recent systematic review and meta-analysis, however, estimated the effect of combined heparin and aspirin therapy compared with aspirin alone in pregnant women with APLAS and recurrent pregnancy losses. The main data showed that the combination of aspirin to heparin (namely unfractionated heparin) improved outcome (live birth) only in patients included because of recurrent early (first trimester) pregnancy losses. On the contrary, when pregnancy losses occurred beyond first trimester (which does not necessarily mean stillbirth), aspirin effect is similar to the combination aspirin plus heparin [46]. Of paramount importance, the same authors concluded that ". . . the efficacy of LMWH plus aspirin remains unproven, highlighting the urgent need for large controlled trials." Indeed, Tulppala [47] showed no benefit of aspirin over placebo in 12 patients with APLAS and history of recurrent fetal loss. Laskin's [48] trial of 88 patients showed prednisone plus aspirin therapy seems worse than no therapy, and Pattison's [49] trial of 40 patients comparing aspirin to placebo also showed no advantage. Cowchock's [50] study of 19 patients also found no advantages of aspirin versus usual care.

In conclusion, low-dose aspirin plus heparin is recommended on the basis of Rai et al. trial [51] where, in a open design, in 90 APLAS patients, pregnancy loss occurred in 13/45 (29%) among those treated with heparin plus aspirin versus 26/45 (48%) in those receiving low-dose aspirin alone. All but 4 out of the 39 losses occurred beyond the first trimester (OR of pregnancy loss 0.50; 95%CI 0.30–0.84). Therefore, these findings (unchallenged vs. placebo) cannot apply to stillbirth.

Conclusion (Table 9.4)

Most of the pregnancy complications related to placental dysfunction including stillbirth and late fetal death have been associated with thrombophilia. Despite the availability of data from several studies, retrospective case–control design (the majority) and populations studied, the heterogeneity of clinical definitions and reduced sample size limit the interpretation of data. Hence, opinions rather than facts still represent today the approach to such an issue.

Unfortunately, long before the "disease" has been discovered, the "cure" is behind the corner. Heparin prophylaxis is implemented by an increasing number of physicians with no rationale, since the lack of any clinical trial able to demonstrate that such an intervention is accompanied by better benefits than placebo. The recent trials published on the ineffectiveness of LMWH prophylaxis in recurrent abortion patients (independently from a thrombophilic trait) just remind us how fundamental are RCTs before establishing any intervention, namely in pregnant women [52, 53].

In the specific case of stillbirth, a statistical association between the event and the presence of maternal mutations of factor V or factor II of the coagulation cascade seems to be confirmed in the present review. Of paramount importance, such an association is confirmed also restricting the inclusion to those cases series where really the term unexplained does mean "several causes have looked for and none found." Moreover, acquired thrombophilia, that is, the presence of antibodies against phospholipids/lupus anticoagulant is associated with an increased rate of unexplained stillbirth. While these findings certainly add to our knowledge, it would be too simple and unrealistic to consider the finding of maternal thrombophilia as a direct, sole cause of intrauterine fetal death.

Table 9.4 Synopsis of this review (Take home messages).

1. Maternal screening for inherited thrombophilia should be restricted to research protocols. Checking for acquired thrombophilia in the postpartum would allow the discovery of APLAS.
2. The evidence of acquired thrombophilia in a woman with a history of stillbirth allows the diagnosis of APLAS. However, despite actual recommendation, there is no evidence to support the use of early thromboprophylaxis for a subsequent pregnancy.
3. There is an association of the history of stillbirth with inherited thrombophilic mutation of either factor V or factor II; however, the strength of such an association is very low. In view of the lack of any randomized controlled trial on this specific topic, there is no data to support the use of antenatal thromboprophylaxis with the aim to reduce recurrence.
4. Antenatal and/or postnatal thromboprophylaxis should be given to women with moderate to high risk factors for the development of VTE, according to current guidelines.

Such a simplistic, reductive approach has also been recently denied by others [54].

The recent renewal of interest toward the subject stimulated the revision of the actual knowledge about stillbirth [55]. The list of events/disorder recognized as a single, unique cause for determining stillbirth is very short (i.e., massive PA, Listeria infection, trisomy 13, etc.) and a recent classification invite to describe both the "supposed" cause of death and the "associated conditions" [56]. In light of this approach we have to consider thrombophilia as an associated condition that may predispose a woman to stillbirth. A support to this approach for clinical interpretations of such findings comes out from the analysis of the strength of the association. Indeed, the odds ratio of either mutations and acquired thrombophilia we here reviewed, ranged 1.5–6.4, as in the most part of the studies published so far [15].

Thus, the management of pregnancy next to stillbirth, also in women presenting with thrombophilia, remains a matter of discussion [57] in view of the absence of evidence-based intervention.

References

1. Kupferminc MJ, Eldor A, Steiman N, et al. Increased frequency of genetic thrombophilia in women with complications of pregnancy. N Engl J Med 1999;340:9–13.
2. Inherited thrombophilias in pregnancy. Practice bulletin ACOG 2010;115:877–87.
3. George D, Erkan D. Antiphospholipid syndrome. Prog Cardiovasc Dis 2009;52:115–25.
4. Lockwood CJ. Heritable coagulopathies in pregnancy. Obstet Gynaecol Surv 1999;54:754–65.
5. Rey E, Kahn SR, David M, et al. Thrombophilic disorders and fetal loss: a meta-analysis. Lancet 2003;361:901–8.
6. Alfirevic Z, Roberts D, Martlew V. How strong is the association between maternal thrombophilia and adverse pregnancy outcome? A systematic review. Eur J Obstet Gynecol Reprod Biol 2002;101:6–14.
7. Völzke H, Grimm R, Robinson DM, et al. Factor V Leiden and the risk of stillbirth in a German population. Thromb Haemost 2003;90:429–33.
8. Said JM, Higgins JR, Moses EK, et al. Inherited thrombophilia polymorphisms and pregnancy outcomes in nulliparous women. Obstet Gynecol 2010;115: 5–13.
9. Gonen R, Lavi N, Attias D, et al. Absence of association of inherited thrombophilia with unexplained third-trimester intrauterine fetal death. Am J Obstet Gynecol 2005;192:742–6.
10. Saade GR, McLintock C. Inherited thrombophilia and stillbirth. Semin Perinatol 2002;26:51–69.
11. Sabadell J, Casellas M, Alijotas-Reig J, et al. Inherited antithrombin deficiency and pregnancy: maternal and fetal outcomes. Eur J Obstet Gynecol Reprod Biol 2010;149:47–51.
12. Robertson L, Wu O, Langhorne P, et al. The Thrombosis: Risk and Economic Assessment of Thrombophilia Screening (TREATS) Study. Thrombophilia in pregnancy: a systematic review. Br J Haematol 2006;132:171–96.
13. Gris JC, Quéré I, Monpeyroux F, et al. Case–control study of the frequency of thrombophilic disorders in couples with late foetal loss and no thrombotic antecedent—the Nîmes Obstetricians and Haematologists Study 5 (NOHA5). Thromb Haemost 1999;81:891–9.
14. Martinelli I, Taioli E, Cetin I, et al. Mutations in coagulation factors in women with unexplained late fetal loss. N Engl J Med 2000;343:1015–8.
15. Ariel I, Anteby E, Hamani Y, et al. Placental pathology in fetal thrombophilia. Hum Pathol 2004;35:729–33.
16. Rodger MA, Paidas M, McLintock C, et al. Inherited thrombophilia and pregnancy complications revisited. Obstet Gynecol 2008;112:320–4.
17. Funai EF. Inherited thrombophilia and preeclampsia: is the evidence beginning to congeal? Am J Obstet Gynecol 2009;200:121–2.
18. Said JM, Brennecke SP, Moses EK, et al. The prevalence of inherited thrombophilic polymorphisms in an asymptomatic Australian antenatal population. Aust N Z J Obstet Gynaecol 2008;48:536–41.
19. Raziel A, Kornberg Y, Friedler S, et al. Hypercoagulable thrombophilic defects and hyperhomocysteinemia in patients with recurrent pregnancy loss. Am J Reprod Immunol 2001;45:65–71.
20. Many A, Elad R, Yaron Y, et al. Third-trimester unexplained intrauterine fetal death is associated with inherited thrombophilia. Obstet Gynecol 2002;99:684–7.
21. Brenner B, Aharon A. Thrombophilia and adverse pregnancy outcome. Clin Perinatol 2007;34:527–41.
22. Alonso A, Soto I, Urgellés MF, et al. Acquired and inherited thrombophilia in women with unexplained fetal losses. Am J Obstet Gynecol 2002;187:1337–42.

23. Gerhardt A, Scharf RE, Mikat-Drozdzynski B, et al. The polymorphism of platelet membrane integrin $\alpha 2\beta 1$ ($\alpha 2807TT$) is associated with premature onset of fetal loss. Thromb Haemost 2005;93:124–9.

24. Nelen WL, Blom HJ, Steegers EA, et al. Hyperhomocysteinemia and recurrent early pregnancy loss: a metaanalysis. Fertil Steril 2000;74:1196–9.

25. Reducing the risk of thrombosis and embolism during pregnancy and the puerperium. 2010. Green-top Guideline No. 37. November 2009. RCOG.

26. Glueck CJ, Kupferminc MJ, Fontaine RN, et al. Genetic hypofibrinolysis in complicated pregnancies. Obstet Gynecol 2001;97:44–8.

27. ACOG Practice Bulletin 68: Antiphospholipid syndrome. Obstet Gynecol. 2005;106:1113–21. ACOG Committee on Practice Bulletins-Obstetrics.

28. Salihu HM, Kinninburgh BA, Aliyu MH, et al. Racial disparity in SB among singleton, twin and triplets gestations in the United States. Obstet Gynecol 2004;104:734–40.

29. Kramer MS, Liu S, Luo Z, et al. Analysis of perinatal mortality and its components: time for a change? Am J Epidemiol 2002;156:493–7.

30. Facchinetti F, Marozio L, Grandone E, et al. Thrombophilic mutations are a main risk factor for placenta abruption. Haematologica 2003;88:785–8.

31. Berghella V. Placenta previa, placenta accreta and vasa previa. Obstetric evidence based guidelines. First Edition. Informa healthcare. 2007, Chapter 24, pp. 187–94.

32. Oyelese Y, Catanzarite V, Prefumo F, et al. Vasa previa: the impact of prenatal diagnosis on outcomes. Obstet gynecol 2004;103:937–42.

33. Baronciani D, Bulfamante G, Facchinetti F. La natimortalità: audit clinico e miglioramento della pratica clinica assistenziale. Il pensiero Scientifico Editore. 2008, Chapter 10, pp. 191–214.

34. Silver RM. Fetal death. Obstet Gynecol 2007;109:153–67.

35. NSW Health Department. Guidelines for investigation of a stillbirth. 1997. Electronic/circular. Sydney: NSW Health Department; 27/10/1997. Report No.: 97/107, Nursing and Midwifery Sub-group SZCSN. Antepartum haemorrhage: Southern Zone Maternity Procedural Guidelines. In; 2003, 104, 108.

36. Smith GCS. Predicting antepartum stillbirth. Curr Opin Obstet Gynecol 2006;18:625–30.

37. Lee YM, Wylie BJ, Simpson LL, et al. Twin chorionicity and the risk of stillbirth. Obstet Gynecol 2006;111:301–8.

38. Geipel A, Berg C, Katalinic A, et al. Prenatal diagnosis and obstetric outcomes in triplet pregnancies in relation to chorionicity. BJOG 2005;112:554–8.

39. Ong SSC, Zamora J, Khan KS, et al. Prognosis for the co-twin following single-twin death: a systematic review. BJOG 2006;113:992–8.

40. Chmait RH, Chavira E, Kontopoulos EV, et al. Third trimester fetoscopic laser ablation of type II vasa previa. J Matern Fetal Neonatal Med 2010;23:459–62.

41. Gris JC, Mercier E, Quere I, et al. Low-molecular-weight heparin versus low dose aspirin in women with one fetal loss and a constitutional thrombophylic disorder. Blood 2004;103:3695–9.

42. Brenner B, Hoffman R, Blumenfeld Z, et al. Gestational outcome in thrombophilic women with recurrent pregnancy loss treated by enoxaparin. Thromb Haemost 2000;83:693–7.

43. Bloomenthal D, von Dadelszen P, Liston R, et al. The effect of factor V Leiden carriage on maternal and fetal health. CMAJ 2002;167:48–54.

44. Walker MC, Ferguson SE, Allen VM. Heparin for pregnant women with acquired or inherited thombophilias (review). Cochrane library, 2009;(1):1–12.

45. Bates SM, Greer IA, Pabinger I, et al. American College of Chest Physicians Venous thromboembolism, thrombophilia, antithrombotic therapy, and pregnancy: American College of Chest Physicians Evidence-Based Clinical Practice Guidelines (8th Edition). Chest 2008;133:844S–886S.

46. Ziakas PD, Pavlou M, Voulgarelis M. Heparin treatment in antiphospholipid syndrome with recurrent pregnancy loss: a systematic review and meta-analysis. Obstet Gynecol 2010;115:1256–62.

47. Tulppala M, Marttunen M, Soderstrom-Anttila V. Low-dose aspirin in prevention of miscarriage in women with unexplained or autoimmune related recurrent miscarriage: effect on prostacyclin and thromboxane A2 production. Hum Reprod 1997;12:1567–72.

48. Laskin CA, Bombardier C, Hannah ME, et al. Prednisone and aspirin in women with autoantibodies and unexplained recurrent fetal loss. N Engl J Med 1997;337:148–53.

49. Pattison NS, Chamley LW, Birdsall M. Does aspirin have a role in improving pregnancy outcome for women with the antiphospholipid syndrome? A randomized controlled trial. Am J Obstet Gynecol 2000;183:1008–12.

50. Cowchock S, Reece EA. Do low-risk pregnant women with antiphospholipid antibodies need to be treated? Am J Obstet Gynecol 1997;176:1099–100.

51. Rai R, Cohen H, Dave M, et al. Randomised controlled trial of aspirin and aspirin plus heparin in pregnant women with recurrent miscarriage associated with phospholipid antibodies (or antiphospholipid antibodies). Br Med J 1997;314:253–7.

52. Kaandorp SP, Goddijn M, van der Post JA, et al. Aspirin plus heparin or aspirin alone in women with recurrent miscarriage. N Engl J Med 2010;362:1586–96.

53. Clark P, Walker ID, Langhorne P, et al. SPIN (Scottish Pregnancy Intervention) study: a multicenter, randomized controlled trial of low-molecular-weight heparin and low-dose aspirin in women with recurrent miscarriage. Blood 2010;115:4162–6167.

54. Rodger MA, Paidas M. 2007. Do thrombophilias cause placenta-mediated pregnancy complications? Semin Thromb Hemost 2007;33:597–603.

55. Facchinetti F, Dekker GA, Baronciani D, Saade G. (Eds.) Stillbirth. Understanding and management. Informa Healthcare. 2010, Chapter 11, pp. 109–13.

56. Flenady V, Frøen JF, Pinar H, et al. An evaluation of classification systems for stillbirth. BMC Pregnancy Childbirth 2009;9:24.

57. Monari F, Facchinetti F. Management of subsequent pregnancy after antepartum stillbirth. A review. J Matern Fetal Neonatal Med, 2010;23(10): 1073–84.

58. Facchinetti F, Marozio L, Frusca T, et al. Maternal thrombophilia and the risk of recurrence of preeclampsia. Am J Obstet Gynecol. 2009 Jan;200(1):46.e1-5. Epub 2008 Oct 9.

CHAPTER 10
Placenta and Cord

Raymond W. Redline, MD

Department of Pathology and Reproductive Biology, Case Western Reserve University School of Medicine,
Cleveland, OH, USA
Department of Pediatric and Perinatal Pathology, University Hospitals Case Medical Center,
Cleveland, OH, USA

Stillbirth, or intrauterine fetal demise (IUFD), is defined as death in utero or lack of cardiac activity at birth after 20 weeks gestational age (GA). The overall prevalence of IUFD is approximately 6/1,000 pregnancies [1, 2]. About half of IUFD occur after 28 weeks and that number has declined about 30% over the past 30 years. Prevalence in the earlier GA group has remained constant. This chapter will not consider the considerable proportion of IUFD attributable to chromosomal/genetic syndromes and lethal congenital anomalies (see Chapters 6 and 11). Risk factors for the non-malformed IUFD have been separated into two groups: those that are common, but associated with only moderately increased risk and those that are rare, but of higher risk. The former include advanced maternal age, non-Hispanic black race, and obesity. Each has a prevalence of about 15% and an associated risk of IUFD of about 1%. The latter group includes mothers with insulin-dependent diabetes, connective tissue disease, or a history of reproductive failure (e.g., infertility requiring artificial reproductive technologies [ARTs], recurrent spontaneous abortion, or prior perinatal morbidity or mortality). Intermediate between these two groups are mothers with underlying medical conditions such as hypertension or hypothyroidism and those who develop preeclampsia.

IUFD are a heterogeneous group of only loosely related conditions. The distinction between cases at greater or less than 28 weeks, mentioned earlier, has little clinical or biologic meaning in contemporary practice. A more useful separation would recognize three categories: (1) previable IUFD (<24 weeks), where conditions triggering labor and delivery alone ensure perinatal death, (2) premature IUFD (24–34 weeks) occurring in immature fetuses who would be subject to the complications of prematurity if delivered early, and (3) term/near-term IUFD (>34 weeks) affecting mature fetuses who would stand an excellent chance of survival if "rescued by birth." Another useful distinction is to separate intrapartum from antepartum IUFD. The former puts the focus on complications of labor and delivery and problems in intrapartum management, while the latter emphasizes sudden unanticipated events and silent intrauterine processes that have escaped antenatal detection. Finally, it is important to separate IUFD associated with fetoplacental abnormalities such as fetal growth restriction (FGR, also see Chapter 7), macrosomia, or congestive heart failure (hydrops fetalis, HF) from IUFD occurring in apparently normal fetuses. IUFD with fetoplacental abnormalities often represent extreme examples of chronically maladaptive gestational disease processes that happen to cause death within the arbitrary time frame of the second half of gestation. These processes can occur at other times during pregnancy, reflecting the continuum

Stillbirth: Prediction, Prevention and Management, First Edition. Catherine Y. Spong.
© 2011 Blackwell Publishing Ltd. Published 2011 by Blackwell Publishing Ltd.

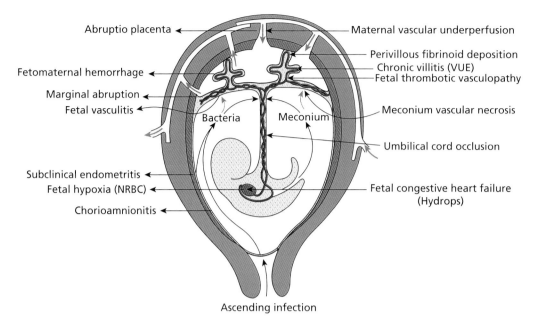

Figure 10.1 Diagram of uterus, placenta, umbilical cord, and fetus showing the anatomic localization of major pathophysiologic processes leading to IUFD: *Maternal vascular perfusion* abnormalities occur due to either global maternal hypotension or intrinsic lesions of centrally located uteroplacental arteries. Rupture of uteroplacental arteries causes *abruptio placenta*, while venous disruption leads to *marginal abruption*. *Chronic villitis* and *perivillous fibrin(oid) deposition* increase the diffusion distance between maternal and fetal blood at the interhemal membrane. *Fetomaternal hemorrhage* occurs due to rupture of fetal villous capillaries. *Fetal thrombotic vasculopathy, fetal vasculitis* associated with chorioamnionitis or villitis, and *meconium-associated vascular necrosis* form a related group of vasodestructive fetoplacental large vessel lesions that have severe effects on placental and fetal circulatory function. *Umbilical cord occlusion* may lead to complete cessation of blood flow, decreased placental venous return (partial obstruction), or ischemia-reperfusion injury (intermittent obstruction). *Fetal hypoxia* leads to ischemic injury to the fetus and an increase in the number of circulating nucleated red blood cells, and *fetal congestive heart failure* is associated with hydrops fetalis. (Figure 2-1, with permission, from Kraus FT, et al. Placental Pathology, AFIP Atlas of Non-tumor Pathology, First Series, American Registry of Pathology, Washington, DC, 2004.)

of perinatal disease, and may complicate future pregnancies by causing infertility, miscarriage, perinatal morbidity, or an increased risk for adult cardiovascular disease related to intrauterine deprivation (fetal origins of adult diseases) [3, 4]. IUFD in normal fetuses, on the other hand, are usually due to exogenous factors such as infection or sudden random events affecting the maternal or fetal circulations.

The underlying mechanisms leading to IUFD in the non-malformed fetus are incompletely understood. There are two broad subgroups; extrinsic factors such as infection (also see Chapter 5), trauma, toxins, drugs of abuse, and severe

psychosocial stress and processes intrinsic to the maternal–placental–fetal unit. The latter include underlying conditions affecting the pregnant mother, inadequate development of the maternal supply line to the placenta (failure of uterine vascular remodeling), intraplacental abnormalities that interfere with gas exchange in the distal villi (thromboinflammatory lesions, also see Chapter 9), processes that obstruct fetal blood flow from the proximal villi through the umbilical cord (UC) (fetoplacental large vessel lesions), and intrinsic problems affecting the fetus (Figure 10.1). In many cases there are abnormalities in more than one of these categories. While no one by itself is sufficient to cause death, these processes can synergize to cause IUFD.

Many classification systems have been devised over the past 25 years in an attempt to better understand IUFD. A handful of recent systems have successfully reduced the numbers of unclassifiable cases, improved interobserver reproducibility, and pinpointed specific areas for further research, quality improvement, and changes in public health policy. Of particular note are the Tulip, ANZAC, and CODAC systems [5]. However, classification is not explanation (for more information on classification of stillbirth, see Chapter 3). The goal of the remainder of this chapter is to concentrate on the pathologist's approach to individual cases in terms of assembling the relevant historical data, evaluating pathologic processes that may progress to IUFD, and assigning cause (or causes) of death (COD), associated conditions, and the most plausible causal pathway [6].

General role of pathologist

Priority number one in the investigation of IUFD is to insure that the placenta is available for examination. It has been estimated that the placenta reveals the primary COD in 60–70% of all IUFD [7, 8]. This should be of no surprise when one considers that the placenta is both the sole mediator of sustenance and homeostasis in utero and the only protection for the fetus from deleterious processes originating in the environment (trauma, toxins, infections) or the mother (disorders of maternal homeostasis, alloimmunity).

The second priority is a careful and timely review of the maternal history, clinical laboratory results, and antenatal imaging studies. This will pinpoint underlying risk factors and evolving gestational problems and guide the selection of appropriate postmortem testing. Minimum and common ancillary samples required to assess IUFD are listed in Table 10.1. It is not outside the pathologist's role to inform clinicians of supplementary parental testing that may be needed based on the initial pathologic findings.

While it is beyond the scope of this chapter to provide a detailed protocol for the fetal autopsy

Table 10.1 Studies to be obtained at the time of initial evaluation.

Critical	Fetal autopsy (permit required) Pathologic examination of placenta and umbilical cord Maternal Kleihauer-Betke/flow cytometry for fetal hemoglobin
Selected cases	Indirect Coombs (antibody screen) Maternal–paternal cross-match TORCH/syphilis serology Parvovirus B19 serology (IgG and IgM) Glycohemoglobin analysis Coagulation profile Maternal thyroid panel Fetal and/or placental karyotype Placental chromosome analysis by CGH Urine toxicology

[9–11], the approach to IUFD varies sufficiently from that of other children and adults that some general comments may be useful. One challenge that stands out above all of the others is severe autolysis (maceration) owing to a prolonged interval between fetal death and delivery which complicates a significant proportion of IUFD [12]. There are at least six common IUFD archetypes encountered upon gross examination by the pathologist, each with a distinct differential diagnosis. Four show recognizable abnormalities: (1) the premature fetus with an UC stricture, (2) the long, thin growth-restricted fetus with a thin UC and markedly reduced subcutaneous fat, (3) the macrosomic fetus with excessive amounts of subcutaneous fat, and (4) the hydropic fetus with serosal effusions (Figure 10.2). The other two are externally normal; the well preserved, structurally normal previable fetus and the normally grown term fetus with only nonspecific findings such as generalized pallor or areas of localized or diffuse plethora.

External examination of the fetus should include liberal use of photographs and X-rays to document gross findings and rule out skeletal abnormalities. Precise fetal measurements to assess intrauterine growth and development are critical. External

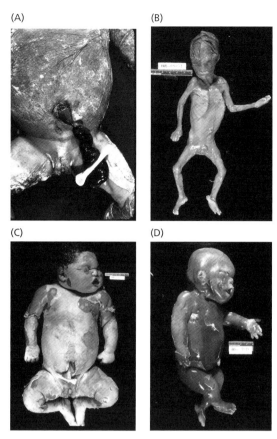

(A) (B)

(C) (D)

Figure 10.2 Common abnormal gross phenotypes associated with IUFD: (A) macerated, premature stillborn fetus with a distinct UC stricture approximately 1–2 cm from the abdominal insertion site. (B) Well-preserved, premature IUFD with marked fetal growth restriction, decreased extracellular fluid volume, decreased subcutaneous fat, and muscle wasting. (C) Macerated, macrosomic term IUFD, born to a diabetic mother, with markedly increased subcutaneous fat. (D) Mildly autolyzed, near-term fetus with hydrops fetalis showing subcutaneous edema, protuberant abdomen (ascites and/or hepatomegaly), and glistening skin (transudation of extracellular fluid).

measurements should include fetal weight, crown-heel length, crown-rump length, head circumference and biauricular arc, foot length, and inner and outer canthal distances. These should be compared to expected values for both birthweight and the clinically estimated GA. Foot and crown-rump lengths

tend to correlate with true GA even in the presence of marked autolysis and/or FGR. The use of postmortem radiographs to estimate GA based on the appearance of epiphyseal centers may also be useful in some instances.

The internal examination should begin with a careful gross inspection of the organs in situ including opening of the heart along the pattern of flow. This screening technique rapidly identifies those fetuses with malformations, which can then be investigated in more detail. Serosal effusions are never an expected finding in IUFD. Even small amounts of fluid in the pleural cavities should raise the issue of HF and prompt an appropriate work up (discussed later). Petechial hemorrhages on the surfaces of thoracic viscera (heart, lungs, thymus) develop as a consequence of negative intrathoracic pressure and suggest a sudden stressful terminal event such as an UC accident or abruptio placenta. They, along with massive aspiration of amniotic fluid squamous cells into the distal airspaces of the lung, are indicators of terminal gasping. Comparing observed versus expected organ weights and relating organ weights to one another are also important components of the autopsy in IUFD. Certain processes such as chronic stress selectively decrease thymus and adrenal weights. Elevated brain to liver weight ratio may suggest FGR, even when severe maceration, unknown GA, and uncertain interval between death and delivery make this assessment problematic [13]. With regard to the latter, timing of death relative to delivery can be accurately assessed in most cases using published tables of gross and histologic changes documented to occur at varying intervals after demise [14–16]. Examination of the brain can be challenging in macerated IUFD, but should never be omitted. Important gross central nervous system abnormalities such as hemorrhages or major malformations may be recognized in even the most autolyzed specimens. Special techniques such as removing the brain under water, prefixation in Bouin's solution, or fetal MRI may be useful in selected cases.

Autopsy bacterial cultures from multiple sites (usually heart, lung, and spleen) should always be performed. This applies even with severely macerated fetuses or after a prolonged postmortem interval. Since the uterus is normally a sterile environment, the identification of any organism may be significant. On the other hand, histology, immunohistochemical staining, and serology are generally more effective methods than culture for the diagnosis of viral infections. Placental bacterial cultures are of limited utility since contamination is frequent and acute chorioamnionitis is a reliable indicator of infection. Placental infection alone would only rarely an acceptable COD (see later) and autopsy cultures will identify those organisms that have escaped from the placenta to enter the fetus.

The final responsibility of the pathologist, in conjunction with the clinical care team, is to determine the COD. COD has been defined as either the initial event in a causal chain of related circumstances or the last significant event in a series of unrelated circumstances [6]. It has been suggested that more than one COD may be assigned for many cases, but that these should be cited in order of likelihood and/or magnitude of effect. It has also been proposed that a COD should have an a priori likelihood of lethality in at least 1/20 affected fetuses (i.e., $p > 0.05$). While the latter suggestion seems reasonable in principle, it may not always be easy to apply. An important concept is that many conditions associated with IUFD are most reliably diagnosed by constellations of findings; the more related abnormalities identified the more certain the final diagnosis. An example would be severe maternal malperfusion of the placenta where FGR, maternal hypertension, high fetoplacental weight ratio, thin UC, and the typical villous changes discussed in the next section would all reinforce one another. In addition to COD, associated conditions including maternal diseases, underlying risk factors, and environmental stressors should be clearly identified and listed along with the COD. Finally, in a summary paragraph the pathologist should characterize the temporal sequence for each insult in terms of weeks (chronic), days (subacute), and hours (acute) before death and provide a plausible narrative of the causal pathway, the potential risk of recurrence, and any further testing required to make a more definitive diagnosis.

Specific conditions

Infections (also see Chapter 5)

Infections occurring during pregnancy account for approximately 10–15% of all IUFD, with increased prevalence at less than 34 weeks GA (Table 10.2) [1]. Purely maternal infections are relatively uncommon causes of IUFD. Circulatory collapse and global hypoperfusion of the fetoplacental unit is one potential mechanism. Gram-negative bacterial sepsis, toxic shock syndrome caused by bacterial superantigens associated with gram-positive organisms such as staphylococci, and H1N1 influenza virus infections are examples of this pathway. A second purely maternal mechanism would be localized infections such as acute appendicitis or pyelonephritis which can

Table 10.2 Infectious causes of IUFD.

Maternal	Bacterial septic shock
	Systemic viral syndromes (e.g., Influenza H1N1)
	Disseminated and/or endometrial tuberculosis
	Urinary tract infections (PTD-previable)
Uterine	Chronic deciduitis (PTD-previable)
	Bacterial vaginosis (PTD-previable)
Placental	Acute chorioamnionitis (PTD-previable)
	Chronic intervillositis (malaria)
Fetoplacental	Viruses:
	CMV
	Other herpesviruses: VZV, HSV, EBV
	Other: rubella, poxviruses
	Protozoans:
	Toxoplasma
	Trypanosoma cruzi
	Bacteria:
	Listeria
	Aerobic: group B streptococci, other streptococci, enteric bacilli
	Anaerobic: Fusobacteria
	Spirochetes: Syphilis
Fetal	Viruses:
	Parvovirus B19, Coxsackie A or B, enteroviruses
	Bacteria:
	B. burgdorfi (Lyme disease)

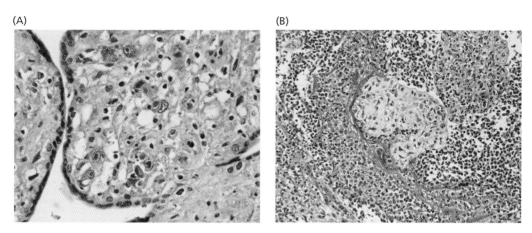

Figure 10.3 Infections associated with IUFD: (A) *Cytomegalovirus* placentitis with numerous viral inclusions, scattered lymphocytes, and degenerating erythrocytes and endothelial cells in the villous stroma (hematoxylin and eosin, 20×). (B) *Listeria monocytogenes* infection with acute (neutrophilic) villitis and intervillous abscess formation (hematoxylin and eosin, 20×).

be associated with high circulating concentrations of pathogen-associated molecular products (PAMPs) that can bind toll-like receptors (TLRs) in the placental membranes triggering preterm labor and delivery in the previable stage.

Chronic hematogenous infections of the placenta are most commonly associated with organisms of the so-called TORCH group (toxoplasmosis, "others," rubella virus, cytomegalovirus [CMV], herpes simplex virus) [17]. These organisms infect both placenta and fetus and generally elicit both maternal and fetal inflammatory responses (chronic placentitis) [18, 19]. CMV is the most common of the TORCH infections and may be detected by typical placental features such as inclusions, villous plasma cells, and prominent fetal capillary damage (Figure 10.3A). Toxoplasmosis and other selected infections (syphilis, varicella zoster, herpes simplex, EBV, and Chagas disease) should also be considered in the appropriate clinical situations. Rubella is vanishingly rare in the postvaccine era. Most TORCH infections occur in previously unexposed mothers and require high viral loads to spread to the placenta, so recurrence is unusual. However, different CMV serotypes are well-documented causes of recurrent fetal infection in previously immune mothers [20]. Acute infection by *Listeria monocytogenes* is a rare cause

of IUFD, usually occurring in the setting of food-borne epidemics. Organisms seed the decidua and spread to adjacent anchoring villi via binding to trophoblast E-cadherin molecules [21]. They can then spread upward within the villous stroma causing an acute villitis with intervillous abscesses (Figure 10.3B). Disseminated fetal infection (granulomatosis infantiseptica) and IUFD develop in most cases of congenital listeriosis. Two hematogenous infections limited to the placenta can lead to IUFD. Placental malaria is a major cause of FGR and stillbirth in mothers exposed to *Plasmodium falciparum* during travels to endemic areas. Primiparous and previously uninfected mothers are at highest risk. These mothers develop massive sequestration of parasites in the intervillous space of the placenta followed by a vigorous host monocytic response that leads to uteroplacental insufficiency [22]. Finally, animal models and recent case reports suggest that bacteria from women with severe periodontal infections may seed the decidua and placental membranes causing a chorioamnionitis indistinguishable from that caused by contiguous infections (discussed later) [23–25].

Contiguous infections of the placenta are usually caused by cervicovaginal bacteria and mycoplasma that inappropriately gain access to the uterine cavity. Risk factors include premature cervical dilatation, premature rupture of the membranes, and colonization of the vagina by abnormal flora (bacterial vaginosis, group B streptococci). Less-common sources of contiguous infection include adjacent structures (bladder, fallopian tube, pelvic abscess) and the uterus itself (chronic endometritis). The placental pathology of all of these infections is indistinguishable: acute inflammation of the membranes (chorioamnionitis) with or without a fetal inflammatory response involving large fetal blood vessels in the UC (umbilical vasculitis or "funisitis") and chorionic plate (chorionic vasculitis). Severe fetal inflammatory responses associated with chorioamnionitis can cause damage to or lead to thrombosis of these placental blood vessels and may also be associated with high levels of systemic fetal cytokines that can contribute to IUFD [26]. Chorioamnionitis should be considered a direct cause of stillbirth in only two situations: (a) when it causes premature delivery of a previable fetus and (b) when there is clear evidence that organisms (and/or PAMPs and other bacterial exotoxins) have breeched the placental barrier to cause fetal circulatory collapse. The latter cases are usually associated with organisms of high pathogenicity such as streptococci, gram-negative bacilli, and fusobacteria. While each episode of contiguous infection is an isolated event, recurrence is common especially for IUFD in the previable period.

This is usually the consequence of underlying predisposing risk factors such as cervical insufficiency or persisting reservoirs of potentially pathogenic flora (e.g., group B streptococcal colonization, bacterial vaginosis, chronic salpingitis).

Finally, some organisms may cross the interhemal barrier leading to fetal infections in the absence of placental involvement. Coxsackie A and B viruses, enteroviruses, and parvovirus B19 are prominent examples causing fetal myocarditis, hepatic necrosis, and red blood cell aplasia, respectively. Parvovirus B19 is further discussed later.

Umbilical cord accidents

UC accidents are estimated to be the cause of IUFD in 2–15% of cases. While they can occur at any GA, they are most frequently implicated after 34 weeks. It is important to accurately identify these cases because they represent random events that are unlikely to occur in subsequent pregnancies. The underlying mechanism of death for UC accidents is compression-related obstruction of umbilical venous blood flow leading to fetal hypoxemia, hypovolemia, and, when intermittent, ischemia-reperfusion injury. Risk factors include hyper-coiling (more than 2–3 coils per 10 cm), long UC (>70 cm), and UC entanglement (Figure 10.4A) [27, 28]. Entanglements (nuchal or body cords) are observed at delivery in 30–40% of pregnancies [29].

(A)

(B)

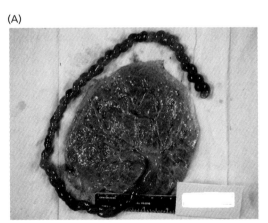
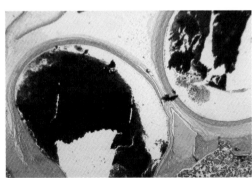

Figure 10.4 Umbilical cord accidents: (A) placenta from a stillborn fetus showing a long, excessively coiled, and macerated umbilical cord. (B) Chorionic plate showing marked dilatation of large veins consistent with upstream umbilical cord occlusion.

However, entanglements at delivery are not considered to be reliable indicators of intrauterine UC compression. Serial ultrasonography in late pregnancy has documented that 60% of mothers have at least one episode of UC entanglement during the last 4 weeks of pregnancy, but that only 8% have persistence on two consecutive examinations [30]. The latter group has been shown to be at increased risk for neurodevelopmental abnormalities at 1 year of age [31]. Entanglements may be especially important in the setting of a previously active fetus with subsequent reduction in amniotic fluid (oligohydramnios) which can both prevent the fetus from becoming disentangled and increase the risk of compression by decreasing the distance between the fetus and the uterine wall. This scenario is commonly observed in postdates pregnancies. Another situation with increased risk is where the placental end of the UC passes under the fetal end. This can result in a true UC knot if the UC loop passes over the fetal head (Type B nuchal UC) [32]. The UC may also, in some cases, precede the presenting fetal part during parturition leading to UC prolapse and intrapartum IUFD. Other UC abnormalities that can act independently or in concert with long, hypercoiled, and/or entangled UC include membranous or furcate placental UC insertion, decreased Wharton's jelly, amnionic tethering of the UC to the fetal surface of the placenta, and encirclement of the UC by amnionic bands [33].

The challenge with UC problems is to distinguish those that critically decrease umbilical blood flow to the fetus from those that are incidental findings. Traditionally, observations such as evidence of UC damage at the site of compression, differences in UC caliber and color between the fetal and placental ends, deformation of fetal structures encircled by the entanglement, and signs of acute fetal hypoxia (massive aspiration of amniotic fluid contents, petechia on the thoracic viscera, increased extramedullary hematopoiesis) and cardiac decompensation (right ventricular dilatation, peripheral congestion, and edema) have been used to support this diagnosis. Unfortunately, these findings are either rare or relatively nonspecific and a diagnosis of UC accident as a cause of IUFD has been

viewed with skepticism by many observers. Recent studies by Boyd and colleagues [34, 35] have made a significant contribution by validating a set of placental criteria that can reproducibly distinguish IUFD secondary to UC accidents from other IUFD. These include marked dilatation of chorionic plate and adjacent stem villous veins (Figure 10.4B) relative to arteries, very recent venous thrombi, and evidence of localized downstream villous changes associated with decreased blood flow (see later). Using these criteria they estimate that 42% of IUFD show evidence of UC accidents. Another finding that can support a diagnosis of prolonged partial/intermittent UC occlusion is an increased number of circulating fetal nucleated red blood cells (NRBCs) within the placental capillaries. Sustained, significant hypoxia of 6–12 or more hours in duration triggers the premature release of red blood cell precursors (NRBCs) from sites of fetal hematopoiesis. A finding of more than one NRBC per high-power field in the placenta has been correlated with an absolute neonatal count of >2,500 $NRBC/mm^3$ and is the only method for assessing this parameter in IUFD, particularly in the absence of a fetal autopsy [36].

UC strictures, predominantly seen in previable IUFD, are a special type of UC anomaly (Figure 10.1A). These strictures are most frequently seen near the fetal insertion site, may be single or multiple, and can in some cases be associated with UC hypercoiling [37, 38]. A few reports suggest that they may recur in subsequent pregnancies. However, recurrence does not seem to have a genetic basis as determined by twin studies [39]. While strictures clearly can occasionally be observed in recent IUFD, they are much more common in the markedly macerated fetus raising the question of whether they may be postmortem artifacts. This is particularly true for isolated strictures at the fetal cord insertion site where there is a well-known physiologic narrowing of the umbilical vein that begins after mid-trimester [40]. Factors supporting a truly significant UC stricture are the same as those listed earlier for UC entanglements (fibrosis, thrombus, old hemosiderin deposits) with emphasis on local changes at the stricture site.

Table 10.3 Chronic placental dysfunction ("uteroplacental insufficiency").

Maternal malperfusion
  Large infarcts
  Severe chronic underperfusion

Thromboinflammatory lesions
  Chronic villitis ("villitis of unknown etiology")
  Massive perivillous fibrin(oid) deposition ("maternal floor infarction")
  Chronic histiocytic intervillositis

Fetal vascular obstruction
  Fetal thrombotic vasculopathy
  Vasodestructive large vessel lesions (inflammatory, toxic)

Chronic peripheral separation ("chronic abruption")
  Developmental abnormalities
  Large or multiple chorangiomas
  Extensive multifocal chorangiomatosis
  Mesenchymal dysplasia
  Dysmorphic villi (?confined placental mosaicism)

Multifactorial (two or more of the above)

Chronic placental dysfunction ("uteroplacental insufficiency")

Chronic placental disorders beginning weeks to months before birth are major causes of FGR and play an important role in many IUFD [41]. These processes can be considered a direct COD in three instances: (1) when sufficiently severe as to exceed placental reserve (estimated at 30–40%), (2) when two or more unrelated severe chronic disorders are observed in the same placenta (estimated to occur in 3% of IUFD) [42], and (3) when associated with catastrophic secondary sequela such as abruptio placenta, occlusive umbilical vein thrombosis, or massive fetomaternal hemorrhage (discussed later). There are five major chronic patterns of placental injury (Table 10.3).

The most common chronic pattern is that of villous findings consistent with maternal vascular malperfusion occurring secondary to inadequate remodeling of the maternal arteries. These findings include villous infarcts, distal villous hypoplasia, increased syncytial knots, excessive intervillous fibrin, and villous agglutination and are observed in approximately 30% of IUFD (Figure 10.5A)

[43]. Maternal arteries in these cases not only lack remodeling, but often develop pathologic changes such as mural hypertrophy, subintimal fibrosis, and, in some cases, fibrinoid necrosis of the vascular wall. The latter lesion, known as acute atherosis, is primarily seen in association with preeclampsia and is strongly associated with rupture of the spiral arteries, presenting clinically as abruptio placenta. Maternal arteriopathy has been reported in 5% of placentas from IUFD.

Although precise numbers are not available, the next most common chronic disorder in IUFD is probably fetal thrombotic vasculopathy (FTV). FTV is defined by the finding of extensive avascular villi (average of more than 15 per section) and is attributable to upstream fetal vascular obstruction (Figure 10.5B) [44]. Obstruction is usually due to large vessel thrombi, which are documented in 30–45% of affected placentas. Earlier villous changes indicating obstruction include stromal vascular karyorrhexis, previously known as hemorrhagic endovasculitis and fibromuscular sclerosis of stem villous vessels. FTV is sometimes a systemic fetal disease with thrombosis or thromboemboli in the liver, kidney, GI tract, or central nervous system [45, 46]. In live-born infants, FTV is also associated with thrombocytopenia [33]. The most common risk factor for FTV is chronic partial/intermittent UC obstruction [33]. Other risk factors include inherited fetal coagulation disorders, circulating maternal antiphospholipid or antiplatelet antibodies, and diabetic pregnancy. FTV must be carefully distinguished from the normal villous involutional changes that accompany IUFD. These latter changes are diffuse, temporally equivalent in all villi, and unassociated with fetal thrombosis.

Chronic villitis (commonly referred to as villitis of unknown etiology, VUE) is caused by maternal lymphocytes gaining access to the placental villi with an accompanying allograft response resembling graft-versus-host disease [47]. Placentas with VUE show focal-diffuse chronic inflammation of the villous stroma with variable amounts of villous agglutination and surrounding fibrin deposition (Figure 10.5C). Although VUE is more common than FTV, affecting approximately 5–7% of all term gestations, it is less commonly extensive enough

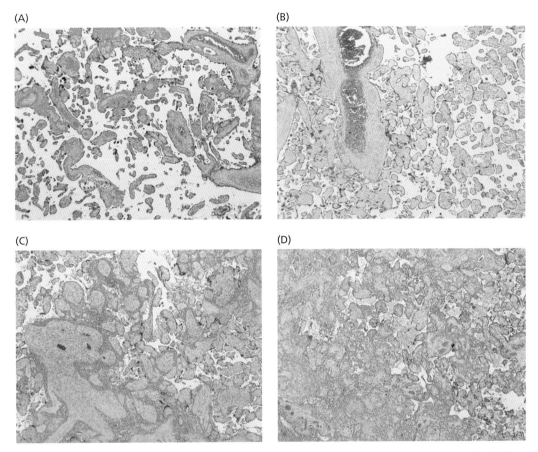

Figure 10.5 Chronic placental dysfunction: (A) *villous changes consistent with severe maternal malperfusion*: distal villous hypoplasia, villous agglutination, increased intervillous fibrin, and focally increased syncytial knots (hematoxylin and eosin, 4×). (B) *fetal thrombotic vasculopathy*: large branching stem villus with fibromuscular sclerosis of large vessels and extensive downstream avascular villi (consistent with upstream thrombosis). Note normally vascularized villi from an adjacent unaffected stem villus on the right (hematoxylin and eosin, 4×). (C) *Diffuse chronic villitis* with associated perivillous fibrin. Large areas of contiguous villi are suffused by a chronic lymphohistiocytic inflammatory infiltrate (hematoxylin and eosin, 4×). (D) *Diffuse perivillous fibrinoid deposition ("maternal floor infarction"):* placental parenchyma with encasement of distal villi by fibrin and extracellular matrix material (hematoxylin and eosin, 4×).

to be considered as a primary COD. A distinct subgroup of women presents with diffuse VUE that accelerates in severity in subsequent pregnancies suggesting maternal priming to fetal alloantigens. This group is most at risk for IUFD. The recurrence risk for diffuse VUE is approximately 25–33% [48]. While some fetal diseases such as neonatal hemochromatosis and biliary atresia have been linked to maternal chimerism, no well-documented case of maternal lymphocyte spread from VUE to

the fetus has been reported [49, 50]. VUE with severe involvement of large placental stem villi may cause fetal vascular occlusion (obliterative fetal vasculopathy) with downstream changes similar to those seen with FTV [44]. It is important to distinguish these entities in IUFD since only VUE has a significant recurrence risk.

Massive perivillous fibrin(oid) deposition (commonly referred to as maternal floor infarction, MFI) is a rare idiopathic condition associated with accumulation of matrix glycoproteins, fibrin, and extravillous trophoblast around large portions of the distal villous tree (Figure 10.5C) [51, 52]. MFI may present alone or as an uncommon complication of severe maternal malperfusion or autoimmune disease. Some studies have linked it to fetal LCHAD deficiency or defects in maternal fibrinolysis [53, 54]. The pathologic findings are most consistent with diffuse villous trophoblast damage leading to both local activation of the maternal clotting cascade and metaplasia of villous cytotrophoblast to a matrix-secreting extravillous phenotype. MFI primarily affects pregnancies of <34 weeks GA, has a high rate of progression to IUFD, and has an extremely high recurrence rate (30–75% in various studies) [55]. An even less-common condition, known as chronic histiocytic intervillositis, is associated with increased perivillous fibrinoid but also shows massive infiltration of the intervillous space by maternal monocyte-macrophages [56]. Findings in this disorder are similar to placental malaria and both are believed to be due to abnormal antigenic stimulation at the interhemal membrane. MFI and chronic histiocytic intervillositis share some clinical features including association with recurrent spontaneous abortion, severe FGR, and very high rates of recurrence in subsequent pregnancies.

The last disorder in this category, chronic peripheral separation (also known as chronic abruption), can be a cause of mild FGR and very early preterm delivery with previable IUFD [57]. Chronic abruption often begins in the first trimester with vaginal bleeding (threatened abortion) and can be detected at that time by ultrasound as a subchorionic hematoma. If bleeding continues, the subchorionic hematoma can give rise to findings consistent with chronic abruption which include organizing marginal hematomas, circumvallate membrane insertion, and rupture into the amniotic cavity with diffuse chorioamnionic hemosiderin deposition. Recurrence of chronic abruption has not been reported.

In addition to the five chronic patterns of placental injury described earlier, primary developmental abnormalities of the placenta can also cause chronic dysfunction contributing to IUFD. These processes include disorders of fetoplacental

vasculogenesis (large chorangiomas or extensive multifocal chorangiomatosis), dysmorphic villous architecture (enlarged edematous stem villi, abnormal villous branching, and shape abnormalities), and diffuse placental mesenchymal dysplasia which can include all of the above features and has been associated in some cases with Beckwith-Wiedmann syndrome [58–62]. There is some evidence suggesting that dysmorphic villi may also be a marker for confined placental mosaicism which has been associated with IUFD [63–65]. Rare families with repetitive IUFD associated with extremely large numbers of placental chorangiomas have been reported [66].

Hemorrhages

Disruptions in the integrity of the maternal circulation are important causes of IUFD. Rarely, in traumatic or spontaneous rupture of a nonuterine maternal vessel, such an aneurysm can cause IUFD secondary to severe hypotension and fetal hypoperfusion. Much more common is premature separation of the uterus from the placenta, so-called abruption. Abruption can be separated into two major categories, abruptio placenta and marginal abruption (also known as peripheral separation) [67]. In abruptio placenta, one or more of the maternal spiral arteries ruptures causing sudden separation of the placenta from its blood supply. Abruptio placenta is distinguished from marginal abruption by its more central location, indentation and/or disruption of the basal plate, and forceful spread of blood within the decidua and behind the membranes (Figure 10.6A). Arterial rupture often occurs in abnormal vessels (e.g., fibrinoid necrosis of the arterial wall in preeclampsia, as discussed earlier) or vessels damaged by ischemia-reperfusion injury (e.g., maternal cocaine, methamphetamine, or nicotine use). Marginal abruptions occur due to rupture of uterine veins, usually at the peripheral edge of the placenta. While these hemorrhages may occasionally be sufficiently extensive to cause IUFD by hypoxia alone, they much more commonly lead to preterm labor and previable IUFD. They are often the final common pathway leading to delivery for other processes such as acute chorioamnionitis, premature cervical dilatation, and

(A)   (B)

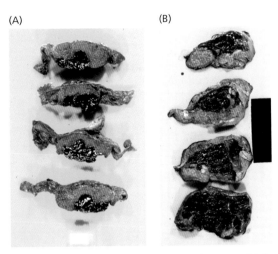

Figure 10.6 Hemorrhages: (A) *abruptio placenta:* multiple cross sections of the placenta show a large retroplacental blood clot indenting the basal plate and extending into the placental parenchyma. (B) *Massive subchorial thrombohematoma:* multiple cross sections of the placenta show a large intervillous blood clot accumulating beneath and raising the chorionic plate.

preterm premature rupture of membranes. All the above mechanisms, maternal hypotension, and disruption of uterine arteries and veins contribute to IUFD in scenarios such as uterine rupture (usually due to dehiscence of a previous C-section scar) and acceleration–deceleration injuries such as motor vehicle accidents.

Significant fetal hemorrhages are less common. They may be sudden and catastrophic when over 20% of blood volume is lost precipitously or more gradual with the progressive onset of fetal anemia and congestive heart failure (HF). Distal villous rupture leading to fetal bleeding into the maternal intervillous space (fetomaternal hemorrhage) has been estimated to occur in 6–14% of IUFD. Most fetomaternal hemorrhages are small and sealed off by the formation of intervillous thrombi, but some remain patent allowing substantial proportions of the total fetal blood volume to escape [68–70]. While placental findings such as multiple large intervillous thrombi, villous edema, and increased circulating NRBCs may be suggestive of fetomaternal hemorrhage, the diagnosis can only be proven

by Kleihauer-Betke or flow cytometric analysis of maternal blood samples for fetal hemoglobin containing cells in the days following delivery. Small numbers of fetal cells are detected by these techniques in up to 50% of pregnancies and 8% of pregnancies have estimated fetomaternal hemorrhages of up to 40 ml. Larger volume hemorrhages occur in less than 1% of pregnancies and are potentially lethal. False-positive tests can occur in maternal hemoglobinopathies which may be associated with persistence of fetal hemoglobin. False negatives can occur with maternal–fetal blood group incompatibility leading to rapid clearance of fetal cells from the maternal circulation. Rupture of an intramembranous fetal placental vessel (ruptured vasa previa) with vaginal bleeding is another rare cause of IUFD. Other intraplacental processes that can potentially sequester large volumes of fetal blood include massive subchorial thrombohematoma (Figure 10.6B) and large subamnionic or intrafunicular (UC) hemorrhages [71]. Significant hematomas can also accumulate within the fetus. Potential sites include liver, adrenals, kidneys, retroperitoneum, and various locations within and adjacent to the calvarium (e.g., germinal matrix, subarachnoid, subdural, subgaleal, cephalohematoma).

Hydrops fetalis

Fetal congestive heart failure, otherwise known as HF, is an uncommon but easily missed contributor to IUFD, particularly in its early stages [72]. Typical early findings include scant pleural effusions, mild cardiomegaly, and right atrioventricular dilatation in the fetus combined with a stereotypical pattern of villous edema with a thickened bilayer of villous trophoblast that is often artifactually separated from the underlying stroma in the placenta (Figure 10.7A). HF can be separated into two broad categories, cases with and without fetal anemia (Table 10.4).

Sensitization to Rh-D was the most common cause of HF and amongst the most common overall causes of IUFD in the era before routine use of Rh immune globulin. More recently, the most common causes of HF with fetal anemia are chronic fetomaternal hemorrhage and parvovirus

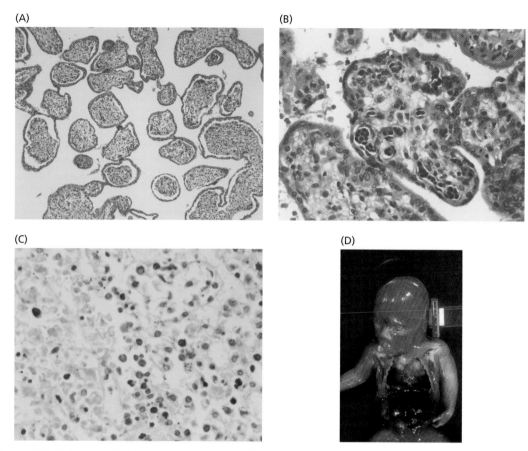

Figure 10.7 Hydrops fetalis: (A) *villous hydrops:* distal villi with diffuse edema and characteristic artifactual detachment of thick villous trophoblast bilayer from the villous stroma (hematoxylin and eosin, 10×). (B) *Erythroblastosis:* fetal villous capillaries are engorged by clusters of immature red blood cell precursors (hematoxylin and eosin, 40×). (C) *human parvovirus B19* infection: erythrocyte inclusions (smudged red glassy center with irregular dark-blue edge) in a section of macerated liver (hematoxylin and eosin, 40×). (D) *mediastinal teratoma:* hydropic fetus with a large obstructing mass within the opened chest cavity.

B19 infection [73]. As discussed earlier, feto-maternal hemorrhages contribute to 6–14% of IUFD. However, the proportion in which chronic hemorrhage leads to severe anemia, high output congestive heart, and HF is much lower. Likewise, it has been stated that 7.5% of IUFD are associated with Parvovirus B19 infection, but in my own experience the number resulting in HF is much lower. While reduced in frequency, blood group incompatibility remains an important cause of HF. In addition to residual cases of Rh-D sensitization, isoimmunization to Rh-C, -c and -e, ABO, Kell,

Duffy, and a handful of other common blood group antigens can also cause HF. When the maternal antibody screen is negative, testing for rare so-called private antigens by performing a maternal–paternal cross-match may also be considered. Other causes of severe anemia with hydrops include G6PD deficiency, alpha thalassemia, and congenital dys-erythropoietic anemia. Cases of HF secondary to severe fetal anemia are often characterized by hepatomegaly due to increased extramedullary hematopoiesis and diffuse erythroblastosis, which can be seen in either fetal or placental capillaries

Table 10.4 Differential diagnosis of hydrops fetalis.

Anemia	
Immune	Rh-D
	Other common antigens (Rh-C,-c, or -e; Kell, Duffy, ABO)
	Rare or "private" antigens
Nonimmune	Parvovirus B19
	Massive fetomaternal hemorrhage
	Hemolysis: alpha thalassemia, G6PD deficiency
	Hypoproliferative (congenital dyserythropoietic)
Other	
Cardiovascular	Decreased venous return: thoracic or abdominal mass lesions, fetoplacental venous thrombosis
	Cardiac arrhythmias: supraventricular tachycardia, congenital heart block
	Right heart malformations: Ebstein anomaly, atrioventricular canal
	Arteriovenous shunts: fetal tumors, placental chorangioma, arteriovenous malformations
	Lymphatic anomalies: Primary lymphangiectasia, Down syndrome, Turner syndrome, Noonan syndrome, Lethal multiple pterygium syndrome
Hepatic	CMV, perinatal hemochromatosis, thrombotic liver disease, metabolic storage disease
Renal	Congenital nephrotic syndromes, renal vein thrombus

(Figure 10.7B). Parvovirus inclusions are occasionally observed in the placenta, but are most reliably found at fetal sites of extramedullary hematopoiesis such as the liver (Figure 10.7C).

Other causes of congestive heart failure leading to HF include decreased venous return due to obstructing mass lesions (e.g., mediastinal teratoma [Figure 10.7D], cystic adenomatoid malformation, peritoneal cyst) or placental venous thrombosis (FTV, umbilical vein thrombus), cardiac arrhythmias (supraventricular tachycardia, congenital heart block), right-sided cardiac malformations (Ebstein anomaly, hypoplastic right ventricle), cardiomyopathies (myocarditis, metabolic storage

diseases, mitochondriopathies), arteriovenous shunts (placental chorangioma, arteriovenous malformations, congenital tumors), and fetal lymphatic anomalies (primary lymphangiectasia, Turner syndrome, other chromosomal abnormalities). Less commonly, diffuse edema with HF can develop secondary to decreased plasma oncotic pressure. Reduced fetal serum total protein concentration due to congenital liver diseases (e.g., CMV infection, metabolic storage disease, perinatal hemochromatosis, thrombotic liver disease) or congenital nephrotic syndromes (Finnish nephropathy, diffuse mesangial sclerosis, Denys-Drash syndrome) are the most common causes.

Placental dysmaturity

The concept of "placental maturation defect," also known as distal villous immaturity, in the context of IUFD was first introduced by Stallmach who found this process in 2.3% of all IUFD at term [74]. The lesion is defined by a constellation of findings including enlarged distal villi with numerous central capillaries, abundant villous stroma, a uniform thick layer of syncytiotrophoblast and, most importantly, a deficiency in the number of vasculosyncytial membranes (Figure 10.8). The latter are specialized regions of close apposition between syncytiotrophoblast and fetal villous capillary endothelium. They are critical for efficient gas exchange in the third trimester as respiratory and metabolic demands accelerate when growth of the fetus outpaces that of the placenta. The villous structural changes all act to increase the diffusion distance across the interhemal membrane decreasing both overall placental efficiency and reserve to withstand acute stress. Placental maturation defect is most commonly observed in placentas from diabetic pregnancies, particularly those from mothers with poor glucose control. Diabetic pregnancies are well known to be at risk for late IUFD and other factors such as the increased demand due to excessive placental and fetal mass, underlying maternal vascular disease, and metabolic derangements associated with the diabetic state may also contribute to this risk. Other conditions associated with placental maturation defects include maternal obesity, excessive pregnancy weight gain, HF,

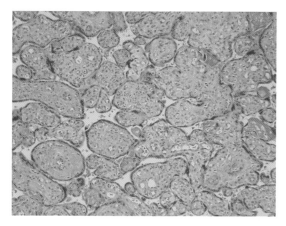

Figure 10.8 Placental maturation defect (distal villous immaturity): enlarged, histologically immature distal villi in the placenta of a term IUFD with a diabetic mother. Villous stroma is excessive. Trophoblast is thickened. Capillaries are predominantly centrally located and there is a deficiency of vasculosyncytial membranes (hematoxylin and eosin, 10×).

hypercoiling of the UC, chromosomal abnormalities, and the group of dysmorphic developmental placental lesions discussed earlier [75].

Intrinsic maternal

Several of the maternal conditions linked to IUFD in the absence of fetoplacental abnormalities including trauma, severe systemic disease, uterine rupture, and cervical insufficiency have already been discussed. Intrahepatic cholestasis of pregnancy, a rare disorder linked to mutations of the MDR3 bile transporter in some cases, has been associated with increased rates of IUFD [76]. This association seems to be restricted to mothers with very high circulating levels of bile acids that may cross the placenta and interfere with fetal cardiomyocyte function [77]. Maternal syndromes associated with episodic hypotension have been implicated in IUFD by other authors [78, 79]. Maternal obesity, advanced maternal age, and infertility constitute a sometimes overlapping group of risk factors implicated in IUFD [80–82]. Interestingly, these same risk factors have been associated with increased IUFD in captive baboon populations [83]. The underlying mechanisms

for IUFD in this scenario are poorly understood, but may relate to abnormal uterine receptivity to placentation and abnormal maternal physiologic accommodation to pregnancy. Markers for poor accommodation to pregnancy including elevated maternal hematocrit due to hemoconcentration, decreased first-trimester maternal serum PAPP-A levels, and increased amniotic fluid activin-A levels have all been associated with IUFD [84–86].

Intrinsic fetal

Amniotic fluid plays a critical role in protecting the fetus and disorders of amniotic fluid volume are important risk factors for IUFD [87]. Amniotic fluid is composed primarily of fetal urine and its volume is regulated by renal function, fetal swallowing, and transepithelial fluid transport across the fetal skin and placental membranes. Decreased fluid volume, oligohydramnios, occurs with premature rupture of membranes, decreased renal perfusion, or intrinsic renal disease and can predispose to UC compression. Increased fluid volume, polyhydramnios, can occur with cardiac failure, abnormalities of swallowing, or, possibly, membrane transport defects and is a risk factor for UC prolapse. However, IUFD in cases of abnormal amniotic fluid volume is not restricted to cases with UC accidents. Fetal stool, meconium, is passed into the amniotic fluid during labor in up to 15% of term gestations. Meconium release prior to labor is much less common and can lead to prolonged exposure to high concentrations of bile acids. These toxic substances can cause vasospasm, vascular necrosis, and sometimes ulceration and vascular rupture in structures with exposed surfaces including the UC, lungs, and chorionic plate [88, 89].

Apart from aneuploidy, genetic syndromes, and major congenital malformations, the question arises as to whether more subtle fetal developmental problems also contribute to IUFD. A variety of observations implicate hidden genetic and epigenetic factors. First, a high proportion of aneuploid fetuses without lethal congenital malformations die in utero without any clear pathologic or physiologic explanation. Second, chromosomally normal fetuses with minor anomalies are at increased risk for IUFD. Third, IUFD is increased in the absence of recognizable anomalies in the offspring of consanguineous unions [90]. These observations suggest that anatomic or physiologic derangements associated with abnormal gene expression may exist that are not detectable with present methods. Noteworthy in this regard are recent reports of a high frequency of anomalous DNA methylation of imprinted genes in male, but not female, IUFD and the identification of neuronal abnormalities in the arcuate nucleus of the medulla oblongata in some IUFD, abnormalities that overlap those described in sudden infant death syndrome [91, 92].

Research priorities

While the search for a COD is important for the understanding and future management of IUFD, identifying a lesion is not equivalent to understanding it, and understanding it does not mean it can be prevented. There are large gaps in our knowledge regarding the basic physiology of successful pregnancy. Minor genetic and epigenetic abnormalities and the genetic background they act upon surely explain many deficiencies in the capacity to form a robust germ cell, support the implantation of a fertilized zygote, and orchestrate the maternal–fetal cross talk required to allow a developing fetus to flourish. Further investigation of these processes is needed to understand how risk factors associated with IUFD such as obesity, ART, advanced maternal age, and recurrent fetal loss act at a mechanistic level. Similarly, the mechanisms of IUFD associated with an abnormal maternal environment in cholestasis of pregnancy, thrombophilia, autoimmunity, environmental exposures, and severe maternal stress are also incompletely understood. With respect to pathology, new methods of genetic testing and structural analysis applied to the fetal autopsy or placental examination have the potential to uncover novel abnormalities. While a large number of placental lesions have been cataloged, we still lack sufficient evidence-based data to assess which lesions or combinations of lesions are most deleterious for fetal well-being. Complete understanding of the underlying causes for some of these lesions is also lacking. Finally, the myriad of new maternal serum and sonographic markers being used for the early prediction of risk for aneuploidy, preeclampsia, and FGR might eventually be useful for identifying women at increased risk for IUFD. All of these gaps in understanding are areas where pathologists with an interest in going beyond identifying a single COD can make a significant contribution in our understanding of IUFD and other adverse pregnancy outcomes.

References

1. Silver RM, Varner MW, Reddy U, et al. Work-up of stillbirth: a review of the evidence. Am J Obstet Gynecol 2007;196(5):433–44.
2. Silver RM. Evaluation of fetal death from nongenetic causes. 2009. www.contemporaryobgyn.net/stillbirth.
3. Getahun D, Lawrence JM, Fassett MJ, et al. The association between stillbirth in the first pregnancy and subsequent adverse perinatal outcomes. Am J Obstet Gynecol 2009;201(4):378e1–6.
4. Byrne CD, Phillips DI. Fetal origins of adult disease: epidemiology and mechanisms. J Clin Pathol 2000;53(11):822–8.
5. Flenady V, Froen JF, Pinar H, et al. An evaluation of classification systems for stillbirth. BMC Pregnancy Childbirth 2009;9:24.
6. Froen JF, Pinar H, Flenady V, et al. Causes of death and associated conditions (Codac): a utilitarian approach to the classification of perinatal deaths. BMC Pregnancy Childbirth 2009;9:22.
7. Korteweg FJ, Erwich JJ, Holm JP, et al. Diverse placental pathologies as the main causes of fetal death. Obstet Gynecol 2009;114(4):809–17.
8. Kidron D, Bernheim J, Aviram R. Placental findings contributing to fetal death, a study of 120 stillbirths between 23 and 40 weeks gestation. Placenta 2009;30(8):700–4.
9. MacPherson T. A model perinatal autopsy protocol. Washington, DC: American Registry of Pathology; 1994.
10. Keeling JW. The perinatal necropsy. In: Keeling JW, Khong TY (eds), Fetal and neonatal pathology, Fourth edition. London, UK: Springer-Verlag; 2007, pp. 20–53.
11. Siebert JR. Perinatal, fetal, and embryonic autopsy. In: Gilbert-Barness E (ed), Potter's pathology of the fetus, infant, and child, Second edition. Philadelphia, PA: Mosby Elsevier; 2007, pp. 695–739.

12. Moore IE. Macerated stillbirth. In: Keeling JW, Khong TY (eds), Fetal and neonatal pathology. London, UK: Springer-Verlag; 2007, pp. 224–39.

13. Mitchell ML. Fetal brain to liver weight ratio as a measure of intrauterine growth retardation: analysis of 182 stillborn autopsies. Mod Pathol 2001;14(1):14–19.

14. Genest DR, Williams MA, Greene MF. Estimating the time of death in stillborn fetuses. 1. Histologic evaluation of fetal organs—an autopsy study of 150 stillborns. Obstet Gynecol 1992;80(4):575–84.

15. Genest DR. Estimating the time of death in stillborn fetuses. 2. Histologic evaluation of the placenta—a study of 71 stillborns. Obstet Gynecol 1992;80(4): 585–92.

16. Genest DR, Singer DB. Estimating the time of death in stillborn fetuses. 3. External fetal examination—a study of 86 stillborns. Obstet Gynecol 1992;80(4): 593–600.

17. Greenough A. The TORCH screen and intrauterine infections. Arch Dis Child 1994;70:F163–5.

18. Bittencourt AL, Garcia AG. The placenta in hematogenous infections. Pediatr Pathol Mol Med 2002;21(4):401–32.

19. Bittencourt AL, Garcia AG. Pathogenesis and pathology of hematogenous infections of the fetus and newborn. Pediatr Pathol Mol Med 2002;21(4):353–99.

20. Yamamoto AY, Mussi-Pinhata MM, Boppana SB, et al. Human cytomegalovirus reinfection is associated with intrauterine transmission in a highly cytomegalovirus-immune maternal population. Am J Obstet Gynecol 2010;202(3):297e1–8.

21. Robbins JR, Skrzypczynska KM, Zeldovich VB, et al. Placental syncytiotrophoblast constitutes a major barrier to vertical transmission of *Listeria monocytogenes*. PLoS Pathog 2010;6(1):e1000732.

22. Rogerson SJ, Pollina E, Getachew A, et al. Placental monocyte infiltrates in response to *Plasmodium falciparum* malaria infection and their association with adverse pregnancy outcomes. Am J Trop Med Hyg 2003;68(1):115–19.

23. Han YW, Redline RW, Li M, et al. *Fusobacterium nucleatum* induces premature and term stillbirths in pregnant mice: implication of oral bacteria in preterm birth. Infect Immun 2004;72(4):2272–9.

24. Han YW, Ikegami A, Bissada NF, et al. Transmission of an uncultivated *Bergeyella* strain from the oral cavity to amniotic fluid in a case of preterm birth. J Clin Microbiol 2006;44(4):1475–83.

25. Han YW, Fardinin Y, Chen C, et al. Term stillbirth caused by oral *Fusobacterium nucleatum*. Obstet Gynecol 2010;115(2, Part 2):1–4.

26. Redline RW. Placental inflammation. Semin Neonatol 2004;9(4):265–74.

27. Machin GA, Ackerman J, Gilbert-Barness E. Abnormal umbilical cord coiling is associated with adverse perinatal outcomes. Pediatr Dev Pathol 2000;3(5): 462–71.

28. Baergen RN, Malicki D, Behling C, Benirschke K. Morbidity, mortality, and placental pathology in excessively long umbilical cords: retrospective study. Pediatr Dev Pathol 2001;4(2):144–53.

29. Hankins GDV, Snyder RR, Hauth JC, et al. Nuchal cords and neonatal outcome. Obstet Gynecol 1987; 70:687–92.

30. Clapp JF, 3rd, Stepanchak W, Hashimoto K, et al. The natural history of antenatal nuchal cords. Am J Obstet Gynecol 2003;189(2):488–93.

31. Clapp JF, 3rd, Lopez B, Simonean S. Nuchal cord and neurodevelopmental performance at 1 year. J Soc Gynecol Investig 1999;6(5):268–72.

32. Collins JH. Nuchal cord type A and type B. Am J Obstet Gynecol 1997;177(1):94.

33. Redline RW. Clinical and pathological umbilical cord abnormalities in fetal thrombotic vasculopathy. Hum Pathol 2004;35(12):1494–8.

34. Boyd TK, Gang DL, Pflueger S. Mechanical umbilical blood flow obstruction predisposes to placental fetal vascular thrombosis and stillbirth. Pediatr Dev Pathol 2006;9:335.

35. Parast MM, Crum CP, Boyd TK. Placental histologic criteria for umbilical blood flow restriction in unexplained stillbirth. Hum Pathol 2008;39(6):948–53.

36. Redline RW. Elevated circulating fetal nucleated red blood cells and placental pathology in term infants who develop cerebral palsy. Hum Pathol 2008; 39(9):1378–84.

37. Blackburn W, Cooley NR. The umbilical cord. In: Stevenson RE, Hall JG, Goodman RM (eds), Human malformations and related anomalies. New York, NY: Oxford University Press; 1993.

38. Peng HQ, Levitin-Smith M, Rochelson B, Kahn E. Umbilical cord stricture and overcoiling are common causes of fetal demise. Pediatr Dev Pathol 2006;9(1): 14–19.

39. Rodriguez JI, Marino-Enriquez A, Suarez-Aguado J, Lapunzina P. Umbilical cord stricture is not a genetic anomaly: a study in twins. Pediatr Dev Pathol 2008; 11(5):363–9.

40. Skulstad SM, Kiserud T, Rasmussen S. Degree of fetal umbilical venous constriction at the abdominal wall in a low-risk population at 20-40 weeks of gestation. Prenat Diagn 2002;22(11):1022–7.

41. Redline RW, Patterson P. Patterns of placental injury: correlations with gestational age, placental weight, and clinical diagnosis. Arch Pathol Lab Med 1994; 118:698–701.

42. Driscoll S. Autopsy following stillbirth: a challenge neglected. In: Ryder O, Byrd M (eds), One medicine. Berlin: Springer-Verlag; 1984, pp. 20–31.

43. Redline RW, Boyd T, Campbell V, et al. Maternal vascular underperfusion: nosology and reproducibility of placental reaction patterns. Pediatr Dev Pathol 2004;7:237–49.

44. Redline RW, Ariel I, Baergen RN, et al. Fetal vascular obstructive lesions: nosology and reproducibility of placental reaction patterns. Pediat Dev Pathol 2004;7:443–52.

45. Dahms BB, Boyd T, Redline RW. Severe perinatal liver disease associated with fetal thrombotic vasculopathy. Pediatr Dev Pathol 2002;5(1):80–5.

46. Leistra-Leistra MJ, Timmer A, van Spronsen FJ, et al. Fetal thrombotic vasculopathy in the placenta: a thrombophilic connection between pregnancy complications and neonatal thrombosis? Placenta 2004; 25(Suppl. A):S102–5.

47. Redline RW. Villitis of unknown etiology: noninfectious chronic villitis in the placenta. Hum Pathol 2007;38(10):1439–46.

48. Redline RW, Abramowsky CR. Clinical and pathologic aspects of recurrent placental villitis. Hum Pathol 1985;16:727–31.

49. Whitington PF, Malladi P. Neonatal hemochromatosis: is it an alloimmune disease? J Pediatr Gastroenterol Nutr 2005;40(5):544–9.

50. Muraji T, Hosaka N, Irie N, et al. Maternal microchimerism in underlying pathogenesis of biliary atresia: quantification and phenotypes of maternal cells in the liver. Pediatrics 2008;121(3):517–21.

51. Andres RL, Kuyper W, Resnik R, et al. The association of maternal floor infarction of the placenta with adverse perinatal outcome. Am J Obstet Gynecol 1990;163:935–8.

52. Katzman PJ, Genest DR. Maternal floor infarction and massive perivillous fibrin deposition: histological definitions, association with intrauterine fetal growth restriction, and risk of recurrence. Pediatr Dev Pathol 2002;5(2):159–64.

53. Matern D, Schehata BM, Shekhawa P, et al. Placental floor infarction complicating the pregnancy of a fetus with long-chain 3-hydroxyacyl-CoA dehydrogenase (LCHAD) deficiency. Mol Genet Metab 2001;72(3): 265–8.

54. Katz VL, DiTomasso J, Farmer R, Carpenter M. Activated protein C resistance associated with maternal

55. Redline RW. Invited commentary—maternal floor infarction and massive perivillous fibrin deposition: clinicopathologic entities in flux. Adv Anat Pathol 2002;9:372–3.

56. Boyd TK, Redline RW. Chronic histiocytic intervillositis: a placental lesion associated with recurrent reproductive loss. Hum Pathol 2000;31:1389–92.

57. Redline RW, Wilson-Costello D. Chronic peripheral separation of placenta. The significance of diffuse chorioamnionic hemosiderosis. Am J Clin Pathol 1999;111(6):804–10.

58. Tonkin IL, Setzer ES, Ermocilla R. Placental chorangioma: a rare cause of congestive heart failure and hydrops fetalis in the newborn. Am J Roentgenol 1980;134:181–3.

59. Ogino S, Redline RW. Villous capillary lesions of the placenta: distinctions between chorangioma, chorangiomatosis, and chorangiosis. Hum Pathol 2000; 31:945–54.

60. Dicke JM, Huettner P, Yan S, et al. Umbilical artery Doppler indices in small for gestational age fetuses: correlation with adverse outcomes and placental abnormalities. J Ultrasound Med 2009;28(12):1603–10.

61. Jauniaux E, Nicolaides KH, Hustin J. Perinatal features associated with placental mesenchymal dysplasia. Placenta 1997;18:701–6.

62. Pham T, Steele J, Stayboldt C, et al. Placental mesenchymal dysplasia is associated with high rates of intrauterine growth restriction and fetal demise: a report of 11 new cases and a review of the literature. Am J Clin Pathol 2006;126(1):67–78.

63. Wilkins-Haug L, Greene MF, Roberts DJ, Morton CC. Frequency of confined placental mosaicism in pregnancies with intrauterine growth retardation. Am J Obstet Gynecol 1992;166:350.

64. Astner A, Schwinger E, Caliebe A, et al. Sonographically detected fetal and placental abnormalities associated with trisomy 16 confined to the placenta. A case report and review of the literature. Prenat Diagn 1998;18(12):1308–15.

65. Kalousek DK, Barrett I. Confined placental mosaicism and stillbirth. Pediatr Pathol 1994;14(1):151–9.

66. Benirschke K. Recent trends in chorangiomas, especially those of multiple and recurrent chorangiomas. Pediatr Dev Pathol 1999;2:264–9.

67. Redline RW. Placental pathology: a systematic approach with clinical correlations. Placenta 2008; 29(Suppl. A):S86–91.

68. Kaplan C, Blanc WA, Elias J. Identification of erythrocytes in intervillous thrombi: a study using

floor infarction treated with low-molecular-weight heparin. Am J Perinatol 2002;19(5):273–7.

immunoperoxidase identification of hemoglobins. Hum Pathol 1982;13:554–7.

69. de Almeida V, Bowman JM. Massive fetomaternal hemorrhage: Manitoba experience. Obstet Gynecol 1994;83(3):323–8.

70. Biankin SA, Arbuckle SM, Graf NS. Autopsy findings in a series of five cases of fetomaternal haemorrhages. Pathology 2003;35(4):319–24.

71. Shanklin DR, Scott JS. Massive subchorial thrombohaematoma (Breus' mole). Br J Obstet Gynaecol 1975;82:476–87.

72. Machin GA. Hydrops revisited: literature review of 1,414 cases published in the 1980s. Am J Med Genet 1989;34(3):366–90.

73. Morey AL, Keeling JW, Porter HJ, Fleming KA. Clinical and histopathological features of parvovirus B19 infection in the human fetus. Br J Obstet Gynaecol 1992;99:566–74.

74. Stallmach T, Hebisch G, Meier K, et al. Rescue by birth: defective placental maturation and late fetal mortality. Obstet Gynecol 2001;97(4):505–9.

75. de Laat MW, van der Meij JJ, Visser GH, et al. Hypercoiling of the umbilical cord and placental maturation defect: associated pathology? Pediatr Dev Pathol 2007;10(4):293–9.

76. Gonzales E, Davit-Spraul A, Baussan C, et al. Liver diseases related to MDR3 (ABCB4) gene deficiency. Front Biosci 2009;14:4242–56.

77. Gorelik J, Patel P, Ng'andwe C, et al. Genes encoding bile acid, phospholipid and anion transporters are expressed in a human fetal cardiomyocyte culture. BJOG 2006;113(5):552–8.

78. Friedman EA, Neff RK. Hypertension-hypotension in pregnancy. Correlation with fetal outcome. JAMA 1978;239(21):2249–51.

79. Kinsella SM, Lohmann G. Supine hypotensive syndrome. Obstet Gynecol 1994;83(5 Pt 1):774–88.

80. Nohr EA, Bech BH, Davies MJ, et al. Prepregnancy obesity and fetal death: a study within the Danish National Birth Cohort. Obstet Gynecol 2005;106(2): 250–9.

81. Reddy UM, Ko CW, Willinger M. Maternal age and the risk of stillbirth throughout pregnancy in the United States. Am J Obstet Gynecol 2006;195(3): 764–70.

82. Jackson RA, Gibson KA, Wu YW, Croughan MS. Perinatal outcomes in singletons following in vitro fertilization: a meta-analysis. Obstet Gynecol 2004; 103(3):551–63.

83. Schlabritz-Loutsevitch NE, Moore CM, Lopez-Alvarenga JC, et al. The baboon model (*Papio hamadryas*) of fetal loss: maternal weight, age, reproductive history and pregnancy outcome. J Med Primatol 2008;37(6):337–45.

84. Stephansson O, Dickman PW, Johansson A, Cnattingius S. Maternal hemoglobin concentration during pregnancy and risk of stillbirth. JAMA 2000; 284(20):2611–17.

85. Smith GC, Stenhouse EJ, Crossley JA, et al. Early pregnancy levels of pregnancy-associated plasma protein a and the risk of intrauterine growth restriction, premature birth, preeclampsia, and stillbirth. J Clin Endocrinol Metab 2002;87(4):1762–7.

86. Petraglia F, Gomez R, Luisi S, et al. Increased midtrimester amniotic fluid activin A: a risk factor for subsequent fetal death. Am J Obstet Gynecol 1999;180 (1 Pt 1):194–7.

87. Aagaard-Tillery KM, Holmgren C, Lacoursiere DY, et al. Factors associated with nonanomalous stillbirths: the Utah Stillbirth Database 1992–2002. Am J Obstet Gynecol 2006;194(3):849–54.

88. Burgess AM, Hutchins GM. Inflammation of the lungs, umbilical cord and placenta associated with meconium passage in utero. Review of 123 autopsied cases. Pathol Res Pract 1996;192(11):1121–8.

89. King EL, Redline RW, Smith SD, et al. Myocytes of chorionic vessels from placentas with meconium associated vascular necrosis exhibit apoptotic markers. Hum Pathol 2004;35:412–17.

90. Stoltenberg C, Magnus P, Skrondal A, Lie RT. Consanguinity and recurrence risk of stillbirth and infant death. Am J Public Health 1999;89(4):517–23.

91. Pliushch G, Schneider E, Weise D, et al. Extreme methylation values of imprinted genes in human abortions and stillbirths. Am J Pathol 2010; 176(3):1084–90.

92. Folkerth RD, Zanoni S, Andiman SE, Billiards SS. Neuronal cell death in the arcuate nucleus of the medulla oblongata in stillbirth. Int J Dev Neurosci 2008;26(1):133–40.

CHAPTER 11
Congenital Anomalies

Michael Varner MD and Janice L.B. Byrne MD

Division of Maternal-Fetal Medicine, Department of Obstetrics and Gynecology, University of Utah Health Sciences Center, Salt Lake City, UT, USA

Division of Maternal-Fetal Medicine, Department of Obstetrics and Gynecology, Division of Medical Genetics, Department of Pediatrics, University of Utah Health Sciences Center, Salt Lake City, UT, USA

When pregnancy results in a live birth, the incidence of recognizable anomalies has historically been estimated at approximately 2–3% [1, 2]. However, the actual frequency of structural anomalies is much higher. Autopsy series reveal overall anomaly rates of 7–18%, most of which would not have historically been recognized at the time of birth [3, 4].

Any discussion of causality with stillbirth must be predicated on accurate diagnoses. Although an ever-increasing number of diagnostic studies are available for the evaluation of stillbirth, autopsy remains critically important for determination of cause of death. More recently, postmortem magnetic resonance imaging has proven quite accurate in settings where autopsy is not possible or permitted [5]. Maximizing the amount of available information obviously maximizes the possibility of correct identification of the cause(s) of fetal death.

Ultrasonographic imaging is performed almost universally during pregnancy in the course of early twenty-first century American prenatal care and has been repeatedly shown to be of value for identification of major fetal anomalies. The fact that the majority of fetal anomalies occur in pregnancies without antecedent risk factors [6] has been one of several motivating forces in this practice trend. More importantly, however, there have been persistent concerns about the sensitivity of routine obstetric ultrasound for detection of fetal anomalies. While contemporary obstetric ultrasound offers acceptable sensitivity for major

malformations of the central nervous system and urinary tract, it remains less sensitive for many other anomalies. Levi [7] reviewed 36 studies involving over 900,000 fetuses and found an overall sensitivity of obstetric ultrasound for the diagnosis of fetal anomalies of 40.4% (range 13.3–82.4%).

The widespread use of ultrasound also confounds cause-specific fetal death rates, as many pregnancies complicated by major fetal anomalies will be terminated and thus not "appear" as fetal deaths. Although this suggests that the most accurate assessment of anomaly-specific perinatal death rates should include both terminations and neonatal deaths together with fetal deaths. The incorporation, or non-incorporation, of this concept will be left to the researchers of the future.

Gordijn and associates [8] reviewed the medical literature through 2002 and reported that autopsies in stillbirths revealed a new diagnosis, made a change in diagnosis, or provided important additional information in 28–75% of cases. They noted that autopsies were more likely to be useful when no clear clinical cause of death was available or if a malformation was present, whether suspected or not. They postulated that the wide ranges were the result of variable stillbirth gestational age definitions, variable rates of pregnancy termination, pathologist expertise, and patient populations.

This also emphasizes the fact that the presence of one or more anomalies does not mean that the anomaly(ies) was(were) responsible for the fetal death. For example, chorioamnionitis may occur in a pregnancy complicated by trisomy 21. Although a detailed discussion of the topic is beyond the scope of this chapter, it should be evident that determination of the pathophysiology behind a fetal death is frequently complex and problematic. Stillbirths may also occur following the confluence of several risk factors. This chapter will focus on those anomalies for which a pathophysiologic cause of death can reasonably be postulated.

Karyotypic abnormalities

In contrast to the roughly 0.3% likelihood of chromosome abnormalities found in live births [9], chromosome abnormalities are found in 6–12% of stillbirths [10]. This is a 20- to 40-fold increase and that is likely a conservative estimate, as karyotyping is frequently unsuccessful, particularly in macerated fetuses.

Aneuploidy

In stillbirths occurring at or beyond 20 weeks gestation, the karyotypic abnormalities are similar to those seen in live births. The most common autosomal trisomies seen in stillbirths are trisomy 21, trisomy 18, and trisomy 13 [11]. Although the estimated contribution of autosomal trisomies to overall fetal death rates is generally estimated at 3–4%, essentially all karyotyped series suffer from a bias resulting from the diagnosis and termination of a substantial percentage of trisomies prior to 20 weeks gestation. It is estimated that 43% of pregnancies complicated by trisomy 21 at the time of chorionic villus sampling would be lost spontaneously prior to term, as compared to 23% diagnosed at the time of amniocentesis that would be lost spontaneously prior to birth [12]. It is estimated that in excess of 90% of pregnancies complicated by Down syndrome diagnosed in the mid-trimester in the United Kingdom end in pregnancy termination and would thus not present as stillbirths [13]. Nonetheless, trisomy 21, trisomy 18, and trisomy 13 still represent the majority of autosomal trisomies seen in stillbirths and have been estimated at 23%, 21%, and 8% of stillbirths with autosomal

trisomies, respectively [11]. While theoretically occurring as frequently as autosomal trisomies, autosomal monosomies are not seen in either live births or stillbirths and are rare in early miscarriages.

Liveborn individuals with trisomy 21 are more likely to have congenital heart disease, leukemia, various developmental bowel abnormalities (duodenal atresia, annular pancreas, imperforate anus, etc.), and instability of the atlanto-axial joint. However, it is not clear that these abnormalities per se increase the rate of stillbirth.

The long-recognized association of maternal serum analyte patterns with fetal aneuploidy is also consistent with abnormal placental function. The placenta in pregnancies complicated by trisomy 21 is known to have abnormal trophoblast fusion and differentiation that is thought to be the result of abnormal human chorionic gonadotropin signaling [14]. Scanning electron microscopy of placental villi from first-trimester pregnancies complicated by trisomies demonstrates changes consistent with these observations [15]. It is likely that this, or similar, placental developmental abnormalities are major contributors to the increased stillbirth rate seen in trisomy 21 pregnancies.

In addition, it has long been recognized that the brains of individuals with trisomy 21 weigh less and have a dramatically decreased number of neurons when compared to matched euploid brains, although this finding seems limited to the third trimester [16]. Recent neurogenetic studies have shown that a number of genes that control neuronal growth and development, particularly the DLX homeobox transcription factors that are required for interneuron development, are virtually absent in both fetal and adult brains of individuals with trisomy 21 [17]. There are also data suggesting that several genes linked to neuronal death, including Cu/Zn superoxide dismutase (SOD1), amyloid-beta precursor protein, and transcription factor ets-2 are all located on chromosome 21, are characteristically overexpressed in the brains of individuals with trisomy 21, and are associated with impaired mitochondrial function leading to chronic metabolic impairment, oxidative stress, and neuronal degeneration [18]. Besides representing a mechanism by which progressive neurologic impairment and eventual dementia are more likely in individuals with trisomy 21, these findings also suggest that generalized central nervous system dysfunction may also play a role in the increased rate of fetal death in pregnancies complicated by trisomy 21.

Over 90% of liveborn individuals with trisomy 18 will have a congenital heart defect, and these infants can also have kidney defects, limb and diaphragm abnormalities. Virtually all individuals with trisomies 13 and 18 will have polyvalvular dysplasia, usually considered nonhemodynamically significant. However, endomyocardial fibroelastosis, myocardial fibrosis, and less commonly, other structural anomalies of the heart may lead to progressive cardiac failure and fetal death. The majority also have characteristic abnormalities of the distal extremities, including overlapping fingers and rocker bottom feet (Figure 11.1). Biologic network analyses performed on amniotic fluid samples from pregnancies complicated by trisomy 18 reveal abnormalities in immune processes and platelet disorders [19]. This same study demonstrated abnormalities in lipid and cholesterol metabolism, adenosine triphosphate metabolism, and energy-coupled protein transport, further suggesting that metabolic disorders—as opposed to structural anomalies—may be the more prominent contributor to the increased stillbirth rates in aneuploid pregnancies. There is a significant skewing of the sex ratio in favor of females in liveborn infants with trisomy 18, consistent with a preferential loss of male conceptions, at least from mid-pregnancy onward [20]. In fetuses with severe growth restriction and clinical features of trisomy 18 but with normal karyotype, the diagnosis of Smith-Lemli-Opitz (SLO) syndrome, an abnormality of cholesterol metabolism, should be considered [21].

Of interest, confined placental mosaicism (CPM) with a substantial euploid cell line in the placenta may represent a mechanism by which fetuses affected with trisomy 18 (and also 13) are less likely to be stillborn [22].

Classic phenotypic features of trisomy 13 include cleft lip and palate, postaxial polydactyly of the hands and feet, malformed and rotated internal organs, congenital heart defects, and severe brain abnormalities (Figure 11.2). The most common congenital heart defects are atrial and ventricular septal defects. Many of the brain abnormalities involve midline craniofacial malformations within the spectrum of the arrhinencephaly–holoprosencephaly complex. While the cause of death in most infants with trisomy 13 is thought to be related to central apnea, the cause in fetal life is less well understood.

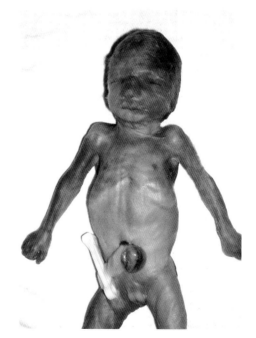

Figure 11.2 Stillborn fetus with trisomy 13 showing characteristic facial features. A prominent, broad nasal root and hypertelorism are evident. In this case, there is no orofacial cleft. Postaxial polydactyly is present but not shown. A small omphalocele can also be seen.

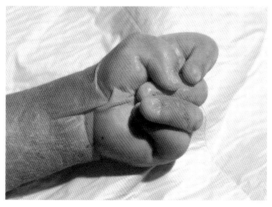

Figure 11.1 Characteristic hand posture of stillborn infant with trisomy 18. Note the overlapping digits, clenched fist, and hypoplastic nails.

Sex chromosome aneuploidy is less common than the autosomal trisomies in stillbirths, a relationship that is reversed in live births [9], where sex chromosome aneuploidy is more common. It is estimated that only 15% of trisomies 13, 18, and 21 survive to term, whereas 75% of sex chromosome trisomies (XXY, XYY, XXX) survive to term.

Klinefelter syndrome (47,XXY) is seen in 4.3–15.0 per 10,000 live births [23, 24] (8.4–29.0 per 10,000 male live births) and 0.2–0.4% of stillbirths [25], suggesting that the majority of fetuses with Klinefelter syndrome result in live births. This is not surprising in view of the generally mild phenotype and the frequent delay in diagnosis until adolescence or adulthood. Likewise, 47,XXX (Trisomy X or Triple X Syndrome) phenotype, while characterized by tall stature and neurodevelopmental delay, has considerable overlap with normal, and is also estimated to occur in only 0.2% of stillbirths [25]. The XYY syndrome is also often diagnosed only when a karyotype is performed for another indication. Individuals with all three of these sex chromosome trisomies have characteristic increased growth velocity in childhood that is thought to be due to the increased gene dosage of three X/Y chromosome SHOX genes [26]. However, there is no evidence to suggest that this abnormality might increase the likelihood of stillbirth.

Monosomy X (Turner syndrome) is an exception to this pattern and represents another 23% of aneuploid stillbirths. In contrast to the sex chromosome trisomies, the likelihood of a 45,X pregnancy surviving to term is less than 1%. Although most pregnancies complicated by 45,X do not survive to 20 weeks, stillbirths occurring at or beyond that point frequently have cystic hygromata, lymphedema, ascites, hydrothorax, and hypoplastic lungs [27] (Figures 11.3 and 11.4). This constellation can lead to fetal death as a result of progressive cardiac compromise. Structural cardiovascular anomalies, in particular left-sided obstructive lesions, are very common, some of which alone, for example, severe postductal coarctation, can also result in fetal death.

Unbalanced translocations/ deletions—chromosomal mosaicism

An essentially infinite variety of unbalanced translocations and deletions as well as chromosome

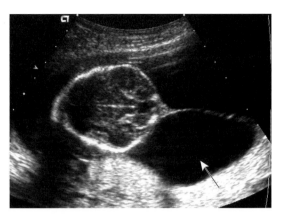

Figure 11.3 Mid-trimester ultrasound of a fetus with Turner syndrome. A typical massive, septate cystic hygroma is seen.

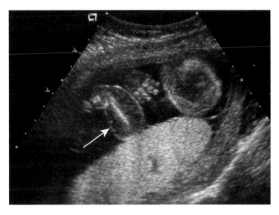

Figure 11.4 Mid-trimester ultrasound of the same fetus with Turner syndrome showing marked extremity edema involving the hands and arms. This pattern of edema is characteristic in Turner syndrome.

mosaicism can be expected more frequently in stillborns. While page limitations preclude an exhaustive review, the subject does reemphasize the importance of a chromosome study in any fetal death, particularly when associated with structural malformations, fetal growth restriction, and/or polyhydramnios.

CPM with fetal growth restriction

Given that the fetus and placenta develop from the same fertilized egg, it is generally assumed that the chromosomal make-up of the placenta and fetus will be identical. However, with the advent of chorionic villus sampling at 10–12 weeks gestation, it has been shown that 1–2% of viable pregnancies will have a cytogenetic abnormality, usually trisomy, that is found only in the placenta. Known as confined placental mosaicism, it was first described in the setting of unexplained fetal growth restriction, and can only be confirmed when the fetus is proven to have a normal karyotype.

CPM can be found in the cytotrophoblast (type I), the chorionic stroma (type II), or both cell lines (type III). CPM is the result of postzygotic mitotic mutations that occurred either in specific placental progenitors (type I or II) or in embryoblasts (type III). This latter situation is consistent with a conception that was originally trisomic and bespeaks the fact that CPM is not always associated with an adverse outcome. In fact, there is evidence that fetuses affected by trisomy 13 or 18 are more likely to be liveborn if associated with an euploid placenta, a phenomenon known as "trisomy rescue" [28].

The clinical impact of CPM is highly variable, ranging from no apparent effect through clinically apparent fetal growth restriction, to fetal death. There is a correlation between the specific involved extra chromosome(s), the timing of the occurrence, the tissue(s) involved, the persistence or nonpersistence of the abnormality, and the likelihood of adverse pregnancy outcomes [10, 22]. A proportion of CPM identified via CVS will not be detectable at term, an occurrence associated with improved better outcomes. Although a number of autosomal trisomies have been described in CPM (chromosomes, 2–3, 7–9, 13–16, 18), evidence suggests that involvement with chromosome 16 is the most likely to lead to fetal death, estimated at over 20% [29].

CPM for autosomal monosomies is extremely rare.

Array comparative genomic hybridization

For years, standard cytogenetic studies have confirmed the association of complex chromosomal rearrangements, duplications, and deletions with stillbirths. However, the more recent development of array comparative genomic hybridization (array CGH) can detect chromosomal gains or losses that are several orders of magnitude smaller than those identifiable by conventional cytogenetic methods. These gains or losses are called copy number variants (CNVs) and are defined as stretches of DNA larger than 1,000 base pairs that are normally found only once on each chromosome but that, in some individuals, may be deleted or present in multiple copies. It has been estimated that CNVs constitute as high as 12% of the human genome [30] and over 40% of identified CNVs overlap with known genes [31], clearly suggesting that CNVs play an important role in gene regulation and expression.

Array CGH testing can now identify specific causes of birth defects and mental retardation that would not be possible by earlier genetic testing and has clearly confirmed the importance of CNVs as a substantial source of human genetic diversity. However, this technology also identifies many areas of uncertain clinical significance in the human genome (so-called benign CNVs and CNVs of uncertain significance), and our understanding of the natural history and range of clinical variability associated with CNVs precludes their widespread clinical use at the time of this writing [32]. At present, multiple databases are actively collecting CNV data (Table 11.1) and the next few years will surely see the identification of numerous confirmed CNV abnormalities that are associated with fetal death. These discoveries will, doubtless, rapidly expand our knowledge of normal and abnormal pregnancy outcomes, although at the time of this writing there have been no published examples of CNV abnormalities presenting as fetal death.

Hydrops fetalis

Hydrops is defined as the presence of excess fluid in two or more body areas, including the pleural or pericardial space, peritoneal cavity, or skin. Hydropic fetuses frequently also have cystic hygromata, polyhydramnios, and placentomegaly. Hydrops can be caused by a number of mechanisms (Table 11.2), including imbalances at a number of checkpoints in the course of extracellular fluid balance (Figure 11.5).

In normal fetal and extrauterine life, a fine balance exists between hydrostatic pressure and plasma

Table 11.1 CNV databases.

Outcome	Database(s)	Website
Normal	Database of Genomic Variants (DGV)	www.projects.tcag.ca/variation
Abnormal	Chromosome Abnormality Database	www.ukcad.org.uk/coccon/ukcad/
	Database of Genomic Structural Variation (dbVar)	www.ncbi.nlm.nih.gov/dbvar
	DECIPHER (Neurodevelopmental Disorders)	www.sanger.ac.uk/PostGenomic/decipher/
	International Standard Cytogenomic Array (ISCA) Consortium	www.isca.genetics.emory.edu/
	European Cytogenetics Association Register of Unbalanced Chromosome Aberrations	www.ecaruca.net

These databases are actively accepting new data with phenotype correlations and will doubtless be reporting phenotype–genotype correlations associated with fetal death in the proximate future.

Table 11.2 Conditions associated with fetal hydrops.

Immunologic	Red cell isoimmunization
Cardiac disease	Structural (obstructive)
	Functional (intrinsic myocardial, arrhythmia, arteriovenous malformation)
Severe anemia	Infection (parvovirus)
	Hemoglobinopathy (alpha-thalassemia)
	Feto-placental or fetal hemorrhage
	Red cell aplasia or dyserthyropoiesis
Aneuploidy	Associated structural anomalies
	Placental dysfunction
Infection	Parvovirus, syphilis, TORCH infections, Lyme disease
Tumors	Teratomas
Skeletal dysplasias	Thanatophoric dwarfism (asphyxiating thoracic dystrophy)
	Osteogenesis imperfecta, type II
	Achondrogenesis, types I and II
	Hypophosphatasia
Syndromic	Clusters of structural malformations
	Inborn errors of metabolism
Monochorionic twins	Twin–twin transfusion syndrome
	Acardiac twin
Pulmonary	Obstructive (diaphragmatic hernia, cystic adenomatoid malformation, teratoma)
Lymphatic	Cystic hygroma
	Congenital lymphedema
Gastrointestinal	Proximal obstruction (atresia, volvulus)
	Peritonitis (meconium, infection)
Genitourinary	Distal obstructions
	Spontaneous perforations
Lysosomal storage disorders	Niemann–Pick type C, mucopolysaccharidosis VII and IVA, Gaucher disease type 2, sialidosis, Farber disease

oncotic pressure, with the former attempting to push fluid out of the vascular compartment into the interstitial space and the latter trying to pull fluid in the opposite direction. This balance can also be affected by the integrity, or nonintegrity, of the vascular endothelium, the compliance of the intravascular space, and the ability of the fetal lymphatic system to drain the interstitial space. The final, but critically important, factor is the function of the fetal heart, and particularly of the

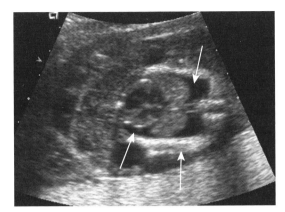

Figure 11.5 Mid-trimester ultrasound of a fetus with hydrops. Bilateral pleural effusions, pericardial effusion, and skin edema can be seen. In addition, the fetus also had massive ascites. The cause was undetermined.

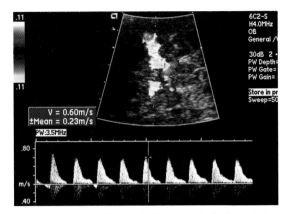

Figure 11.6 Surveillance of a fetus at risk for hemolytic disease due to rhesus alloimmunization by the use of middle cerebral artery peak systolic velocity (MCA-PSV) assessment. The Doppler cursor is on the middle cerebral artery and the waveform below shows a velocity of 60 cm/s, mildly elevated for this gestation.

right side of the fetal heart [33]. If a fetus develops acute or sustained increased right ventricular afterload, hydrops may develop. Once established, the increased hydrostatic pressure on lymphatic drainage and cardiac function tends to maintain or accelerate the pathophysiology.

Although the cause of death in many cases of nonimmune hydrops will be suspected or confirmed based on prenatal ultrasound or autopsy findings, many other cases will require specific laboratory testing for confirmation. In particular, fetal aneuploidy, including autosomal and sex chromosomal differences, may be associated with fetal hydrops and death. Some metabolic disorders such as sialidosis may also present as nonimmune hydrops and fetal death.

Although less common since the advent of Rh-D immune globulin prophylaxis, hydrops may also be immune in origin, reported in 13–24% of hydrops cases in a recent systematic review [34]. Thus, all women with a hydropic stillbirth should have an indirect Coombs test performed to exclude isoimmunization. It must be remembered that other forms of alloimmunization (Kell, Kidd, Duffy, etc.) occur and are not prevented by the administration of Rh-D immune globulin (Figure 11.6).

Autosomal recessive disorders

A number of autosomal recessive disorders are seen in stillbirths. There is no doubt that the actual contribution of this mechanism to fetal death is higher than currently known, in part because of the current difficulties in identifying new cases and in part because the phenotype seen in fetal deaths may be different from that seen in live births. Many known stillbirths resulting from single-gene disorders present clinically with nonimmune hydrops.

Alpha-thalassemia with hydrops

In populations in which alpha-thalassemia has a high prevalence (Africa, Middle East, India, South East Asia, southern China), homozygous fetal involvement often presents with hydrops [35, 36]. These infants have hemoglobin that cannot deliver oxygen to tissues and is unstable, leading to shortened red cell survival. They are usually severely anemic and characteristically have massive hepatosplenomegaly. Both the anemia and the secondary effects of extramedullary hematopoiesis (mechanical compression, hypoproteinemia) reliably lead to fetal death. The associated hypoxia also interferes with organogenesis and development, leading to an increased risk of associated anomalies.

The placentomegaly increases the risk of concurrent preeclampsia and obstetric hemorrhage. Although beyond the scope of this chapter, several excellent reviews are available for further reference [37, 38].

Lysosomal storage diseases causing hydrops

Lysosomal storage diseases result from inherited deficiencies or one or more catabolic lysosomal enzymes. More than 50 specific conditions have been described. While each of these conditions alone is rare, the combined incidence is approximately 1 in 1,500 births [39]. The majority are autosomal recessive, although two (Hunter disease and Fabry disease) are X-linked. Although these conditions are generally thought to first become symptomatic after birth, an increasing number of them are now recognized as causes of hydrops fetalis (Table 11.2) and subsequent stillbirth [39]. Affected infants and children are frequently described as having coarse facies and often have hepatosplenomegaly, contractures, dislocated hips, or club feet [40]. Although the precise mechanism(s) of fetal hydrops are not always clear, common presumptive mechanisms include heart failure from direct myocardial involvement, anemia, and/or hypoproteinemia resulting from hepatic involvement [39]. Common placental findings are highly vacuolated cells and an absence of edema despite concurrent fetal hydrops. Maternal peripheral leukocytes often contain abnormal cytoplasmic granules [41]. These findings should lead to enzymatic testing. The diagnosis of lysosomal storage diseases should also be considered in any setting of possible consanguinity or recurrent hydrops fetalis [39].

Amino acid disorders

Amino acid disorders in the fetus are not generally thought to increase the risk of fetal death. However, poorly controlled amino acid disorders in women of reproductive age, primarily phenylketonuria, have been associated with stillbirth [42].

Peroxisomal disorders

Zellweger syndrome, or cerebrohepatorenal syndrome, was the first described peroxisomal biogenesis disorder, although a number of others have subsequently been described [43]. It represents the most severe phenotype, and some of its multiple congenital anomalies can manifest prenatally. Fetal hypokinesia, renal hyperechogenicity, macrocephaly, and cerebral ventricular enlargement are the most common reported fetal features.

Smith-Lemli-Opitz syndrome

This autosomal recessive syndrome, characterized by multiple congenital anomalies [44], is the result of a deficiency in 7-dehydrocholesterol reductase that catalyzes the conversion of 7-dehydrocholesterol (7-DHC) to cholesterol [45]. Thus, elevated levels of 7-DHC are diagnostic of the syndrome. SLO was the first multiple congenital anomaly syndrome recognized to be caused by a biochemical enzymatic defect [46]. Characteristic abnormalities include severe growth restriction, cardiac defects, holoprosencephaly, unilobate lungs, polydactyly, and syndactyly (Figure 11.7). Cystic hygromata and skin edema have also been reported in the first trimester in pregnancies at risk.

The gene encoding for the 7-dehydrosterol reductase enzyme, DHCR7, has been cloned [47] and has over 80 different mutations [48]. The most common mutation in North American and western European populations is IVS8-1G→C [48, 49], accounting for 29% of DHCR7 abnormalities in surviving patients [48, 49] and is present in 1.13% of the Caucasian population. Thus, if all mutations in the DHCR7 gene are considered, and there are no deviations from the Hardy–Weinberg equilibrium, 3.9–4% of Caucasians are expected to carry a DHCR7 mutation [48]. This should result in a homozygote frequency of 1/2,500. However, the gene frequency in liveborn infants is only about 1/20,000 [48]. This infers that over 85% of homozygotes die before birth and could represent up to 5–7% of stillbirths. To date, no population-based study has evaluated this possibility.

X-linked disorders

There are a number of X-linked disorders that can result in the in utero death of male fetuses. The most commonly cited example is incontinentia

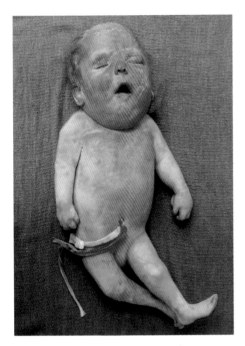

Figure 11.7 Stillborn preterm infant with SLO syndrome. The infant is severely growth restricted and edema of the head, neck, and body is evident. The eyes are small and wide-spaced and the nasal tip is short and upturned. The mouth is small and down-turned. Extremities are short with limited flexion of the joints and the genitalia are ambiguous. Polydactyly (not shown is also present).

pigmenti (IP), a disorder of the skin, eye, and central nervous system that occurs primarily in females despite being caused by hypomorphic mutations in the inhibitory kappaB kinase gamma (IKBKG) gene located on the X chromosome [50]. The precise mechanism of male lethality is not known, although experimental animal models suggest that the cause of death is liver failure [51].

Another example is Rett syndrome, a neurodevelopmental disorder caused by mutations in the methyl DNA binding protein 2 (MeCP2) [52], which is also located on the X chromosome. Like IP, Rett syndrome is seen predominantly in females. It has commonly been thought to be an X-linked condition that is lethal in affected males, although some series suggest that the sex ratios in affected families are normal [53].

In both of these examples, live births consist of approximately one-third unaffected females, one-third affected females, and one-third unaffected males. A positive family history should suggest further testing in the setting of a stillborn male fetus.

Structural anomalies without obvious chromosomal abnormalities

The following discussion reviews a number of structural anomalies seen more commonly with stillbirth which have not been invariably associated with conventional karyotypic abnormalities such as aneuploidy, unbalanced translocation, deletions, duplications, etc. As mentioned previously, the rapidly evolving area of array CGH may well identify submicroscopic abnormalities in the human genome associated with many of these anomalies in the coming years. In addition, the identification of one structural anomaly, whether in the setting of a prenatal ultrasound study or an autopsy, should also trigger a search for other anomalies, chromosome abnormalities, and possible diagnostic syndromes.

Cardiac anomalies

As previously intimated in the "Autosomal Recessive Disorders" section, nonimmune hydrops fetalis represents a "final common pathway" for multiple pathophysiologies (Table 11.2) and cardiac anomalies, both structural and functional, are common causes of this syndrome. However, fetuses with known congenital heart defects but no obvious hydrops are also at increased risk for intrauterine death, estimated in the range of 8% [54]. Not surprisingly, these fetuses are more likely to have other structural or chromosomal abnormalities than are those fetuses with congenital heart defects that are liveborn (Figure 11.8; Table 11.3).

Structural (obstructive)

Although structural heart defects complicate 0.4–0.8% of live births, they are found an order of magnitude more commonly in stillbirths [59, 60]. In a large fetal autopsy series [61], 7% of stillbirths

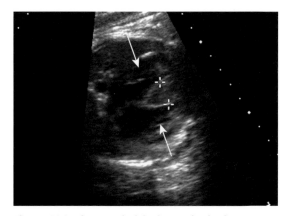

Figure 11.8 Ultrasound of the heart of a third-trimester fetus of a poorly controlled diabetic mother. Note the massively thickened interventricular septum (calipers) as well as the thickened ventricular free walls in this diabetic cardiomyopathy. The heart is markedly enlarged.

were found to have congenital heart defects. This series also noted that congenital heart defects were present in 9% of spontaneous abortions and 22% of induced abortions, suggesting that in a truly unselected population (i.e., without pregnancy terminations) the rate of congenital heart defects amongst stillbirths would doubtless be higher. The most commonly seen defects were ventricular septal defects, atrioventricular septal defects, hypoplastic left heart, and double-outlet right ventricle, comprising 72% of all cases [61]. The majority of these cases had associated extracardiac malformations (66%) and many also had chromosome anomalies (33%).

Structural cardiovascular anomalies per se can lead to stillbirth. The continuously increasing in utero cardiac output requirements for the rapidly developing fetus require ongoing remodeling of

Table 11.3 Selected syndromes associated with cardiac anomalies.

Additional finding	Syndrome	Comment
Skeletal dysplasias	Short rib—polydactyly syndromes	Cardiac defects most common with Saldino-Noonan syndrome
	Chondroectodermal dysplasia (Ellis-van Creveld syndrome)	Cardiac defects, particularly common atrium, in 50–60% [55]
	Campomelic dysplasia	One-third have heart defects (tetralogy of Fallot, VSD, ASD)
Radial aplasia/hypoplasia	Thrombocytopenia—absent radius syndrome	15–30% with cardiac defects, mainly septal defects [56]. Affected individuals have absent radii but preserved thumbs
	Cornelia de Lange syndrome	15–30% with cardiac defects, most commonly VSD
	Holt-Oram syndrome	90% have cardiac defects, most commonly ASD [57]
Multiple organ systems	VACTERL*	75% with cardiac defects
	CHARGE#	75–80% with cardiac defects, particularly conotruncal malformations and tetralogy of Fallot
Hydrops+	SLO syndrome	Cardiac defects in 40%, primarily septal defects
	Noonan syndrome	Pulmonary valve abnormalities, hypertrophic cardiomyopathy
Teratogens	Lithium	Ebstein's anomaly
	Anticonvulsants, particularly valproic acid	VSD [58]
Macrosomia	Undiagnosed or poorly treated diabetes	VSD, transposition of the great arteries

*A syndrome of unknown etiology comprising multiple anomalies, including V = vertebral, A = anal atresia, C = cardiac, TE = tracheoesophageal fistula/atresia, R = renal, and L = limb.
#A syndrome comprising multiple anomalies, including C = coloboma, H = heart, A = atresia of choanae, R = retardation of growth or development, G = genital, E = ear (the diagnosis requires at least four of the six components).
+See Table 11.2.

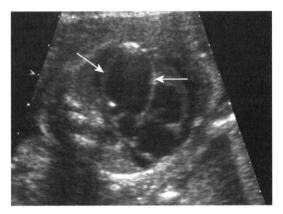

Figure 11.9 Ultrasound of the heart of a third-trimester fetus with critical aortic stenosis. The heart is massively enlarged and hypokinetic. The left ventricle in particular is enlarged with echogenic walls due to endocardial fibroelastosis. A pericardial effusion is also seen.

cardiac anatomy and function. In fetuses with critical obstructive lesions, cardiac anatomy changes during fetal life and cardiac output can become progressively inadequate leading to hypoxia and death (Figure 11.9). This latter course is most commonly seen in postductal coarctations or malformations, intracardiac tumors, or functionally univentricular hearts. Severe regurgitation may also lead to a similar outcome, particularly in the setting of atrioventricular valve regurgitation [62]. Severe Ebstein's anomaly is also associated with an increased risk of stillbirth. The mechanism is presumed due to obstruction to outflow, but dysrhythmias are also seen. Any number of arteriovenous malformations in either the fetus or the placenta can lead to high-output heart failure.

Fetal cardiac tumors can also lead to fetal death, occurring in 6% of fetal cardiac tumor cases in a recent review [63]. Although rhabdomyomas are the most common fetal cardiac tumors, stillbirth was most likely to occur in the presence of a cardiac teratoma, presumably because of their frequent large size and subsequent greater propensity to vascular obstruction. The identification of a fetal cardiac tumor should also raise suspicion for other genetic disorders, particularly tuberous sclerosis, neurofibromatosis, and familial myxoma syndrome [63]. These latter conditions generally have additional physical findings.

The foramen ovale and ductus arteriosus have both been reported to constrict or close in utero. In utero closure of the ductus arteriosus has most commonly been associated with medications, particularly nonsteroidal anti-inflammatory drugs [64]. In utero ductus closure results in right ventricular failure and is commonly associated with hydrops. In utero restriction or closure of the foramen ovale has been reported primarily in fetuses with congenital heart defects that result in left-to-right atrial shunting and/or left atrial hypertension [65], although it has been reported to be associated with stillbirth in the setting of a structurally normal heart [66].

Congestive heart failure, as manifested by ventriculomegaly, is an ominous prenatal finding and is frequently associated with stillbirth or early neonatal death [62, 67]. Cardiomyopathy may be the result of a number of metabolic or infectious (particularly viral, such as cytomegalovirus, and enteroviruses) origins.

Both fetal bradydysrhythmias and tachydysrhythmias have been associated with in utero heart failure and hydrops [67] (Figure 11.10). The history of fetal complete heart block should raise suspicion of either complex congenital heart disease or maternal anti-Ro autoantibodies. These autoantibodies, which can then cross the placenta, cross-react with the fetal bundle of His, leading

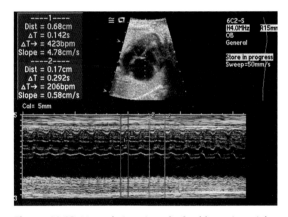

Figure 11.10 M-mode imaging of a fetal heart in atrial flutter. The atrial rate is 423 beats per minute and the ventricular rate is 206 beats per minute, characteristic of 2:1 conduction.

to fibrosis and bradycardia. They can also cause autoimmune injury to cardiac contractile elements, resulting in autoimmune myocarditis [68, 69]. Premortem fetal heart rates less than 55 beats per minute are generally associated with a worse prognosis [68]. Although the diagnosis of complete heart block may not be obvious after death, fibrosis of the bundle of His on postmortem examination should warrant maternal antibody screening, particularly in the setting of in utero heart failure in the absence of other plausible explanation(s).

Fetal tachycardias result in significant peripartum mortality, particularly when associated with nonimmune hydrops. In a series of 127 consecutively diagnosed fetal tachycardias at a single fetal cardiology center [70], the incidence of nonimmune hydrops was 41%, with an overall stillbirth rate of 4.7%. Not unexpectedly, the stillbirth rate was higher in the hydropic fetuses (7.7%). With reasonable certainty these figures substantially underestimate the stillbirth rate with this condition, as many affected fetuses will succumb before a diagnosis is ever established or else prior to evaluation in a referral center.

The long-QT syndrome has been associated with recurrent third-trimester stillbirths. While generally inherited as an autosomal dominant trait, it has also been described in the setting of maternal germ-line mosaicism [71].

Intrathoracic anomaly with hydrops

Congenital cystic adenomatoid malformation (CCAM) is a congenital hamartomatous lung lesion [72]. Three distinct types have been described by Stocker, whose categorization is based on cyst size and microscopic appearance. Type I has large cysts of varying size (>2 cm in diameter), type II has macroscopic cysts of more uniform size (<2 cm in diameter), and type III has microscopic cysts and frequently appears solid in nature on imaging and gross inspection. Although most CCAMs are asymptomatic at birth, they may on occasion cause neonatal respiratory distress, presumably due to air trapping. They may cause stillbirth via external compression of the heart, particularly when the heart occupies less than 20% of the chest area [73]. The development of hydrops in a fetus with a CCAM predicts virtual 100% lethality without

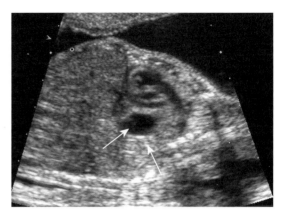

Figure 11.11 Mid-trimester ultrasound of a fetus with a left-sided congenital diaphragmatic hernia. The gastric fundus is seen posterior to the fetal heart in the thorax. Echogenic bowel is also noted posterior to the stomach.

intervention. In the previable fetus, the mortality rate can be halved by surgical removal of the mass. Prenatal surgical removal of CCAMs has been successfully performed and has resulted in resolution of hydrops and subsequent survival, confirming the mechanism of fetal death [74].

Congenital diaphragmatic hernia is seen in 1/3,000 to 1/4,000 births (Figure 11.11). It is an isolated defect in approximately 50–60% of cases, with the remainder occurring in association with other malformations or abnormalities [75, 76]. A detailed list of associated conditions is found in the recent review by Pober [75] but includes chromosome abnormalities, single-gene disorders (Cornelia de Lange syndrome [77], Fryns syndrome [78], etc.) and other associated malformations (particularly cardiovascular, limb, and central nervous system). Fetal death with congenital diaphragmatic hernia is a result of mechanical compression and resultant impaired cardiac function [79]. Both stillbirth and neonatal mortality rates are higher in the multiple anomaly group [80].

Urogenital anomaly causing severe oligohydramnios or anhydramnios

Because the placenta performs the metabolic functions of the kidneys in utero, intrauterine growth and viability can occur in the structural or functional absence of kidneys. However, because the substantial majority of amniotic fluid, at least beyond 20 weeks, is produced via fetal urination, severe oligohydramnios or anhydramnios can be reliably anticipated. These latter conditions result in a "vulnerable umbilical cord" that increases the risk fatal cord compression before birth. Anhydramnios also results in characteristic lung hypoplasia and soft tissue deformities that include low-set ears, wide-set eyes, micrognathia, and limb contractures [81] (Figure 11.12). Severe oligohydramnios or anhydramnios may be prerenal, renal, or postrenal in origin (Table 11.4). Unilateral renal disease (agenesis, multicystic kidney disease) is not

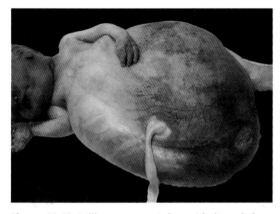

Figure 11.12 Stillborn preterm infant with distended abdomen due to a massively enlarged fetal bladder from urethral atresia in a female. A similar presentation is seen in males with severe obstruction from posterior urethral valves. Lethal pulmonary hypoplasia is usually the cause of death.

Table 11.4 Fetal renal causes of severe oligohydramnios or anhydramnios.

Category	Examples
Prerenal	Severe placental insufficiency
	Twin–twin transfusion syndrome
	Maternal medications (NSAIDs*)
Renal	Bilateral renal agenesis
	Bilateral multicystic dysplastic kidneys
	Bilateral polycystic kidney disease
Postrenal	Lower urinary tract obstruction
	Prune belly syndrome
	Posterior urethral valves
	Urethral atresia

*NSAIDs = nonsteroidal anti-inflammatory drugs.

per se a cause of stillbirth when accompanied by a contralateral normal kidney.

Multicystic dysplastic kidney disease, whether unilateral or bilateral, has a high rate of associated anomalies, 26% and 67%, respectively [82]. The condition also has an interesting gender distribution, being more commonly unilateral in males and more commonly bilateral in females. Females are also more likely to have associated structural and chromosomal abnormalities [81].

Autosomal recessive polycystic kidney disease is frequently associated with progressive oligohydramnios, markedly enlarged echogenic kidneys, and pulmonary hypoplasia (Figure 11.13).

Likewise, horseshoe kidney per se is not associated with an increased risk of fetal death. However, in a series of fetal, perinatal, and infant deaths associated with congenital renal anomalies, over half of the perinatal deaths associated with a horseshoe kidney had a chromosomal abnormality, most commonly trisomy 18 and Turner syndrome [83].

Lethal skeletal dysplasia

The skeletal dysplasias are a heterogeneous group of disorders that have in common significant shortening of the long bones and variable other structural abnormalities. They are thought to occur in 2–3 per 10,000 births [84]. Several forms are usually lethal in the early neonatal time period, the most

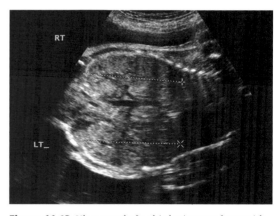

Figure 11.13 Ultrasound of a third-trimester fetus with autosomal recessive polycystic kidneys. Bilateral massive enlargement of the kidneys is noted (calipers). The chest is also small and associated with lethal pulmonary hypoplasia in this case.

common being thanatophoric dwarfism, osteogenesis imperfecta (type II), and achondrogenesis (types I and II). These are all severe micromelic dwarfing conditions associated with severe shortening of the ribs, restricted lung volume, and acute neonatal respiratory failure.

Thanatophoric dysplasia (TD) is the most common prenatally diagnosed lethal skeletal dysplasia and is the result of a mutation of the fibroblast growth factor receptor 3 gene located on the short arm of chromosome 4 [85]. Fetuses with type II TD have megalencephaly, mainly involving the temporal lobes [86], resulting in a characteristic "cloverleaf skull." These fetuses frequently have platybasia and foramen magnum stenosis with resultant restricted cerebrospinal fluid flow and ventriculomegaly. They also have straighter femora than that seen in type I TD which has a normal skull shape and curved "telephone receiver" femora (Figures 11.14 and 11.15). Various other central nervous system abnormalities have also been described, including dysplasia of the hippocampus, abnormal cerebral lamination, brain stem hypoplasia, and agenesis of the corpus callosum [87], suggesting that central nervous system dysfunction could increase the risk of fetal death.

These dwarfing conditions are frequently associated with other pregnancy complications, including severe polyhydramnios, premature labor, and malpresentation, that predispose to intrapartum demise.

Other skeletal dysplasias may, or may not, be lethal in the neonatal time period. Several of these, notably Jeune syndrome and Ellis-van Creveld syndrome, often have other associated anomalies (specifically renal and cardiac, respectively) that may increase their likelihood of antepartum or neonatal death.

It is important to emphasize that even nonlethal skeletal dysplasias may be associated with stillbirth. The most commonly recognized of these is heterozygous achondroplasia. Fetal deaths occurring in such affected fetuses should generally warrant a search for other associated causes, although the

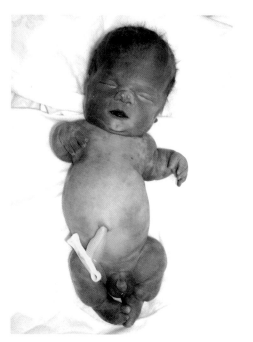

Figure 11.14 Stillborn preterm infant with type I TD. Note the severely shortened limbs (micromelia) and small chest. The calvarium, which is normally shaped, is disproportionately large for the body.

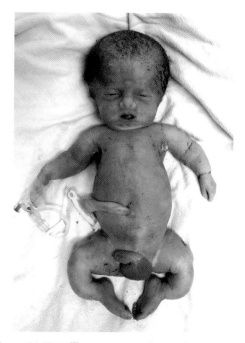

Figure 11.15 Stillborn preterm infant with perinatal lethal type II osteogenesis imperfect. Short limbs and a small chest are apparent. The apparent curvature of the lower extremities is due to multiple fractures.

risk of sudden death in individuals with hetero-zygous achondroplasia is increased as a result of cervical cord or brain stem compression and result-ant interference with respiratory control centers [88]. Similar acute compromise could presumably also occur in utero. Homozygous achondroplasia should also be excluded in this circumstance when both parents have achondroplasia.

Fetal tumors

Tumors in the fetus comprise a spectrum of dis-orders quite different from that seen in children. Although many are histologically benign, they fre-quently prove lethal because of either their location or their size. Given the rapid cell division and dif-ferentiation that occurs in the normal fetus, tumors frequently arise from a failure to completely differ-entiate with resultant unrestricted growth. Large tumors have been reported within weeks following normal fetal ultrasounds [89]. This again empha-sizes the importance of autopsy, as such findings might well not otherwise be identified.

Teratomas are the most common fetal tumor [90, 91], and they can be seen in almost every organ system. All teratomas contain elements of all three germ cell layers, with neural elements most often predominating in fetal tumors. Prognosis is gener-ally associated with the differentiation of the neural tissue. Although occasionally associated with other structural anomalies, teratomas are not associated with an increased risk of aneuploidy. They are gener-ally found in the midline and can appear anywhere from the brain to the coccyx, although sacrococ-cygeal teratomas are by far the most common site (70–80%) [92] (Figure 11.16). Sacrococcygeal ter-atomas are usually primarily solid, but may have a prominent cystic component, and are highly vascular. The amount of invasion into the pelvis is highly variable. When primarily cystic, they can be confused with meningomyeloceles. The vascularity frequently functions as an arteriovenous malfor-mation and these cases may present with hydrops. Prenatal resection of sacrococcygeal teratomas effec-tively resolves the high-output heart failure and has resulted in utero resolution of hydrops [93].

Teratomas are also seen in more cephalad locations. The head and neck is the second most

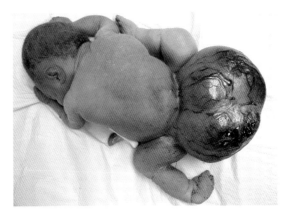

Figure 11.16 Neonatal demise with large sacrococcygeal teratoma and hydrops due to high-output heart failure. Note the prominent vascularity of the tumor.

common location for fetal teratomas. They are commonly associated with polyhydramnios as a result of direct mass effects.

Although neuroblastomas are second only to ter-atomas in frequency amongst fetal tumors, they are relatively uncommonly associated with fetal death [94]. Most fetal neuroblastomas arise from the adrenal gland and are more commonly right sided. Unlike neuroblastomata presenting in infancy or childhood, prenatal onset neuroblastoma may spontaneously regress after birth without sequelae.

Although leukemia is the most common malig-nancy amongst children, it is uncommon in stillborn fetuses. These fetuses frequently present with hepat-osplenomegaly and hydrops. Leukemia is 10–20 times more common in fetuses with trisomy 21, so the diagnosis of fetal leukemia should always prompt analysis of the karyotype [95].

Fetal liver tumors can lead to hydrops and fetal death several mechanisms, including mass effect, high-output cardiac failure, or rapid fluid shifts into tumor spaces [96]. The most common intrin-sic hepatic malignancies seen in stillbirths are hemangioendotheliomas, hepatoblastomas, and mesenchymal hamartomas.

Intracranial tumors can also cause fetal death. Large tumors have obvious secondary compression and distortion effects on surrounding structures and can also disrupt normal brain development. Unlike childhood tumors, which are more commonly infratentorial in location, fetal brain tumors are more commonly supratentorial in location. The most common histopathology is a teratoma, followed by astrocytoma.

Abdominal wall defects

Abdominal wall defects consist primarily of either gastroschisis or omphalocele, although other rarer types exist.

Gastroschisis is a full-thickness abdominal wall defect characteristically located to the right of a normal umbilical cord insertion and associated with variable evisceration of the fetal intestines (Figure 11.17). The etiology of gastroschisis remains uncertain but likely involves abnormality in early body wall folding. However, its epidemiology is unique in that it occurs predominantly in young, frequently nulliparous, women and seems to be encountered more commonly in the past several decades [97, 98]. Unlike omphalocele,

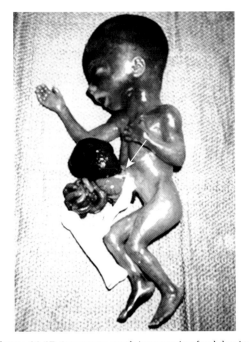

Figure 11.17 Seventeen week intrauterine fetal demise with gastroschisis. Note the typical location of the defect to the right of the normally inserted umbilical cord. The defect is large with extrusion of the liver, stomach, and bowel.

gastroschisis is less commonly associated with aneuploidy or abnormalities of other organ systems, the exception being a 10–20% association with segmental bowel obstruction [99]. Population-based series describe an increased risk of still-birth, in the range of 5–10% [97, 98]. These fetal deaths are characteristically in the third trimester and have thus far not been predicted by antepartum fetal surveillance. Gastroschisis is associated with an increased risk of oligohydramnios and growth restriction and fetal death has been reported more commonly when amniotic fluid volume is decreased [97], suggesting that cord compression may play a role. Alternatively, gastroschisis is associated with an increased protein loss (as confirmed by maternal serum and amniotic fluid alpha-fetoprotein levels that are characteristically higher than with omphalocele) that may lead to hypovolemia and cardiovascular compromise [100, 101]. An association between cytokine-mediated inflammation in gastroschisis-associated preterm birth and stillbirth has also been proposed [102] and may explain, at least in part, the failure of antepartum surveillance to prevent these fetal deaths. Of interest, maternal genitourinary infection in early pregnancy has also been associated with an increased risk of gastroschisis [103].

Omphalocele is characterized by herniation of bowel and other organs into the umbilical cord, with the tissues being covered by peritoneal membranes. Although seen in approximately 1 per 5,000 live births [104], it is seen in approximately 1 per 1,000 late first-trimester ultrasounds [105]. In contrast to gastroschisis, omphaloceles, particularly when located centrally rather than epigastric [104], are commonly associated with other structural and/or chromosomal abnormalities. As a result, the likelihood of fetal death in omphalocele, even when restricted to pregnancies that decline pregnancy termination, is 26% [106].

Although neonatal omphalocele series report sex ratios of approximately 1:1 [107], prenatally diagnosed series demonstrate female:male ratios approaching 1:2 [104], suggesting that affected male fetuses are more likely to be stillborn than females.

Aneuploidy, particularly trisomy 18, is very common with omphalocele, particularly when associated with other anomalies, when only bowel is present in the defect [108], and when the defect is relatively smaller [109]. Other associated syndromes, particularly Beckwith-Wiedemann syndrome, should also be considered. Beckwith-Wiedemann syndrome should specifically be considered in the setting of an omphalocele also associated with fetal overgrowth, macroglossia, and placentomegaly. In addition, an uncommon placental finding, called placental mesenchymal dysplasia and characterized by enlarged stem villi with loose connective tissue and cyst formation but absent trophoblast proliferation, is seen more commonly in Beckwith-Wiedemann syndrome [110]. The chromosome locus for Beckwith-Wiedemann syndrome is 11p15, a location shared with IGF2. This association has been hypothesized as the common link between these two findings [111].

Neural tube defects

Neural tube defects are the result of failed closure of the neural tube at 26–28 days after conception (Figure 11.18). The advent of mid-trimester maternal serum and ultrasound screening programs has substantially reduced the contribution of anencephaly to stillbirth statistics as a result of pregnancy termination [112]. However, a recent report from Ireland, where pregnancy termination is illegal, described amongst 26 cases a 23%

prelabor death rate (6/26) and a 35% intrapartum death rate (9/26) [113].

Fetuses with spina bifida also have predictable abnormalities of the brain and brain stem, many of which are the result of a characteristic herniation of the posterior fossa contents into the foramen magnum. This can result in sufficient compromise of vital brain stem functions to result in fetal death.

Pentalogy of Cantrell/ectopia cordis

Pentalogy of Cantrell is characterized by five features: a midline anterior abdominal wall defect, a cleft (usually distal) sternum, a diaphragmatic defect, a diaphragmatic pericardial defect, and cardiac defects [114]. In clinical practice, the diagnosis is frequently applied even when individuals have only three or four of these findings. A classification system for the complete and incomplete syndrome has been presented by Toyama [115]. A literature review by van Hoorn and associates [116] demonstrates a high frequency of other associated anomalies, monozygotic twinning, and aneuploidy. Although case reports overemphasize successful interventions and diagnoses, this review does identify several stillbirths [116] and it is highly likely that many other stillbirths go unreported. Many of these infants were identified in early pregnancy by the combination of an omphalocele plus a marker of cardiac dysfunction (pericardial effusion and/or thickened nuchal translucency). Although some debate on the issue exists in the literature [116, 117], perinatal survival does seem to correlate with the extent of the cardiac defect. It is likely that cardiac dysfunction in utero is also a common contributor to fetal death.

Neuromuscular disorders

A number of neuromuscular disorders, such as Walker-Warburg syndrome, congenital myasthenia gravis, congenital muscular dystrophies, and spinal muscular atrophy, are classically diagnosed in the early neonatal period because of generalized poor muscle tone. However, these conditions can also be sufficiently severe, and can also have other associated structural abnormalities, to result in fetal death.

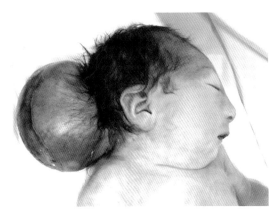

Figure 11.18 Stillborn term infant with large posterior encephalocele.

Walker-Warburg syndrome is the most severe congenital muscular dystrophy. It is an autosomal recessive disorder that is commonly associated with brain abnormalities, including lissencephaly, hydrocephalus, cerebellar hypoplasia, brain stem maldevelopment, and occipital encephalocele. Anterior eye abnormalities are also common [118]. A knockout mouse model for *O*-mannosyl-transferase, the gene responsible for this condition, results in predictable embryonic lethality [119] suggesting that the condition could well be under-diagnosed in humans.

Congenital myasthenia gravis can result in multiple fetal contractures (arthrogryposis multiplex congenital) and can result in fetal death. It is caused by transplacental transfer of maternal antibodies and is usually associated with known maternal myasthenia gravis, although it has been reported in women who themselves were asymptomatic [120].

Congenital myotonic dystrophy is an autosomal dominant condition and affected pregnancies are characteristically complicated by polyhydramnios and frequently accompanied by fetal club feet and ventriculomegaly [121]. It has long been known to be associated with an increased risk of fetal death, and pregnant women with the disease are also at increased risk for dysfunctional labor and postpartum hemorrhage as a result of poor uterine contractility [122]. This constellation of maternal and fetal complications should particularly warrant consideration of this complication, as the condition is a trinucleotide repeat abnormality that may be amplified in the fetus of a previously undiagnosed woman [123].

Amniotic band syndrome

Amniotic band syndrome is a sporadic abnormality that is the result of the entrapment of the developing fetus by disrupted amnion. The amnion disruption is thought to be a very early first-trimester phenomenon. The syndrome is quite variable in presentation but can include amputations, deformities, constrictions, and clefts (Figure 11.19). The abnormalities do not characteristically follow anticipated embryologic or vascular disruptions.

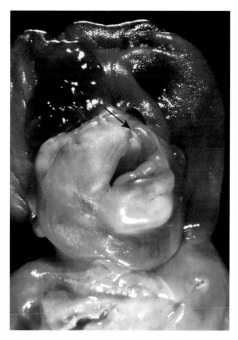

Figure 11.19 Stillborn preterm infant with severe disruption defects from amniotic bands. Most of the fetal face is missing, along with the calvarium. Note the asymmetric lip cleft.

Fetal metabolic disorders

Inborn errors of metabolism

(Storage diseases—sialidosis, Gaucher's disease, Niemann–Pick disease, gangliosidosis, type I)

Fetuses affected by long-chain fatty acid oxidation disorders may present with cardiomyopathy and/or arrhythmias. These pregnancies are also frequently complicated by severe preeclampsia and the combination of functional fetal heart disease and maternal preeclampsia, HELLP syndrome, or acute fatty metamorphosis should suggest this diagnosis [124].

References

1. Williams Obstetrics, 23rd edition. Cunningham FG, Leveno KJ, Bloom S, Hauth JC, Rouse DJ, Spong CY (eds). New York: McGraw-Hill; 2010.

2. Nikkila A, Rydhstroem H, Kallen B, Jorgensen C. Ultrasound screening for fetal anomalies in Southern Sweden: a population-based study. Acta Obstet Gynecol Scand 2006;85:688–95.

3. Newton D, Coffin CM, Clark EB, Lowichik A. How the pediatric autopsy yields valuable information in a vertically integrated health care system. Arch Pathol Lab Med 2004;128:1239–46.

4. Friederici HH, Sebastian M. Autopsies in a modern teaching hospital. A review of 2537 cases. Arch Pathol Lab Med 1984;108:518–21.

5. Woodward PG, Sohaey R, Jackson DP, et al. Post mortem MR imaging: comparison with findings at autopsy. Am J Roentgenol 1997;168:41–6.

6. Long G, Sprigg A. A comparative study of routine versus selective fetal anomaly ultrasound scanning. J Med Screen 1990;5:6–10.

7. Levi S. Ultrasound in prenatal diagnosis: polemics around routine ultrasound screening for second trimester malformations. Prenat Diagn 2002;22:285.

8. Gordijn SJ, Erwick JJHM, Khong TY. Value of the perinatal autopsy: critique. Pediatr Dev Pathol 2002;5:480–8.

9. Hassold T, Abruzzo M, Adkins K, et al. Human aneuploidy: incidence, origin and etiology. Environ Mol Mutagen 1996;28:167–75.

10. Wapner RJ, Lewis D. Genetics and metabolic causes of stillbirth. Semin Perinatol 2002;26:70–4.

11. Pauli RM, Reiser CA. Wisconsin stillbirth service program II. Analysis of diagnoses and diagnostic categories in the first 1,000 referrals. Am J Med Genet 1994;50:135–53.

12. Morris JK, Wald NJ, Watt HC. Fetal loss in Down syndrome pregnancies. Prenat Diagn 1999;19:142–5.

13. Britt DW, Risinger ST, Miller V, et al. Determinants of parental decisions after the prenatal diagnosis of Down syndrome: bringing in context. Am J Med Genet 1999;93:410–16.

14. Malassine A, Frendo JL, Evain-Brion D. Trisomy 21-affected placentas highlight prerequisite factors for human trophoblast fusion and differentiation. Int J Dev Biol 2010;54:475–82.

15. Rockelein G, Ulmer R, Schwille R. Surface and branching of placental villi in early abortion: relationship to karyotype. Scanning electron microscopic study. Virchows Arch A Pathol Anat Histopathol 1990;417:151–8.

16. Becker LE, Mito T, Takashima S, Onodera K. Growth and development of the brain in Down syndrome. Prog Clin Biol Res 1991;373:133–52.

17. Lockstone HE, Harris LW, Swatton JE, et al. Gene expression profiling in the adult Down syndrome brain. Genomics 2007;90:647–60.

18. Helguera P, Pelsman A, Pigino G, et al. ets-2 promotes the activation of a mitochondrial death pathway in Down's syndrome neurons. J Neurosci 2005;25:2295–303.

19. Wang TH, Chao AS, Chen JK, et al. Network analyses of differentially expressed proteins in amniotic fluid supernatant associated with abnormal human karyotypes. Fertil Steril 2009;92:96–107.

20. Parker MJ, Budd JLS, Draper ES, Young ID. Trisomy 13 and trisomy 18 in a defined population: epidemiological, genetic and prenatal observations. Prenat Diagn 2003;23:856–60.

21. Pinar H. Postmortem findings in term neonates. Semin Neonatol 2004;9:289–302.

22. Kalousek DK, Vekemans M. Confined placental mosaicism. J Med Genet 1996;33:529–33.

23. Buckton KE, O'Riordan ML, Ratcliffe S, et al. A G-band study of chromosomes in liveborn infants. Ann Hum Genet 1980;43:227–39.

24. Hamerton JL, Canning N, Ray M, Smith S. A cytogenetic survey of 14,069 newborn infants. I. Incidence of chromosome abnormalities. Clin Genet 1975;8:223–43.

25. Jacobs PA, Hassold TJ. The origin of numerical chromosome abnormalities. Adv Genet 1995;33:101–33.

26. Thomas NS, Harvey JF, Bunyan DJ, et al. Clinical and molecular characterization of duplications encompassing the human *SHOX* gene reveal a variable effect on stature. Am J Med Genet Part A 2009;149A:1407–14.

27. Canki N, Warburton D, Byrne J. Morphological characteristics of monosomy X in spontaneous abortions. Ann Genet 1988;31:4–13.

28. Kalousek DK, Barrett IJ, McGilliary BC. Placental mosaicism and intrauterine survival of trisomies 13 and 18. Am J Hum Genet 1989;44:338–43.

29. Benn P. Trisomy 16 and trisomy 16 mosaicism: a review. Am J Med Genet 1988;79:121–33.

30. Redon R, Ishikawa S, Fitch KR, et al. Global variation in copy number in the human genome. Nature 2006;444:444–54.

31. Henrichsen CN, Chaignat E, Reymond A. Copy number variants, diseases and gene expression. Hum Mol Genet 2009;18:R1–8.

32. Friedman JM. High-resolution array genomic hybridization in prenatal diagnosis. Prenat Diagn 2009;29:20–8.

33. Kleinman CS, Nehgme RA. Cardiac arrhythmias in the human fetus. Pediatr Cardiol 2004;23:234–51.

34. Bellini C, Hennekam RCM, Fulcheri E, et al. Etiology of non-immune hydrops fetalis: a systematic review. Am J Med Genet Part A 2009;149A:844–51.

35. Hirst JE, Arbuckle SM, Do TM, et al. Epidemiology of stillbirth and strategies for its prevention in Vietnam. Int J Gynaecol Obstet 2010 May 27 [Epub ahead of print] PMID: 20553788.

36. Taweevisit M, Thorner PS. Hydrops fetalis in the stillborn: a series from the central region of Thailand. Pediatr Dev Pathol 2010 Mar 16 [Epub ahead of print] PMID: 20233068.

37. Chui DHK, Waye JS. Hydrops fetalis caused by alpha-thalassemia: an emerging health care problem. Blood 1998;91:2213–22.

38. Leung WC, Leung KY, Lau ET, et al. Alpha-thalassaemia. Semin Fetal Neonatal Med 2008;13: 215–22.

39. Stone DL, Sidransky E. Hydrops fetalis: lysosomal storage disorders in extremis. Adv Pediatr 1999;46:409–40.

40. Piraud M, Froissart R, Mandon G, et al. Amniotic fluid for screening of lysosomal storage diseases presenting in utero (mainly as non-immune hydrops fetalis). Clin Chim Acta 1996;248:143–55.

41. Stangenberg M, Lingman G, Roberts G, Ozand P. Mucopolysaccharidosis VII as cause of fetal hydrops in early pregnancy. Am J Med Genet 1992;44:142–4.

42. Naughten E, Saul IP. Maternal phenylketonuria—the Irish experience. J Inherit Metab Dis 1990; 13:658–64.

43. Powers JM, Moser HW. Peroxisomal disorders: genotype, phenotype, major neuropathologic lesions, and pathogenesis. Brain Pathol 1998;8:101–20.

44. Smith DW, Lemli L, Opitz JA. A newly recognized syndrome of multiple congenital anomalies. J Pediatr 1964;64:210–17.

45. Irons M, Elias ER, Salen G, et al. Defective cholesterol biosynthesis in Smith-Lemli-Opitz syndrome. Lancet 1993;341:1414.

46. Kelley RI, Hennekam RC. The Smith-Lemli-Opitz syndrome. J Med Genet 2000;37:321–35.

47. Moebius FF, Fitzky BU, Lee JN, et al. Molecular cloning and expression of the human delta7-sterol reductase. Proc Natl Acad Sci USA 1998;95: 1899–902.

48. Opitz JM, Gilbert-Barness E, Ackerman J, Lowichik A. Cholesterol and development: the RSH ("Smith-Lemli-Opitz") syndrome and related conditions. Pediatr Pathol Mol Med 2002;21:153–81.

49. Nowaczyk MJ, Nakamura LM, Waye JS. DHCR7 and Smith-Lemli-Opitz syndrome. Clin Invest Med 2001;24(6):311–17.

50. Scheuerle A, Nelson DL. Incontinentia pigmenti. In: Pagon RA, Bird TC, Dolan CR, Stephens K (eds), GeneReviews (Internet). Seattle, WA: University of Washington, Seattle; 1993–1999 June 8 [updated 2008 Jan 28].

51. Rudolph D, Yeh WC, Wakeham A, et al. Severe liver degeneration and lack of NF-kappaB activation in NEMO/IKKgamma-deficient mice. Genes Dev 2000;14:854–63.

52. Hite KC, Adams VH, Hansen JC. Recent advances in MeCP2 structure and function. Biochem Cell Biol 2009;87:219–27.

53. Fyfe S, Leonard H, Dye D, Leonard S. Patterns of pregnancy loss, perinatal mortality, and postneonatal childhood deaths in families of girls with Rett syndrome. J Child Neurol 1999;14:440–5.

54. Boldt T, Andersson S, Eronen M. Outcome of structural heart disease diagnosed in utero. Scand Cardiovasc J 2002;36:73–9.

55. Katsouras CS, Thomadakis C, Michalis LK. Cardiac Ellis-van Creveld syndrome. Int J Cardiol 2003; 87:315–16.

56. Toriello HV. Thrombocytopenia absent radius syndrome. In: Pagon RA, Bird TC, Dolan CR, Stephens K (eds), Gene reviews. Seattle: University of Washington, Posted online December 8, 2009.

57. Bruneau BG, Logan M, Davis N, et al. Chamber-specific cardiac expression of Tbx5 and heart defects in Holt-Oram syndrome. Dev Biol 1999;211:100–8.

58. Kozma C. Valproic acid embryopathy: report of two siblings with further expansion of the phenotypic abnormalities and a review of the literature. Am J Med Genet 2001;98:168–75.

59. Hoffmann JIE, Christianson R. Congenital heart disease in a cohort of 19,502 births with long-term follow-up. Am J Cardiol 1978;42:641–7.

60. Mitchell SC, Corones SB, Berendes HW, et al. Distribution of congenital heart malformations in an autopsied child population. Int J Cardiol 1985; 8:235–50.

61. Tennstedt C, Rhaoui R, Korner H, Dietel M. Spectrum of congenital heart defects and extracardiac malformations associated with chromosomal abnormalities: results of a seven year necropsy study. Heart 1999;82:34–9.

62. Eronen M. Outcome of fetuses with heart disease diagnosed in utero. Arch Dis Child 1997;77: F41–6.

63. Isaacs H. Fetal and neonatal cardiac tumors. Pediatr Cardiol 2004;23:252–73.

64. Shehata BM, Bare JB, Denton TD, et al. Premature closure of the ductus arteriosus: variable response among monozygotic twins after in utero exposure to indomethacin. Fetal Pediatr Pathol 2006;25:151–7.

65. Donofrio MT, Bremer YA, Moskowitz WB. Diagnosis and management of restricted or closed foramen ovale in fetuses with congenital heart disease. Am J Cardiol 2004;94:1348–51.

66. Porcelli PJ, Saller DN, Duwaji M, Cowett RM. Nonimmune fetal hydrops with isolated premature restriction of the foramen ovale. J Perinatol 2002;12:37–40.

67. Groves AMM, Allan LD, Rosenthal E. Outcome of isolated congenital complete heart block diagnosed in utero. Heart 1996;75:190–4.

68. Schmidt KG, Ulmer HE, Silverman NH, et al. Perinatal outcome of fetal complete atrioventricular block a multicenter experience. J Am Coll Cardiol 1991;17:1360–6.

69. Horsfall AC, Li JM, Maini RN. Placental and fetal cardiac laminin are targets for cross-reacting autoantibodies from mothers of children with congenital heart block. J Autoimmun 1996;9:561–8.

70. Simpson JM, Sharland GK. Fetal tachycardias: management and outcome of 127 consecutive cases. Heart 1998;79:576–81.

71. Miller TE, Estrella E, Myerburg RJ, et al. Recurrent third-trimester fetal loss and maternal mosaicism for long-QT syndrome. Circulation 2004;109:3029–34.

72. Rosado-de-Christenson ML, Stocker JT. From the archives of the AFIP: congenital cystic adenomatoid malformation. RadioGraphics 1993;11:865–86.

73. Mahle WT, Rychik J, Tian ZY, et al. Echocardiographic evaluation of the fetus with congenital cystic adenomatoid malformation. Ultrasound Obstet Gynecol 2000;16:620–4.

74. Adzick NS, Harrison MR, Flake AW, et al. Fetal surgery for cystic adenomatoid malformation of the lung. J Pediatr Surg 1993;28:806–12.

75. Pober BR. Genetic aspects of human congenital diaphragmatic hernia. Clin Genet 2008;74:1–15.

76. Colvin J, Bower C, Dickinson JE, Sokol J. Outcomes of congenital diaphragmatic hernia: a population-based study in Western Australia. Pediatrics 2005;116:e356–63.

77. Marino T, Wheeler PG, Simpson LL, et al. Fetal diaphragmatic hernia and upper limb anomalies suggest Brachmann-de Lange syndrome. Prenat Diagn 2002;22:144–7.

78. Fryns JP. Fryns syndrome: a variable MCA syndrome with diaphragmatic defects, coarse face, and distal limb hypoplasia. J Med Genet 1987;24:271–4.

79. Baumgart S, Paul JJ, Huhta JC, et al. Cardiac malposition, redistribution of fetal cardiac output, and left heart hypoplasia reduce survival in neonates with congenital diaphragmatic hernia requiring extracorporeal membrane oxygenation. J Pediatr 1998; 133:57–62.

80. Skari H, Bjornland K, Haugen G, et al. Congenital diaphragmatic hernia: a meta-analysis of mortality factors. J Pediatr Surg 2000;35:1187–97.

81. Vanderheyden T, Kumar S, Fisk NM. Fetal renal impairment. Semin Neonatol 2003;8:279–89.

82. Lazebnik N, Bellinger MF, Ferguson JE II, et al. Insights into the pathogenesis and natural history of fetuses with multicystic dysplastic kidney disease. Prenat Diagn 1999;19:418–23.

83. Scott JES. Fetal, perinatal, and infant death with congenital renal anomaly. Arch Dis Child 2002; 87:114–17.

84. Spirt BA, Oliphant M, Gottlieb RH, Gordon LP. Prenatal sonographic evaluation of short-limbed dwarfism: an algorithmic approach. RadioGraphics 1990;10:217–36.

85. Miller E, Blaser S, Shannon P, Widjaja E. Brain and bone abnormalities of thanatophoric dwarfism. AJR 2009;192;48–51.

86. Hevner RF. The cerebral cortex malformation in thanatophoric dysplasia: neuropathology and pathogenesis. Acta Neuropathol 2005;110:208–21.

87. Kalache KD, Lehmann K, Chaoui R, et al. Prenatal diagnosis of partial agenesis of the corpus callosum in a fetus with thanatophoric dysplasia type 2. Prenat Diagn 2002;22:404–7.

88. Hecht JT, Butler IJ. Neurologic morbidity associated with achondroplasia. J Child Neurol 1990;5:84–97.

89. Schlembach D, Bonnemann A, Rupprecht T, Beinder R. Fetal intracranial tumors detected by ultrasound: a report of two cases and review of the literature. Ultrasound Obstet Gynecol 1994;14: 407–18.

90. Purkos SE, Muir KR, Southern L, et al. Neonatal tumours: a thirty-year population-based study. Med Pediatr Oncol 1994;22:309–17.

91. Werb P, Scuery J, Ostor A, et al. Survey of congenital tumors in perinatal necropsies. Pathology 1992;24:247–53.

92. Woodward PJ, Sohaey R, Kennedy A, Koeller KK. A comprehensive review of fetal tumors with pathologic correlation. RadioGraphics 2005;25:215–42.

93. Schmidt KG, Silverman NH, Harrison MR, Callen PW. High-output cardiac failure in fetuses with large sacrococcygeal teratoma: diagnosis by echocardiography and Doppler ultrasound. J Pediatr 1989;114: 1023–8.

94. Bjorge T, Engeland A, Tretli S, Heuch I. Birth and parental characteristics and risk of neuroblastoma in a population-based Norwegian cohort study. Br J Cancer 2008;99:1165–9.

95. Robertson M, De Jong G, Mansvelt B. Prenatal diagnosis of congenital leukemia in a fetus at 25 weeks gestation with Down syndrome: case report and review of the literature. Ultrasound Obstet Gynecol 2003;21:486–9.

96. Isaacs H Jr. Fetal and neonatal hepatic tumors. J Pediatr Surg 2007;42:1797–803.

97. Reid KP, Dickinson JE, Doherty DA. The epidemiologic incidence of congenital gastroschisis in Western Australia. Am J Obstet Gynecol 2003; 189:764–8.

98. Santiago-Munoz PC, McIntire DD, Barber RG, et al. Outcomes of pregnancies with fetal gastroschisis. Obstet Gynecol 2007;110:663–8.

99. Brantberg A, Blaas HGK, Salvesen KA, et al. Surveillance and outcome of fetuses with gastroschisis. Ultrasound Obstet Gynecol 2004;23:4–13.

100. Carroll SG, Kuo PY, Kyle PM, Soothill PW. Fetal protein loss in gastroschisis as an explanation of associated morbidity. Am J Obstet Gynecol 2001;184:1297–301.

101. Palomaki GE, Hill LE, Knight GJ, et al. Second-trimester maternal serum alpha-fetoprotein levels in pregnancies associated with gastroschisis and omphalocele. Obstet Gynecol 1988;71:906–9.

102. Luton D, de Lagausie P, Guibourdenche J, et al. Prognostic factors of prenatally diagnosed gastroschisis. Fetal Diagn Ther 1997;12:7–14.

103. Feldkamp ML, Reefhuis J, Kucik J, et al. Case–control study of self reported genitourinary infections and risk of gastroschisis: findings from the national birth defects prevention study, 1997–2003. BMJ 2008;336:1420–3.

104. Brantberg A, Blaas HGK, Haugen SE, Eik-Nes SH. Characteristics and outcomes of 90 cases of fetal omphalocele. Ultrasound Obstet Gynecol 2005;26: 527–37.

105. Snijder RJ, Brizot ML, Faria M, Nicolaides KH. Fetal exomphalos at 11 to 14 weeks of gestation. J Ultrasound Med 1995;14:569–74.

106. Fratelli N, Papageorghiou AT, Bhide A, et al. Outcome of antenatally diagnosed abdominal wall defects. Ultrasound Obstet Gynecol 2007; 30:266–70.

107. Baird PA, MacDonald EC. An epidemiologic study of congenital malformations of the anterior abdominal wall in more than half a million consecutive live births. Am J Hum Genet 1981;33: 470–8.

108. Nicolaides KH, Snijder RJ, Cheng HH, Gosden C. Fetal gastro-intestinal and abdominal wall defects: associated malformations and chromosomal abnormalities. Fetal Diagn Ther 1992;7:102–15.

109. Lakasing L, Cicero S, Davenport M, et al. Current outcome of antenatally diagnosed exomphalos: an 11 year review. J Pediatr Surg 2006;41:1403–6.

110. Cohen MC, Roper EC, Sebire NJ, et al. Placental mesenchymal dysplasia associated with fetal aneuploidy. Prenat Diagn 2005;25:187–92.

111. Jauniaux E, Nicolaides KH, Hustin J. Perinatal features associated with placental mesenchymal dysplasia. Placenta 1997;18:701–6.

112. Velie EM, Shaw GM. Impact of prenatal diagnosis and elective termination on prevalence and risk estimates of neural tube defects in California, 1989–1991. Am J Epidemiol 1996;144:473–9.

113. Obeidi N, Russell N, Higgins JR, O'Donoghue K. The natural history of anencephaly. Prenat Diagn 2010;30:357–60.

114. Cantrell JR, Haller JA, Ravitch MM. A syndrome of congenital defects involving the abdominal wall, sternum, diaphragm, pericardium and heart. Surg Gynecol Obstet 1958;107:602–14.

115. Toyama WM. Combined congenital defects of the anterior abdominal wall, sternum, diaphragm, pericardium, and heart: a case report and review of the syndrome. Pediatrics 1972;50:778–92.

116. van Hoorn JHL, Moonen RMJ, Huysentruyt CJR, et al. Pentalogy of Cantrell: two patients and a review to determine prognostic factors for optimal approach. Eur J Pediatr 2008;167:29–35.

117. Zidere V, Allan LD. Changing findings in pentalogy of Cantrell in fetal life. Ultrasound Obstet Gynecol 2008;32:835–7.

118. Vajsar J, Schachter H. Walker-Warburg syndrome. Orphanet J Rare Dis 2006;1:29. Published online 2006 August 3. Doi: 10.1186/1750-1172-1-29.

119. Willer T, Prados B, Falcon-Perez JM, et al. Targeted disruption of the Walker-Warburg syndrome gene Pomt1 in mouse results in embryonic lethality. Proc Natl Acad Sci USA 2004;101:14126–31.

120. Vincent A, Newland C, Brueton L, et al. Arthrogryposis multiplex congenita with maternal

autoantibodies specific for a fetal antigen. Lancet 1995;346:24–5.

121. Zaki M, Boyd PA, Impey L, et al. Congenital myotonic dystrophy: prenatal ultrasound findings and pregnancy outcome. Ultrasound Obstet Gynecol 2007;29:284–8.

122. Hilliard GD, Harris RE, Gilstrap LC, Shoumarker RD. Myotonic muscular dystrophy in pregnancy. South Med J 1977;70:446–7.

123. Turner C, Hilton-Jones D. The myotonic dystrophies: diagnosis and management. J Neurol Neurosurg Psychiatry 2010;81:358–67.

124. Rakheja D, Bennett MJ, Rogers BB. Long-chain L-3-hydroxyacyl-coenzyme A dehydrogenase deficiency: a molecular and biochemical review. Lab Invest 2002;82:815–24.

125. Vidaillet HJ. Cardiac tumors associated with hereditary syndromes. Am J Cardiol 1988;61:1355–9.

PART III

Management of the Patient with a Stillbirth

CHAPTER 12

Workup of the Patient with a Stillbirth

Robert M. Silver, MD and Michael L. Draper, MD

Division of Maternal-Fetal Medicine, Department of Obstetrics and Gynecology, University of Utah Health Sciences Center, Salt Lake City, UT, USA

Stillbirth is emotionally difficult for families and physicians. It is also common, affecting about 1:160–1:200 pregnancies in the United States and a higher proportion in many parts of the world. One of the most helpful things clinicians can do for families is to facilitate a thorough evaluation for potential causes of stillbirth. First, determining an etiology for the stillbirth can greatly facilitate grieving and help with emotional "closure." Even if a cause of death is not ascertained, the process of simply trying to identify a "reason" is emotionally valuable. Families need to believe that people in the health care system acknowledge their grief and want to do everything possible to help avoid a recurrence. Also, identifying the cause of stillbirth (whether a sporadic cause or one with a potential for recurrence) may allow couples to avoid unnecessary tests and interventions in subsequent pregnancies. Second, determining an etiology is invaluable in counseling patients regarding both the risk of another stillbirth as well as other adverse pregnancy outcomes in subsequent pregnancies. The majority of couples at least consider another pregnancy after suffering a stillbirth. Finally, in select cases it may be possible to improve outcomes in subsequent pregnancies. For example, medical interventions may improve perinatal outcome in patients with diabetes, hypertensive disease, and antiphospholipid syndrome (APS).

Evaluations for potential causes of stillbirth are often inadequate or incomplete [1]. For example, the rate of perinatal autopsy in the United States is estimated at considerably less than 50% in all but a few dedicated centers [2]. There are many contributing factors. In some instances, the clinician may be unaware of the appropriate "work-up" for stillbirth. Many times they will attribute a fetal death to a "cord accident," often on the basis of a nuchal cord noted at delivery. Nuchal cords are common, found in approximately 25% of deliveries and ordinarily result in no harm, thus this (often) false assumption prevents investigation into other potential etiologies for the stillbirth. In other cases, some tests such as perinatal autopsy may not be available. Clinicians, especially obstetricians, who usually have favorable outcomes often feel awkward or uncomfortable spending time with grieving families. Also, the clinician may worry that the family will not approve of or accept testing. Finally, in some cases, clinicians are reluctant to investigate stillbirths for fear of medicolegal liability. They are worried about uncovering suboptimal practice that may have contributed to the stillbirth.

Families also may be resistant to an evaluation for potential causes of stillbirth. They are grieving and may be angry with physicians and the entire medical system for "failing" them. Families often

Stillbirth: Prediction, Prevention and Management, First Edition. Catherine Y. Spong.
© 2011 Blackwell Publishing Ltd. Published 2011 by Blackwell Publishing Ltd.

verbalize that a "work-up" will not change anything and will not bring their child back to life. Many parents inappropriately blame themselves and often feel guilty about what happened and there is usually anxiety about their ability to have a healthy pregnancy in the future. They may have misconceptions about testing, especially autopsy and genetic testing. In addition, cultural and religious beliefs may influence their desire and/or willingness to proceed with a stillbirth evaluation. It is the role of the clinician to take the time needed to explore these issues and to counsel patients in a supportive and nonjudgmental manner. Clearly explaining the rationale behind an evaluation for causes of stillbirth and the potential short- and long-term benefits for families is critical. Families should be encouraged to allow an evaluation within the boundaries of their personal and cultural values. Finally, in most circumstances, the cost of testing must be considered prior to initiating a comprehensive and often expensive evaluation for potential causes of stillbirth.

It may be difficult to ascertain a definitive cause of stillbirth, even after a "complete" work-up. Fetal death may be associated with multiple factors in some cases, and it may be impossible to tell which disorder was most directly responsible for the loss. For example, infection and aneuploidy may be present concurrently, with neither being the clear sole cause of stillbirth. Other conditions, such as well-controlled diabetes mellitus, may be associated with stillbirth without directly causing it. Such conditions may be considered risk factors, rather than causes of stillbirth. In some cases, stillbirth is associated with not only multiple risk factors but also with multiple etiologies. This problem illustrates the need for unbiased and thorough investigation. Also, it is likely that many causes of stillbirth remain to be discovered, and investigation into previously unrecognized causes of stillbirth has been limited. Finally, even in referral centers using systematic and extensive evaluations for recognized potential etiologies of stillbirth, the proportion of stillbirths not convincingly attributable to a specific cause ranges from 10% to 85% [1, 3–7]. This percentage varies with the classification scheme [6, 7]

(see Chapter 3) as well as the thoroughness of the work-up.

Because of these limitations, the optimal evaluation of stillbirth remains controversial and is influenced by medical and nonmedical factors including cost. We recognize that the generally accepted evaluation of stillbirth differs among experts and that clear data are lacking. A rational approach to deciding which tests are most useful might rely on the consideration of several principles. First, it is most cost-effective to test for the more common causes of stillbirth. Second, certain tests such as autopsy and placental histopathology can provide diagnostic information for numerous rather than single causes of stillbirth. Accordingly, such tests are a good use of resources. Third, testing for relatively uncommon conditions should be guided by clues in the clinical history and initial round of testing. Finally, an argument could be made for identifying treatable conditions that predispose to recurrent stillbirth. Although preference should be given to common, recurrent, and preventable disorders, there is value to the identification of sporadic conditions. Until data from ongoing studies are available for stronger recommendations on the appropriate work-up, clinicians need to do the best they can with available information.

Components of evaluation for possible causes of stillbirth

Clinical history and evaluation

Perhaps the most important starting point in the evaluation of stillbirth is a comprehensive clinical evaluation. This should include a maternal interview and careful review of the medical record. A clinical evaluation allows one to direct a focused and cost-effective work up. Clinicians are strongly encouraged to document ultrasound findings, pathologic examination, and other data pertinent to distinguishing among types of pregnancy losses. Elements of the history may suggest the etiology of the fetal death. This is especially helpful when considering whether to test for uncommon conditions or if resources are limited. It is important to gather information regarding the specific events pertaining to the stillbirth in question. One should determine the gestational age at the time of demise, whether it was antepartum or intrapartum, and whether there were symptoms such as bleeding, contractions, or evidence of viral or bacterial infection that preceded the demise.

A complete review of the prenatal record is indicated, including an appraisal of the first prenatal examination, blood pressures, assessment of proteinuria, prepregnancy body mass index, weight gain during pregnancy, and laboratory values and ultrasound findings. For instance, in addition to an aneuploidy risk, an abnormal maternal serum screen may suggest an increased risk for placental compromise [8, 9]. Other prenatal laboratory values that may be useful include antibody screens, serologic tests for syphilis such as an rapid plasma reagin (RPR) or venereal disease laboratory test (VDRL), tests for chlamydia or gonorrhea, and a screen for gestational diabetes.

Ultrasound findings may be useful in a variety of ways. They can help establish accurate gestational dating, a critical factor in determining if the fetus had impaired growth. A lack of abnormalities on a quality mid-trimester sonogram substantially decreases the odds of abnormal fetal karyotype and genetic syndromes. Obstetric sonogram also provides important data regarding abnormal placentation, conditions of the cervix, abnormal interval growth, and amniotic fluid volume, and the chorionicity of multiple gestations.

One might also discover signs, symptoms, or evidence of previously unrecognized maternal acute or chronic medical disease (such as those suggestive of diabetes, hypertension, lupus, thyroid disease, viral infection, or intrahepatic cholestasis of pregnancy). Obstetric complications should also be emphasized with attention to first- or second-trimester bleeding, preterm uterine contractions, leaking amniotic fluid, fetal movement, evidence of cervical insufficiency, etc. If possible, records of antepartum hospitalizations or emergency department visits should be reviewed. Assessment of medical and environmental exposures, recent travel and trauma should also be performed.

A thorough social history may also identify risk factors of stillbirth such as smoking or substance abuse, while a family history might suggest genetic etiologies. Demographic and other risk factors for fetal death that can be obtained from the history include race, low socioeconomic status, limited prenatal care, less education, advanced maternal age, and obesity. A careful obstetric history is also important. The risk of stillbirth (and other adverse pregnancy outcomes) is considerably higher in subsequent pregnancies in cases of recurrent fetal death or adverse pregnancy outcomes [10, 11]. It is important to be careful when discussing risk factors for stillbirth with families. On the one hand, it is worthwhile to encourage smoking cessation or weight loss in obese women. On the other hand, it is important to stress that most women who smoke or are obese do not suffer stillbirth and the patient should be reassured that these behaviors were unlikely to directly cause her loss. Key elements of the clinical history as recommended in ACOG practice bulletin number 102 are shown in Box 12.1 [12].

Perinatal autopsy

Fetal autopsy is probably the single most useful diagnostic test in determining the cause of fetal loss [13]. Indeed, the vast majority of potential etiologies of stillbirth have an associated autopsy finding. Abnormalities such as birth defects, dysmorphic features, and major conditions such as amniotic band syndrome (Figure 12.1) can be identified. The postmortem examination can confirm infection, anemia, hypoxia, and metabolic abnormalities, and has been found to provide new information that influences counseling about subsequent pregnancies in 26–80% of cases [14–16].

Measurements such as foot length and body weight taken as part of an autopsy are helpful because these may identify a small for gestational age fetus; a major risk factor for fetal death. The use of customized, rather than generic growth curves may improve the utility of fetal growth assessment. A population-based study from Sweden illustrates that the use of customized, rather than population-based growth curves is better for predicting stillbirth (odds ratio of 6.1 for small for gestational age fetuses using customized

---

Box 12.1 Essential components of history

Details of the current pregnancy
- Maternal age
- Gestational age (supportive evidence including sonograms)
- Medical conditions complicating pregnancy
  - Pregnancy-induced hypertension
  - Gestational diabetes
  - Cholestasis of pregnancy; pruritis
  - Viral illness
- Multifetal gestation
- Known pregnancy complications
  - Preterm labor
  - Rupture of membranes
  - Cervical insufficiency
  - Fetal structural or chromosomal abnormalities including abnormal serum screening
  - Infections
  - Trauma
  - Abruption
- Maternal symptoms suggestive of above complications
- Maternal serum marker screen
- Antenatal sonograms (fetal anatomic surveys)
- Genetic testing such as amniocentesis or chorionic villous sampling
- Antenatal testing such as nonstress tests

Maternal medical history
- Chronic illnesses
  - Diabetes

- Thyroid disease
- Autoimmune disease
- Hypertension
- Cardiopulmonary disease
- Renal disease
- History of pertinent acute conditions
  - Prior venous thromboembolism
- Substance use
- Known genetic abnormalities
  - Balanced translocations
  - Single-gene mutations

Pregnancy history
- Recurrent miscarriages
- Previous stillbirth or neonatal demise
- Previous pregnancy complicated by
  - Growth restriction
  - Hypertension
  - Fetal anomalies
  - Abruption

Family history
- Developmental delay or mental retardation
- Stillbirth or recurrent miscarriage
- Genetic syndromes
- Significant medical illnesses (pulmonary embolism, severe hypertension)

Modified from Ref. [60] ACOG Technical bulletin No. 102: Management of Stillbirth. Obstet Gynecol 2009; 112.

---

growth charts, compared with 1.2 for small for gestational age fetuses determined by population-based curves) [17].

When a full autopsy is performed, published guidelines should be followed [18, 19]. It is appropriate to take photographs of the whole body, face, extremities, and any abnormalities to allow for subsequent consultation. Whole body X-rays are important to exclude possible skeletal dysplasias. Autopsy can also provide clues as to the timing of intrauterine death, another important consideration when determining fetal growth.

A complete postmortem evaluation is recommended in all cases of stillbirth, yet, unfortunately, autopsy is underutilized. Rates vary throughout the country, but perinatal autopsy is performed in significantly less than 50% of cases, with the exception of a few dedicated centers [2]. The use of fetal autopsy is often limited by cost or a lack of trained pathologists. When local expertise is not available, some referral centers may be willing to perform the autopsy for stillbirths that did not deliver at their own institution, or at least evaluate tissue blocks sent from outside pathologists. In all cases, the responsible clinician should communicate details of the case to the pathologist prior to the postmortem examination. Such communication not only has the potential to raise interest and increase quality, but it also promotes the most appropriate work-up, and allows one to request tissue collection that may be needed for additional analysis.

There may be discomfort on the part of the physician or patient to perform, or even discuss

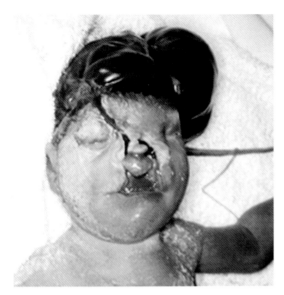

Figure 12.1 Third-trimester fetal death with acalvarium. On ultrasonography, there was suspicion of possible neural tube defect. However, autopsy demonstrated amniotic band syndrome. (Courtesy of Dr. Janice L.B. Byrne.)

autopsy. Similarly, patients may have reservations due to cultural or individual concerns. Often, patients are unaware of the potential benefits of autopsy. In addition, they may have misconceptions about the procedure itself. For example, many families believe that their infant will be disfigured or unavailable for a prolonged period of time, potentially delaying rituals such as burial. It is important for clinicians to strongly encourage autopsy in a fashion that is not overbearing and is sensitive to the concerns of the family. Often, patients reconsider the procedure when they are made aware of the benefits and once they have their logistical concerns addressed. If families are uncomfortable with a complete autopsy, partial autopsy, gross examination, and various imaging modalities, such as X-ray and magnetic resonance imaging (MRI), can all provide meaningful information [20, 21]. External examination is most useful when accomplished by a trained pathologist and/or a physician skilled in genetics and dysmorphology, especially if the family refuses autopsy all together. Patients and families should be allowed ample time to see and hold the baby and perform

any religious or cultural activities prior to sending the fetus to the pathologist.

Placental pathology

Gross and histologic evaluation of the placenta, umbilical cord, and fetal membranes is an essential component of the evaluation. In contrast to autopsy, families rarely refuse to allow an evaluation of the placenta. Placental evaluation is increasingly advised in all cases of adverse perinatal outcome, including stillbirth [22].

A trained pathologist should perform the evaluation and published guidelines should be followed. Placental weight should be documented and noted in relation to the norms for gestational age. As with autopsy, the value of placental pathology cannot be overemphasized because it provides information regarding a broad array of potential causes of stillbirth. In one series of stillbirth, evaluation of the placenta contributed to a diagnosis in almost half the cases [23].

Gross evaluation may reveal conditions specific to gestational tissues that may cause or contribute to fetal death such as abruption (Figure 12.2), umbilical cord thrombosis, velamentous cord

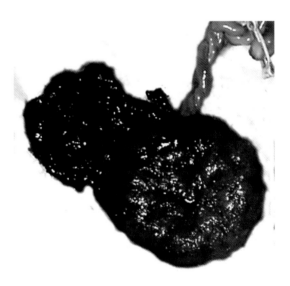

Figure 12.2 Large clot adherent to approximately one-third of the placenta. (Courtesy of Dr. Janice L.B. Byrne.)

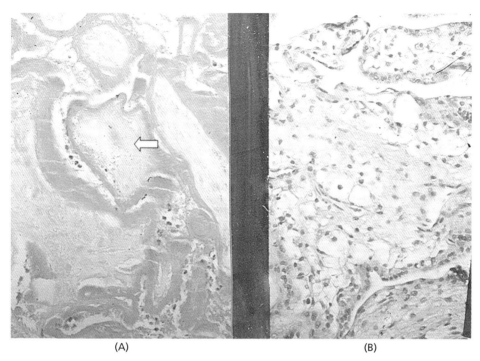

(A)   (B)

Figure 12.3 Placenta demonstrating villous infarction from a case of second-trimester fetal death in a patient with antiphospholipid syndrome (A). (B) Normal placenta is shown for comparison. A: ×40, original magnification. B: ×100, original magnification. (Courtesy of Dr. Robert M. Silver.)

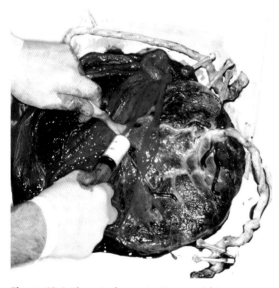

Figure 12.4 Placenta demonstrating arterial-to-venous anastomoses after injection of milk in a pregnancy complicated by twin–twin transfusion syndrome. (Courtesy of Dr. Janice L.B. Byrne.)

insertion, and vasa previa. Placental evaluation also provides information about infection, genetic abnormalities, fetal anemia, hypoxia, APS (Figure 12.3), and thrombophilias. Examination of the placental vasculature and membranes can be particularly helpful in multifetal gestations. Chorionicity can be established and vascular anastomoses identified (Figure 12.4).

Umbilical cord knots or tangling should be noted but interpreted with caution. Perhaps no other single etiology is purported to be the cause of stillbirth as often as umbilical cord accidents. This is especially true for cases near term and is thought to be due to cord compression with cessation of blood flow to the fetus in the setting of a nuchal or "true knot" in the umbilical cord. Because cord entanglement occurs in about 30% of uncomplicated pregnancies and "true knots" in the cord usually result in live births, it is impossible to confidently attribute a fetal death to a cord accident on the basis of nuchal cord alone. Ideally, stillbirth should only be considered to be likely due to cord accidents if (1) other recognized causes of still-birth are excluded and (2) there is accompanying evidence on autopsy and placental evaluation that the cord accident is the cause. Examples include histologic examination showing evidence of cord occlusion (chorionic villous edema, thrombus in fetal vessels, and intervillous karyorrhexis) and/or fetal hypoxia. Parast and colleagues [24] suggest specific histologic criteria for the diagnosis of cord occlusion. Minimal histologic criteria for cord accident include vascular ectasia and thrombosis within the umbilical cord, chorionic plate, and/or stem villi [24]. A probable diagnosis requires those findings as well as regional distribution of avascular villi or villi showing stromal karyorrhexis. It is noteworthy that a variety of other cord abnormalities are also associated with stillbirth (Figure 12.5) [25].

Karyotype and genetic evaluation

Genetic evaluation by karyotype should be encouraged in all cases of fetal death. An abnormal fetal karyotype has been noted in 8–13% of all stillbirths and greater than 30% of those with structural anomalies or intrauterine growth restriction [12, 26, 27]. However, these numbers are likely an underestimate because karyotype is often unsuccessful due to cell culture failure. The most common abnormalities are monosomy X (23%) (Figure 12.6), trisomy 21 (23%), trisomy 18 (21%), and trisomy 13 (8%) [26]. Alternatively, the risk of chromosomal abnormalities in stillbirths with no dysmorphic features (especially if no abnormalities were noted on antepartum ultrasound) and normal growth is probably less than 2%. This can be especially important when cost is an issue, thus when the fetus appears normal and is appropriately grown, omitting the fetal karyotype may be appropriate.

Unfortunately, attempts at cell culture in cases of stillbirths are successful in only about one half of cases. Acceptable cytologic specimens include amniotic fluid, a placental block taken from below the cord insertion site that includes the chorionic plate, an umbilical cord segment, or internal fetal tissues that thrive under low oxygen tension such as costochondral or patellar tissue.

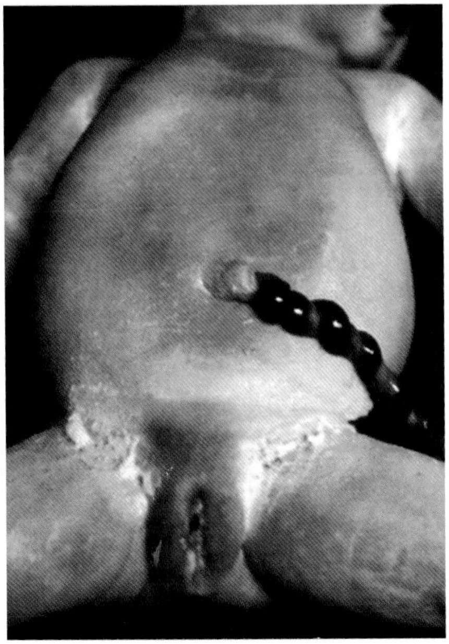

Figure 12.5 Stillbirth with umbilical cord stricture and thrombosis. (Courtesy of Dr. Janice L.B. Byrne.)

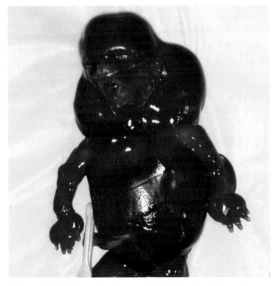

Figure 12.6 Second-trimester fetal death with cystic hygroma and nonimmune hydrops. The fetus had Turner's syndrome. (Courtesy of Dr. Janice L.B. Byrne.)

Fetal skin is suboptimal but sometimes suffices. Tissues should be placed in sterile tissue culture medium of lactated ringers at room temperature, and the temptation to send these specimens in formalin should be strictly rejected. If necessary, the tissue can be placed in a sterile container without fluid. Cultured amniocytes have the highest yield and amniocentesis prior to delivery should be strongly considered. This is acceptable to many patients given the minimal risk, and can even be accomplished after epidural placement when the patient desires this method of pain relief for induced labor.

If culture is unsuccessful, fluorescent in situ hybridization (FISH) or array-based comparative genomic hybridization (CGH) may be helpful in identifying structural chromosome abnormalities [28]. FISH can be used to test for the most common aneuploidies but will not detect more subtle chromosome abnormalities. CGH will detect small deletions or duplications, termed copy number changes, which may be too small to be detected even with traditional karyotype. Also, it does not require live cells from culture. However, CGH has some limitations. First, many small copy number changes will be of uncertain clinical significance. Second, it will not detect cytogenetic abnormalities, such as translocations, that do not result in copy number changes. Third, it requires high-quality DNA that may be hard to obtain from macerated tissues. Finally, insurance carriers may not cover the test [29]. In addition to not requiring successful cell culture, array CGH may identify genetic abnormalities responsible for pregnancy loss that are not ascertained with traditional karyotype. This was the case in 13–14% of two recent series of fetal deaths [30, 31]. As array CGH technology becomes less expensive and more widely available and as we become better at determining which copy number changes are clinically important, it likely will become a very useful tool in the evaluation of stillbirth.

Many fetal deaths have genetic abnormalities that are not detected by conventional cytogenetic analysis or CGH. Malformations, deformations, syndromes, or dysplasias have been reported in up to 35% of fetal losses undergoing perinatal autopsy [5, 26]. Although up to 25% of these fetuses are aneuploid, most will have normal karyotypes. The best current diagnostic approach for these cases is perinatal autopsy with input from a geneticist. However, continued developments in molecular genetic technology such as CGH should greatly facilitate our ability to determine previously unrecognized genetic conditions associated with fetal death.

Rare cases of stillbirth are caused by a handful of single-gene disorders such as alpha thalassemia. Genetic analysis to assess for these disorders should not be routinely used, but guided by clinical suspicion, family history, or autopsy and placental evaluation. Currently unrecognized single-gene disorders probably cause or serve as risk factors for stillbirth, notably those that are not associated with obvious malformations. These include autosomal recessive disorders like glycogen storage disorders or metabolic disorders. At present, testing for such conditions remains investigational. Confined placental mosaicism (complete or partial placental aneuploidy in the presence of a euploid fetus) has also been implicated as a possible etiology for stillbirth [32]. As with widespread testing for single-gene disorders and microdeletions, routine testing is not advised at present.

Testing for fetal–maternal hemorrhage

Fetal–maternal hemorrhage (FMH) has been reported to account for 1.5–14% of stillbirths [33–36], a meaningful proportion, and routine screening for this potential cause is advised. The Kleihauer-Betke test can detect fetal erythrocytes in maternal blood, based on elution of adult hemoglobin from adult red cells. The more acid-resistant fetal hemoglobin remains intact in fetal red cells, and the remaining hemoglobin is subsequently visualized by staining with erythrosine (Figure 12.7). A limitation of this test is that a small amount of fetal cells may be detected in uncomplicated pregnancies, so results must be interpreted in the setting of the clinical and pathologic findings. The manual Kleihauer-Betke (used by most laboratories) is limited by statistical

(A) (B)

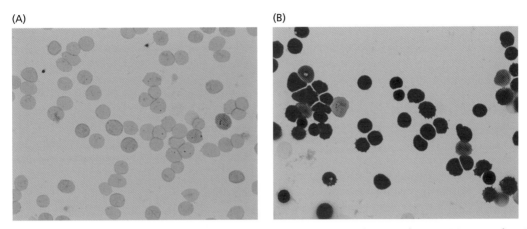

Figure 12.7 Kleihauer-Betke stain. Fetal cells stain dark red. (A) Negative control, ×100 oil. (B) Positive control ×100 oil. (Courtesy of Dr. William A. Brooks III.)

imprecision in quantifying large-volume FMH as it only involves the assessment of a small number of cells and may result in underestimation in cases of large FMH [37]. Flow cytometry may be a more accurate alternative to the Kleihauer-Betke and is used by some centers to identify fetal red cells in the maternal circulation. Both tests are useful for the assessment of stillbirth because only massive hemorrhage (e.g., >20% of the fetal circulation) is likely to cause fetal death.

In cases of antepartum stillbirth, assessment of fetal blood in the maternal circulation should preferably be accomplished prior to delivery as delivery itself may cause FMH. However, given that stillbirth is likely only due to massive FMH, it is probably useful to assess for FMH up to a few weeks after delivery [38]. Delivery-associated FMH greater than 30 ml likely occurs in only 0.23–1.0% of live births [38–41]. Truly massive hemorrhage of greater than 150 ml probably occurs in only about one in 2,800 live births [42]. Owen and colleagues [43] attempted to address this issue by assessing pre- and post-delivery Kleihauer-Betke stains in 66 cases of stillbirth. Three (4.6%) had massive fetomaternal hemorrhage with positive tests both pre- and post-delivery. There were no cases of false-positive results postdelivery in the other 63 cases [43].

There is no clear consensus as to the definition of a blood volume to identify FMH severe enough to cause stillbirth, and no one threshold will pertain to all situations. For example, one factor that substantially influences the clinical impact of fetal bleeding is whether the hemorrhage is acute or chronic. Acute hemorrhage can lead to cardiovascular decompensation, stroke, disseminated intravascular coagulation, and death. In contrast, chronic bleeding may allow the fetus to adapt to a lower hematocrit and potentially survive. An approach to identifying chronic bleeding may be through the identification of increased production of erythroblasts and reticulocytes (which seems to require 1–2 days or more of anemia) in fetal blood using flow cytometry [38]. Another consideration is gestational age. Fetal blood volume at earlier gestational ages is lower and, consequently, a smaller blood loss from an earlier fetus represents a larger percentage of blood than in a fetus of more advanced gestational age (i.e., a 30 ml loss in a 60 g fetus represents 42% of the total fetal blood volume while the same bleed in a 3,600 g fetus is only 7%) [44].

A threshold of 30 ml has been used to define "massive" or "severe" FMH, chosen in part because it identifies RhD-negative women requiring more than the standard dose of RhD immune globulin to prevent RhD red cell alloimmunization. Sebring [38] noted a 50% mortality rate in fetuses with acute bleeds of 20% or more of their total blood volumes. Others have noted death after 40% [45].

Rubod and colleagues [33] have taken a systematic approach to the issue. They assessed all cases (48) of severe FMH over an 8-year period in a cohort of 45,180 deliveries (rate of 1.1 per 1,000). A threshold of 20 ml/kg of fetal bleeding was associated with an increased risk for stillbirth, induced preterm delivery, neonatal intensive care unit admission, and neonatal anemia requiring transfusion [33]. Although there is no gold standard for attributing fetal death to FMH, using greater than 20 ml/kg as a threshold for attributing this as a cause of fetal death is reasonable. Autopsy confirmation of fetal anemia and hypoxia should be used to corroborate the Kleihauer-Betke or flow cytometry results when considering fetal death to be a result of FMH.

Indirect Coombs'/antibody screen

Testing for maternal antibodies that may result in red cell alloimmunization during pregnancy is generally performed at the initial prenatal visit. Alloimmunization is a recognized, albeit uncommon, cause of stillbirth and will usually be associated with specific clinical and pathologic findings, such as fetal hydrops. Sensitization during the current pregnancy is very unlikely to result in stillbirth if testing was initially normal. Thus, it need not be repeated if it was obtained during the pregnancy. However, an indirect Coombs' should be assessed if it was not previously obtained.

Toxicology screen

A maternal urine toxicology screen is generally recommended as part of the initial evaluation of stillbirth (also see Chapter 4). Although in some populations it may be decreasing, maternal substance use is associated with a meaningful proportion of stillbirths. As an alternative to maternal urine screen, it is possible to measure stable metabolites of recreational drugs in fetal meconium, hair, and homogenized umbilical cord. However, at present such testing is not widely available. Although maternal recreational drug use is associated with an increased risk of stillbirth, it may be difficult to confirm that it is a cause of fetal death. The most convincing link is between cocaine and stillbirth. Cocaine use during pregnancy is associated with a sixfold increased risk of stillbirth, primarily as a result of fetal growth restriction and/or abruption [46]. The relationship between stillbirth and other illicit drugs is less clear.

Testing for infections

Infections are a generally accepted cause of stillbirth, accounting for about 10–25% of cases in developed countries (see Chapter 5) [47] and an even higher proportion in developing countries. In developed countries, infections are more common in stillbirths occurring relatively early in gestation. Indeed, infection has been implicated as a cause of stillbirth in up to 20% of cases occurring at less than 28 weeks of gestation [48]. Infectious agents may cause stillbirth by direct fetal infection, placental damage, and severe maternal illness. While an evaluation for infection is warranted in cases of stillbirth, it is important to be cautious when attributing fetal death to infection. Mothers often have vaginal infection or colonization, or systemic viral infections that may have nothing to do with a stillbirth. *Fetal autopsy and histologic evaluation of the placenta, membranes, and umbilical cord provide the most convincing proof of infection being truly the cause of stillbirth* (see also Chapter 10). For instance, a positive culture of group B *Streptococcus* in fetal lungs is convincing evidence of causality, while positive vaginal group B streptococcal culture alone is not.

Viral infections

Since the most common viral infection that has been linked to fetal death is parvovirus B19, maternal serology for this virus is often recommended. It has been implicated in up to 8% of fetal deaths in one study based on the identification of viral nucleic acid in the placenta [49], although in the United States, parvovirus is associated with less than 1% of stillbirths [47]. Finding viral nucleic acid in the fetus or placenta without histologic evidence of viral infection may represent a false-positive result; yet in cases at increased risk, may be worthwhile, because viruses are difficult to culture and nucleic acid testing probably identifies cases that would have been otherwise missed. Parvovirus is more likely to be associated with fetal death if a careful history reveals that infection

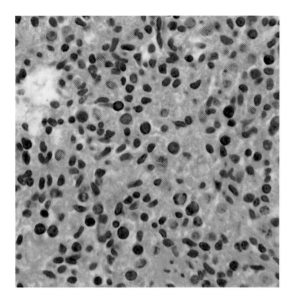

Figure 12.8 Fetal spleen from a case of parvovirus B19-associated fetal death in the second trimester. Erythroblasts show marginated chromatin and typical amphophilic intranuclear inclusions. Hematoxylin and eosin stain. (×1,000, original magnification.) (Courtesy of Dr. Janice L.B. Byrne.)

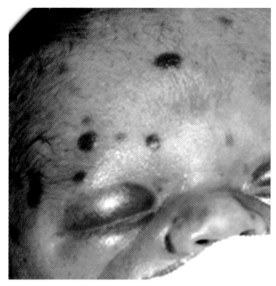

Figure 12.9 Extramedullary hematopoiesis in an infant with CMV infection. (Courtesy of Dr. Janice L.B. Byrne.)

occurred during the first two trimesters of pregnancy. When parvovirus is suspected, specific questions of exposure to "fifth disease" (erythema infectiosum) in children they have contact with is warranted, because infection may be asymptomatic in adults. When parvovirus is responsible for fetal death, the mechanism is most often destruction of erythropoietic tissue leading to severe anemia and hydrops (Figure 12.8). However, direct myocardial damage has also been implicated as contributing to fetal death. Again, results of serologic testing must be interpreted in the context of the clinical and histopathologic findings, as most pregnancies complicated by parvovirus infection do not result in fetal death.

Other viral infections may also contribute to or cause fetal death. Pathogens include enteroviruses, such as coxsackie A and B, echoviruses, and cytomegalovirus (CMV). The coxsackie viruses, like parvovirus, can cause fetal death through placental inflammation, myocarditis, and hydrops. While CMV is the most commonly acquired

congenital viral infection, it only rarely causes stillbirth. Testing for CMV serology is not routinely advised unless there is clinical (Figure 12.9) or histopathologic suspicion for the disease. The same is true for a variety of other viruses that are uncommon causes of stillbirth. Although human immunodeficiency virus (HIV) has been linked to stillbirth, HIV-positive women usually have other risk factors, making it difficult to document an independent association between HIV and fetal death.

Bacterial infection

Bacterial pathogens implicated in stillbirth include *Escherichia coli*, group B streptococci, *Ureaplasma urealyticum*, and less frequently *Klebsiella*, *Mycoplasma hominus*, and *Bacteroides* from ascending infection. Most of these organisms are vaginal flora that reaches the amniotic sac and the fetus through the cervix. However, *Listeria monocytogenes* can reach the fetus through hematogenous transmission. Some organisms cause clinically apparent intra-amniotic infection, while other indolent organisms such as *Mycoplasmas*, *Ureaplasmas*, and *Listeria* may cause vague symptoms that are difficult to diagnose. In cases of suspected bacterial infection, the most reliable test is culture of normally sterile neonatal body sites such as the lung. Culture of the placenta is likely to be contaminated with vaginal flora. In theory, culturing "in between" layers of the amniotic sac to avoid vaginal contamination may avoid vaginal bacteria, but utility has not been proven.

Other infections

The risk of stillbirth from syphilis increases with advancing gestation as the responsible spirochete, *Treponema pallidum*, may cross the placenta and directly infect the fetus. Syphilis is a major cause of fetal death in developing countries and persists in some parts of the United States. In fact, there has been a 23% increase in the rate of congenital syphilis in the United States between 2005 and 2008. The increase is primarily in non-Hispanic black women in the Southern United States [50]. In low-risk populations, negative screening with routine prenatal laboratory evaluation in the first trimester likely suffices. However, repeat screening at the time of fetal death should be considered in high-risk populations. A reasonable alternative approach would be to reserve assessment of serology for cases wherein congenital syphilis is suspected on the basis of clinical history, autopsy, or placental pathology. Other spirochetes such as *Borrelia burgdorferi* (the causative agent in Lyme disease) produce sporadic stillbirths. Testing for this organism should be reserved for cases with clinical suspicion of maternal Lyme disease (e.g., history of a tick bite and rash).

Malaria may be a cause of fetal death in women who contract a primary infection during pregnancy. Other less common organisms associated with fetal death include *Toxoplasma gondii*, and leptospira. Toxoplasmosis is a parasitic disease transmitted through undercooked meat or cat feces, and may directly infect the fetus via transplacental passage. This occurs in around 40% of cases of maternal infection. It has been linked to sporadic death, which may occur in up to 5% of pregnancies after infection between 10 and 24 weeks [51]. It is an uncommon cause of stillbirth in the United States, and routine testing in the absence of clinical suspicion (e.g., fetal hydrocephalus, intracranial calcifications, hepatosplenomegaly, or identification of the parasite in fetal tissues) is not advised.

Infectious work-up

Testing for these various pathogens should be guided by the clinical history, as well as findings on autopsy, placental pathology, or imaging. If autopsy, pathology, or history is suggestive of an infectious etiology, an evaluation should be undertaken. This may include maternal or neonatal serology, special tissue stains, and/or testing for bacterial or viral nucleic acids, which may be more sensitive than culture, but may also lead to false-positive results. *However, if clinical or histologic evidence is lacking, testing for infection is of questionable utility.* Although assessment of "TORCH" (toxoplasmosis, rubella, CMV, herpes simplex) titers has been traditionally advised for the evaluation of stillbirth, routine testing is of unproven utility. As stated earlier, routine culture of the placental membranes should be considered experimental and is not recommended at present.

Testing for antiphospholipid syndrome and heritable thrombophilias

APS is an acquired autoimmune condition characterized by the production of moderate to high levels of antiphospholipid antibodies and specific clinical features. Although one fetal death is considered sufficient to satisfy the clinical criteria for APS, a diagnosis of APS is based on a combination of both clinical and laboratory criteria [52]. APS is responsible for a small, yet meaningful percentage of stillbirths (estimated at 2–3%). Screening is advised because it poses a very high risk for recurrent fetal death and treatment can improve outcomes in subsequent pregnancies. Laboratory testing is performed by testing for lupus anticoagulant as well as IgG and IgM for both anticardiolipin and anti-beta2-glycoprotein antibodies. A moderate to high IgG or IgM titer (greater than 40 MPL/GPL or greater than 99th percentile) is considered positive but must be confirmed with repeat testing 6–12 weeks later. Lower titers, as well as a positive test of the IgA isotype, are of uncertain clinical significance. Women who suffer a stillbirth that is accompanied by growth restriction, severe preeclampsia, or other evidence of placental insufficiency, or who have systemic lupus erythematosus (SLE) or thrombosis are more likely to test positive for APS than women who suffer stillbirths without these features. In addition, placental pathology may show inflammation, thrombosis, and/or infarction (Figure 12.3) in cases where APS is responsible for the stillbirth.

Routine testing for heritable thrombophilias is controversial (also see Chapter 9). Most case–control studies show an association between heritable thrombophilias and late fetal loss [53]. However, the association is modest with odds ratios of about 2–3 [53]. Also, thrombophilias were not associated with stillbirth in several large prospective cohort studies [54–56]. Finally, thrombophilias are extremely common in normal healthy individuals and the vast majority of women with thrombophilias have uncomplicated pregnancies. At worst, thrombophilias are a modest risk factor for, rather than a cause of stillbirth.

Testing for thrombophilias may be most appropriate in cases with evidence of placental insufficiency (placental infarction, fetal growth restriction, oligohydramnios, or preeclampsia), recurrent losses, or a personal or strong family history of thrombosis. The thrombophilias most strongly linked to stillbirth include the Factor V Leiden mutation, G20210A prothrombin gene mutation, and deficiencies of antithrombin III, protein C, and protein S. The latter three conditions are rare in the absence of a family history of thrombosis. It is important to note that reliable testing for protein C and S activity cannot be obtained during pregnancy and should be delayed until at least 6 weeks after delivery. In theory, positive results for thrombophilias could affect future pregnancy management since thromboprophylaxis may improve outcome [57]. However, other studies showed no benefit from thromboprophylaxis [58, 59]. Therefore, in the absence of the aforementioned complications, routine testing is not indicated and may lead to unnecessary interventions. The associations between other thrombophilias such as the methylenetetrahydrofolate reductase mutations and stillbirth are unclear and testing is not recommended.

Testing for maternal medical conditions

Clinically apparent maternal conditions including diabetes, thyroid disease, asthma, SLE, cholestasis of pregnancy, and renal disease have all been associated with stillbirth. On balance, approximately 10% of stillbirths are associated with maternal medical disorders. In many cases, these conditions should be considered risk factors for, rather than causes of stillbirth since most women with these disorders do not have stillbirths. It is sometimes difficult to evaluate the contribution of medical disorders to stillbirth since good medical care may dramatically influence the risk.

Pregestational diabetes carries a relative risk of about 2.5 for stillbirth [12]. However, some women with gestational diabetes mellitus (GDM) diagnosed during pregnancy actually have undiagnosed type 2 diabetes. These women have the same risk of fetal loss as women with type 2 diabetes. Diabetes is more likely to be the cause of stillbirth when there is evidence of poor glycemic control, fetal macrosomia, or placental vasculopathy of diabetes. Patients with lupus or renal disease may have an increased risk of stillbirth that approaches 20–30 times the risk of the general population [12]. Pregnancy loss in the setting of these conditions typically occurs in women with clinically apparent and severe disease. However, the association of more subtle maternal medical conditions with stillbirth is controversial, and testing for subclinical disease is of uncertain utility. For example, stillbirth is unlikely to be secondary to mild glucose intolerance, subclinical thyroid disease, or renal disease with a mildly elevated serum creatinine. Similarly, a positive test for antinuclear antibodies in the absence of other findings of lupus is likely of no significance. Therefore, testing should be guided by maternal medical history, physical examination, and clinical circumstances. Assessment of bile acids is appropriate in cases of pruritis or elevated liver function tests in an attempt to diagnose intrahepatic cholestasis of pregnancy. Routine testing for other subclinical maternal diseases is not recommended.

Uterine abnormalities

Losses associated with cervical insufficiency, preterm labor and preterm premature rupture of membranes, and abruption raise suspicion for possible uterine malformations. Such conditions, as well as prior fetal malpresentation, should prompt consideration for sonohysterogram or other imaging of the uterine cavity. Stillbirths in these settings tend to be intrapartum and occur at previable or periviable gestations. In cases of uterine septums, surgical revision may improve outcome in subsequent pregnancies.

Summary

Recommendations for the diagnostic evaluation of stillbirth are summarized in Box 12.2. It is uncertain whether it is preferable to test for potential causes of stillbirth in a sequential, rather than comprehensive manner. Sequential testing has the potential benefit of cost savings and the avoidance of positive results that may cause anxiety yet not identify a true etiology of stillbirth (e.g., positive serology for CMV with no evidence of fetal infection). However, some cases may be due to more than one cause or the interaction of several causes or risk factors that may only be recognized through comprehensive testing. The answer may lie in a modified combination of the two approaches. Because clinical history, perinatal autopsy, placental evaluation, karyotype, and screening for FMH (such as Kleihauer-Betke) identify a cause in a significant number of stillbirths, they are recommended in all cases. Autopsy, placental evaluation, karyotype, screen for FMH, and toxicology screen are all time-dependent studies and are either less reliable or cannot be done long after delivery, so it is best to do these as part of the initial evaluation. Other tests should be considered after this baseline assessment in selected situations when a diagnosis is suggested by the clinical history, autopsy, or placental pathology.

When evaluated in a thorough, systematic fashion, many cases of stillbirth can be assigned an etiology. This process can facilitate grieving and emotional closure for families, counseling about subsequent pregnancies and, in some cases, obstetric interventions that improve outcome in subsequent pregnancies. Ongoing research, such as that being conducted by the Stillbirth Collaborative Research Network of the National Institute of Child Health

---

Box 12.2 Suggested evaluation of stillbirth

Recommended in all cases
- Autopsy
- Placental pathology
- Karyotype
- Kleihauer-Betke or other screen for fetal–maternal hemorrhage

Helpful in some cases when condition is suggested by clinical history, autopsy, placental pathology, or other data source.
- Syphilis serology (if not performed early in pregnancy; consider repeating in high-risk populations)
- Indirect Coombs' (if not performed earlier in pregnancy)
- Parvovirus B19 IgG and IgM
- Lupus anticoagulant, IgG and IgM anti-cardiolipin and anti-beta-2-glyprotein-I antibodies
- Toxicology screen
- Factor V Leiden, Prothrombin gene mutation, Antithrombin III, Protein C & S levels (must be done at least 6 weeks postpartum)
- Glucose screening test, glycohemoglobin
- Thyroid stimulating hormone
- Maternal serology or other testing such as fetal tissue culture or stains for other infectious etiologies
- Bile acids
- Sonohysterogram

Not generally useful
- Routine TORCH titers
- ANA testing
- Cultures of placental membranes
- Testing for MTHFR mutations

Modified from Ref. [61] Silver et al. Am J Obstet Gynecol 2007; 110 with permission from Elsevier.

---

and Human Development, will help to further clarify the optimal "work-up" of stillbirth.

References

1. Walsh CA, Vallerie AM, Baxi LV. Etiology of stillbirth at term: a 10-year cohort study. J Matern Fetal Neonatal Med 2008;21:493–501.
2. Silver RM. Fetal death. Obstet Gynecol 2007;109: 153–67.

3. Petersson K. Diagnostic evaluation of fetal death with special reference to intrauterine infections. [Dissertation]. Sweden, Stockholm: Department of Clinical Science, Division of Obstetrics and Gynecology, Karolinska Institutet; 2002.

4. Horn LC, Langner A, Stiehl P, et al. Identification of the causes of intrauterine death during 310 consecutive autopsies. Eur J Obstet Gynecol Reprod Biol 2004;113:134–8.

5. Pauli RM, Reiser CA. Wisconsin Stillbirth Service Program: II. Analysis of diagnoses and diagnostic categories in the first 1,000 referrals. Am J Med Genet 1994;50:135–53.

6. Lu JR, McCowan L. A comparison of the Perinatal Society of Australia and New Zealand-Perinatal Death Classification system and relevant condition at death stillbirth classification systems. Aust N Z J Obstet Gynecol 2009;49:467–71.

7. Vergani P, Cozzolino S, Pozzi E, et al. Identifying the causes of stillbirth: a comparison of four classification systems. Am J Obstet Gynecol 2008;199:319e1–4.

8. Dugoff L, Hobbins JC, Malone FD, et al. Quad screen as a predictor of adverse pregnancy outcome. Obstet Gynecol 2005;106:260–7.

9. Smith GC, Stenhouse EJ, Crossley JA, et al. Early pregnancy levels of pregnancy-associated plasma protein a and the risk of intrauterine growth restriction, premature birth, preeclampsia, and stillbirth. J Clin Endocrinol Metab 2002;87:1762–7.

10. Frias AE Jr, Luikenaar RA, Sullivan AE, et al. Poor obstetric outcome in subsequent pregnancies in women with prior fetal death. Obstet Gynecol 2004; 104:521–6.

11. Rasmussen S, Irgens LM, Skjaerven R, Melve KK. Prior adverse pregnancy outcome and the risk of stillbirth. Obstet Gynecol 2009;114:1259–70.

12. ACOG Practice Bulletin No. 102: management of stillbirth. Obstet Gynecol 2009;113:748–61.

13. Silver RM, Varner MW, Reddy U, et al. Work-up of stillbirth: a review of the evidence. Am J Obstet Gynecol 2007;196:433–44.

14. Faye-Petersen OM, Guinn DA, Wenstrom KD. Value of perinatal autopsy. Obstet Gynecol 1999;94: 915–20.

15. Michalski ST, Porter J, Pauli RM. Costs and consequences of comprehensive stillbirth assessment. Am J Obstet Gynecol 2002;186:1027–34.

16. Bonetti LR, Ferrari P, Trani N, et al. The role of fetal autopsy and placental examination in the causes of fetal death: a retrospective study of 132 cases of stillbirths. Arch Gynecol Obstet 2010;Jan 6:Epub.

17. Clausson B, Gardosi J, Francis A, Cnattingius S. Perinatal outcome in SGA births defined by customised versus population-based birthweight standards. BJOG 2001;108:830–4.

18. Bove KE. Practice guidelines for autopsy pathology: the perinatal and pediatric autopsy. Arch Pathol Lab Med 1997;121:368–76.

19. Valdes-Depena M, Huff DS. Perinatal autopsy manual. Washington, DC: Armed Forces Institute of Pathology; 1983.

20. Thayyil S, Cleary JO, Sebire NJ, et al. Post-mortem examination of human fetuses: a comparison of whole-body high-field MRI at 9.4 T with conventional MRI and invasive autopsy. Lancet 2009;374: 467–75.

21. Woodward PJ, Sohaey R, Harris DP, et al. Postmortem fetal MR imaging: comparison with findings at autopsy. AJR Am J Roentgenol 1997;168:41–6.

22. Khong TY. From delivery suite to laboratory: optimizing returns from placental examination in medico-legal defence. Aust N Z J Obstet Gynaecol 1997;37:1–5.

23. Heazell AE, Martindale EA. Can post-mortem examination of the placenta help determine the cause of stillbirth? J Obstet Gynaecol 2009;29:225–8.

24. Parast MM, Crum CP, Boyd TK. Placental histologic criteria for umbilical blood flow restriction in unexplained stillbirth. Hum Pathol 2008;39:948–53.

25. Tantbirojn P, Saleemuddin A, Sirois K, et al. Gross abnormalities of the umbilical cord: related placental histology and clinical significance. Placenta 2009; 30:1083–8.

26. Wapner RJ, Lewis D. Genetics and metabolic causes of stillbirth. Semin Perinatol 2002;26:70–4.

27. Kortweg FJ, Bouman K, Erwich JJ, et al. Cytogenetic analysis after evaluation of 750 fetal deaths: proposal for a diagnostic workup. Obstet Gynecol 2008; 111:865–74.

28. Benkhalifa M, Kasakyan S, Clement P, et al. Array comparative genomic hybridization profiling of first-trimester spontaneous abortions that fail to grow in vitro. Prenat Diagn 2005;25:894–900.

29. ACOG Committee Opinion Number 446. Comparative genomic hybridization in prenatal diagnosis. Obstet Gynecol 2009;114:1161–3.

30. Warren JE, Turok DK, Maxwell TM, et al. Array comparative genomic hybridization for genetic evaluation of fetal loss between 10 and 20 of weeks gestation. Obstet Gynecol 2009;114:1093–102.

31. Raca G, Artzer A, Thorson L, et al. Array-based comparative genomic hybridization (aCGH) in the genetic evaluation of stillbirth. Am J Med Genet A 2009;149A:2437–43.

32. Kalousek DK, Barrett I. Confined placental mosaicism and stillbirth. Pediatr Pathol 1994;14:151–9.

33. Rubod C, Derulle P, Le Gouf F, et al. Long-term prognosis for infants after massive fetomaternal hemorrhage. Obstet Gynecol 2007;110:256–60.

34. Laube DW, Schauberger CW. Fetomaternal bleeding as a cause for "unexplained" fetal death. Obstet Gynecol 1982;60:649–51.

35. Marions L, Thomassen P. Six cases of massive fetomaternal bleeding causing intra-uterine fetal death. Acta Obstet Gynecol Scand 1991;70:85–8.

36. Samadi R, Greenspoon JS, Gviazda I, et al. Massive fetomaternal hemorrhage and fetal death: are they predictable? J Perinatol 1999;19:227–9.

37. Pelikan DM, Mesker WE, Scherjon SA, et al. Improvement of the Kleihauer-Betke test by automated detection of fetal erythrocytes in maternal blood. Cytometry B Clin Cytom 2003;54:1–9.

38. Sebring ES, Polesky HF. Fetomaternal hemorrhage: incidence, risk factors, time of occurrence, and clinical effects. Transfusion 1990;30:344–51.

39. Bowman JM. Controversies in Rh prophylaxis: who needs Rh immune globulin and when should it be given? Am J Obstet Gynecol 1985;151:289–94.

40. Stedman CM, Baudin JC, White CA, Cooper ES. Use of the erythrocyte rosette test to screen for excessive fetomaternal hemorrhage in Rh-negative women. Am J Obstet Gynecol 1986;154:1363–9.

41. Ness PM, Baldwin ML, Niebyl JR. Clinical high risk designation does not predict excess fetal-maternal hemorrhage. Am J Obstet Gynecol 1987;156:154–8.

42. de Almeida V, Bowman JM. Massive fetomaternal hemorrhage: Manitoba experience. Obstet Gynecol 1994;83:323–8.

43. Owen J, Stedman CM, Tucker TL. Comparison of predelivery versus postdelivery Kleihauer-Betke stains in cases of fetal death. Am J Obstet Gynecol 1989;161:663–6.

44. Dziegiel MH, Nielsen LK, Berkowicz A. Detecting fetomaternal hemorrhage by flow cytometry. Curr Opin Hematol 2006;13:490–5.

45. Giacoia GP. Severe fetomaternal hemorrhage: a review. Obstet Gynecol Surv 1997;52:372–80.

46. Lutiger B, Graham K, Einarson T, Koren G. Relationship between gestational cocaine use and pregnancy outcome: a meta-analysis. Teratology 1991;44:405–14.

47. McClure EM, Goldenberg RL. Infection and stillbirth. Semin Fetal Neonatal Med 2009;14:182–9.

48. Copper RL, Goldenberg RL, DuBard MB, Davis RO. Risk factors for fetal death in white, black, and Hispanic women. Collaborative Group on Preterm Birth Prevention. Obstet Gynecol 1994;84:490–5.

49. Skjöldebrand-Sparre L, Tolfvenstam T, Papadogiannakis N, et al. Parvovirus B19 infection: association with third trimester intrauterine fetal death. BJOG 2000; 107:476–80.

50. Centers for Disease Control and Prevention (CDC). Congenital syphilis—United States, 2003–2008. MMWR Morb Mortal Wkly Rep 2010;59:413–17.

51. Montoya JG, Remington JS. Management of *Toxoplasma gondii* infection during pregnancy. Clin Infect Dis 2008;47:554–66.

52. Miyakis S, Lockshin M, Atsumi T, et al. International consensus statement on an update of the classification criteria for definite antiphospholipid syndrome (APS). J Thromb Haemost 2006;4:295–306.

53. Robertson L, Wu O, Langhorne P, et al. Thrombophilia in pregnancy: a systematic review. Br J Haematol 2006;132:171–96.

54. Dizon-Townson D, Miller C, Sibai B, et al. The relationship of the factor V Leiden mutation and pregnancy outcomes for mother and fetus. Obstet Gynecol 2005;106:517–24.

55. Silver RM, Zhao Y, Spong CY, et al. Prothrombin gene G20210A mutation and obstetric complications. Obstet Gynecol 2010;115:14–20.

56. Said JM, Higgins JR, Moses EK, et al. Inherited thrombophilia polymorphisms and pregnancy outcomes in nulliparous women. Obstet Gynecol 2010; 115:5–13.

57. Gris JC, Mercier E, Quere I, et al. Low-molecular-weight heparin versus low-dose aspirin in women with one fetal loss and a constitutional thrombophilic disorder. Blood 2004;103:3695–9.

58. Warren JE, Simonsen E, Branch DW, et al. Thromboprophylaxis and pregnancy outcomes in asymptomatic women with inherited thrombophilias. Am J Obstet Gynecol 2009;200:281e1–5.

59. Kaandorp SP, Goddijin M, van der Post JAM, et al. Aspirin plus heparin or aspirin alone in women with recurrent miscarriage. N Engl J Med 2010;362: 1586–96.

60. ACOG practice bulletin. Clinical management guidelines for obstetrician-gynecologists. Number 46, September 2003. (Replaces technical bulletin number 222, April 1996). Obstet Gynecol 2003;102:647–58.

61. Silver RM, Varner MV, Reddy U, et al. Work-up of stillbirth: a review of the evidence. Am J Obstet Gynecol 2007;196:433–44.

CHAPTER 13
Psychosocial Care

Joanne Cacciatore, PhD, FT, LMSW
Center for Loss and Trauma, Arizona State University, Phoenix, AZ, USA

ATTEND: toward a relationship-based, patient-centered model of psychosocial intervention

The image of a woman reaching down to bring her baby onto her breast at the moment of birth is a powerful one. She birthed her baby, and every cell in her body knows and shows her strength. At the end of hours of pain and emotions felt more intensely than at any other time in life, she is exultant. To know the exhilaration, euphoria, and power that comes with the exhaustion and pain of giving birth is truly empowering [1].

Stillbirth: the collision of birth and death

Maggie just concluded her last visit with the obstetrician before the birth of her new baby. She has waited 10 long months for the baby's arrival. The nursery is complete. Diapers are neatly stacked near the powder-scented wipes. Her tiny clothes sit patiently in the white dresser. The family purchased a Doppler so that every morning they could listen to her heartbeat. For nearly 10 long months, Maggie has changed the way she eats, the way she dresses, her sleep patterns, and even the movies she watches and the music she listens to—all in preparation for their new child. She has parented this baby long before birth, nurturing her within the safety of her womb. The family has already named her "Grace."

Grace's brother and sister sit patiently in the waiting room anticipating the arrival of their new sister, their father already glowing. Any moment now they know that this new addition to their family will change their lives forever; and that she does. The nurse ushers the whole family into a small room. "What is going on?" he asks. As he watches tears streaming down his wife's cheeks, Grace's father hears those three most dreaded words as the nurse replies, "I'm so sorry . . ." And their nightmare begins.

Maggie endures 17 hours of grueling labor, and at the end of her 40-week journey through motherhood, she gives birth and death simultaneously to a beautiful 9-pound baby girl. Though she has not yet begun to process the trauma of this experience, only hours later, she leaves the hospital without Grace, walking past a nursery of healthy newborns on her way. What was to be the happiest day of their lives, the zenith they would celebrate every year, would become their worst nightmare.

Tomorrow, Maggie's breasts will become engorged, and she will wander the hallways of her home yearning to comfort her newborn, her arms literally burning to hold the baby. Primal maternal urges will drive her to the place where Grace is buried, and day after day, she will question, mourn, and, often, blame herself. Maggie has a long, harrowing road ahead.

Stillbirth is a traumatic experience that may incite long-term psychopathology which meets the criteria for anxiety, depression, and posttraumatic stress disorder (PTSD). While no amount of compassionate provider care can bring Grace back to her

---

family, interactions with medical staff during the acute crisis as well as postvention services, such as psychotherapy and ritualization, may significantly influence the degree, range, and intensity of her emotional angst and long-term psychological outcomes. Those individual effects then ripple outward, affecting her partner, children, family, friends, coworkers, and even the community.

It is the responsibility of providers to be knowledgeable, wise, and compassionate. Professionals need to understand that stillbirth, for most women, represents a traumatic and abiding loss on many levels, including biological, psychological, emotional, cognitive, social, and, for some, even spiritual. A multisystemic approach "draws on and expands individual, family, and community resources that are critical components" for patient integration in the aftermath of traumatic loss [2] and provides the necessary infrastructure for increased resiliency.

The Multidimensional Integrative Stillbirth Systems model

Giving birth and death simultaneously is an inexplicable loss for women that elicits cascading psychobiological reactions including symptoms of traumatic stress. Assuming each of the approximately 25,000 babies stillborn in the United States is survived, on average, by two parents, two grandparents, and one sibling, about 125,000 family members are directly affected during the course of 1 year. These profound effects are often both cumulative and intergenerational [3]. While all child deaths are widely accepted as painful and traumatic, stillbirth, due to its relative historic silence, is one of the few manners of death that has been least examined in clinical practice, postmortem data collection, academic research, and public policy, particularly given its frequency in both the Western world and globally. But this historical trend is evolving, and increasing numbers of stakeholders are becoming actively involved in this public health issue that is truly one of the last great mysteries of obstetrics.

The Multidimensional Integrative Stillbirth Systems (MISS) model (see Appendix on page 251)

is a map through which a provider can examine the variables within each system. This model provides a more holistic understanding of a patient, and, thus, better-informed care that recognizes nuance in each individual's experience. The *macro system* is the overarching sociopolitical system in a society, often influenced by culture, values, power, and history. The *mezzo system* relates to more localized, smaller systems within communities that interact directly with the patient, and can include peripheral family, schools, churches, providers, agencies, and workplace and housing communities. The *micro system* is the individual and their family of origin, and it lives within the mezzo system.

The larger, sociopolitical system (macro system) shapes attitudes, values, and beliefs about a social problem through legislation, semantical structuring, and policy. It is also influenced by the overarching cultural and demographic trends. That realm, then, influences public policy administration, social service programming and delivery, management of care, research, and agency formation related to the social problem at the mezzo level. The mezzo level includes academic, philanthropic, and faith-based institutions, hospitals, grassroots organizations, healthcare workers, mental health practitioners, and service delivery agencies. These systems also shape the ways in which society talks about (or silences) a social issue, language formation, including nomenclature and pedagogy. The micro system consists of the individual and immediate family members.

There is a continuous colloquy between the systems, and research has offered evidence to suggest that the influences of both the macro and mezzo systems on the individual and family can have long-term, deleterious—or protective—effects. The outcomes in the MISS model range from diminished functioning and compromised mental and emotional well-being to neutrality to transcending loss through posttraumatic growth. Providers who are relationally attuned to their patients help to buffer the negative effects of traumatic losses, thus affecting the outcome variables in the model. This paradigm provides a framework through which the proposed model of care, ATTEND (attunement, trust, therapeutic touch, egalitarianism, nuance, and death education), can emerge.

The unspeakable: macro trends in stillbirth

At some point in history, stillbirth became the unspeakable. Copious misinformation about stillbirth in society has led to false assumptions about the nature of this tragedy. Despite the fact that many babies are stillborn beyond viability, their deaths are often nosologically identified as a pregnancy or reproductive loss. Many academic journal articles and books discuss stillbirth in the context of miscarriage or abortion, failing to recognize its uniqueness in terms of emotional attachment, physiology, economics, and social factors. Even full-term intrapartum deaths are not counted in infant mortality data.

Until recently, while the actual deaths are recognized through each state's vital records office and final disposition mandated, no official record of birth was available to parents until 2001 when Arizona passed the first law in the nation allowing a Certificate of Birth Resulting in Stillbirth (CBRS). Since then, 26 other states have followed suit [3]. But these legislative changes have not come without great cost. Lobbying Goliaths around the nation have worked at halting the bill's success in many states such as California, New York, and Pennsylvania, where the grassroots efforts of mothers and fathers and grandparents have been stalled due to abortion politics. What are the effects of this grassroots movement?

A search of news articles regarding stillbirth for the 20-year period between 1980 and 2000 revealed that very little media attention was given to stillbirth, resulting in between one to 11 stillbirth related stories in the media each year. Over that same 20-year period, the topic of stillbirth was featured in the print media a total of 78 times. Of those, 9 of the 11 stories were related to fetal death and legal issues such as drug abuse or domestic violence during pregnancy and the other two were related to inadequate medical care. Since the inception of the CBRS legislative movement in 2001 through mid-2007, over the course of the 6 years, stillbirth has been featured in media articles around the country more than 300 times, most of them centered on abortion politics and the CBRS. Because of the wrongfully perceived connection to abortion rights, feminist organizations have a standing history of circumventing, and now even fighting against, this uniquely feminine public health problem.

For the first time in history, this social policy movement has thrust stillbirth into the public light, and now grieving mothers and their stillborn babies are being used as political pawns in the minefield of reproductive rights debates. Yet, the movement has received monumental attention, being featured in some of the most prolific media venues in the world, sometimes making front-page headlines including the: *New York Times, Los Angeles Tribune, Boston Globe, San Francisco Chronicle, Los Angeles Monitor, San Diego Tribune, Arizona Republic, Sacramento Bee, Mothering*, and the pop-culture giant, *People Magazine*. Local news stations in Arizona, California, New York, Texas, Rhode Island, Washington, Florida, and many other states have aired stories on families experiencing stillbirth. CNN's flagship show *American Morning* and *National Public Radio* featured the legislative push for stillborn birth certificates. There are aggregate corollaries from the political and legal quarrelling: It is an important time for stillbirth. Finally, public attention is turning toward this very tragic loss for women and their partners. Though, much of the attention, at least until very recently, has been focused on the controversy instead of issues related to support, appropriate psychosocial care, or research.

The insidious seeping into the psyche

These contentious macro factors affect parents of stillborn babies at the mezzo and micro levels. Rando [4] identifies all child deaths as complicated and traumatic, yet many of the common misconceptions about stillbirth at a macro level contradict, and thus can complicate, a woman's lived experiences. Social and political factors such as the degree of perceived social support and validation are important factors influencing normal and protracted grief reactions. Doka [5] describes disenfranchised grief as that which "persons experience when they incur a loss that is not or cannot be openly acknowledged, publicly mourned, or socially supported." This may hinder the grief process, increasing feelings of isolation and despair. Stillbirth is considered a socially stigmatized loss, similar to suicide, AIDS, or the death of a disabled child, and thus, grieving mothers often feel disenfranchised [6], making them more vulnerable to painful, existential emotions that may jeopardize mental and emotional health. This marginalization, as well as death anxiety on the part of providers and individuals, may also affect the ways in which others, at the mezzo level, interact with grieving families following stillbirth. Providers need to truly understand the connection between those influences and the psychological experiences of stillbirth on a grieving family.

In the case of stillbirth, "the bereavement of the mother . . . is unique in that she is grieving the loss of a part of the self" [7]. She has lost, in a very tangible sense, material immortality. Rubin et al. [8] acknowledge deficits in the previous empirical criterion for PTSD noting another potential marker which exacerbates trauma and often goes unrecognized. This parallel feature is uniquely stressful because it "attacks the very coherence and association" of the decedent in the mind of the mourner. In this trauma marker, the mental image of and the expectations associated with the person who died is in complete incongruence with the mourner's cognitive representation of them and the experience. Thus, "the task of working through loss can become overwhelming, and the task of reorganization of the relationship to the deceased can depart from its natural course" [8]. For example, some obstetricians tend to experience "an abrupt cut off in the identity construction process" as soon as they discover the baby's death, and that "denial of the baby's existence was expressed" both explicitly and implicitly to the mother. In a swift and dramatic instant, there is a resultant "unraveling . . . and rapid deconstruction of her motherhood" [9], potentially intensifying the traumatic experience.

The commonly held rejection of stillbirth as the death of child arouses a discrepancy in the mother's reality and may delegitimize grief responses after the death of a stillborn child [10]. Providers,

family members, and friends often mourn the death of a stillborn baby differently, since the baby was intangible to them; whereas, if a 10-year old child died, an entire community—friends, neighbors, teachers—would likely share in the mourning. Mothers experience "social pressure to forget . . . with the fact that the person being remembered was known to so few" [11]. Even responses from spiritual leaders can be invalidating. For example, the standard practice of refusing baptism to a stillborn baby implicitly devalues the baby's worth. This may further heighten the sense of aloneness after stillbirth, intensifying and complicating grief and sometimes causing protracted grief and social withdrawal [12]. Thus, as both the intensity and validity of a grief emotions go unrecognized, and even shamed, by others, the bereaved mother may find herself "at odds with the social milieu and . . . forced to rely solely on her own resources to negotiate grief resolution" [10]. Social reactions perceived as abandoning by providers, family members, or even partners may result in tremendous exogenous stress on the woman, her family, and even the marital dyad as women suffer losses related to their sense of self.

Few human experiences are as unnatural as giving birth to a dead baby, a death out of order, and survivor guilt is not uncommon. The mother, often plagued with self-doubt, wonders about her role in the baby's death. She may also wonder about her worthiness as a mother to her surviving or subsequent children. Because women often experience their unborn babies as an integral extension of the self, to "abandon" the baby is to abandon the mother. To deny the baby's worth is to also refute the woman's worth. That implicit denial of her worthiness does not come without significant risk. Many women feel like failures, and sometimes, even murderous [11]. After all, "what kind of woman kills her own child while in the womb?" [13]. As one mother said, "That baby was a part of me . . . I blamed and hated myself for allowing it to happen" [14]. These feelings can hinder healing for both parents. Bereaved parents who perceived themselves as unworthy suffered more intensely and for longer periods than those whose esteem was intact [15]. Thus, this damaging blow to self-esteem may significantly compromise posttraumatic growth and emotional reconciliation.

Individual and familial challenges: micro systems

Families are confronted with many challenges when a child dies. This is due to "(1) the unnaturalness of the death, (2) parents' failure as protectors, (3) the need for reorganization of the family, (4) the need to adjust roles, and (5) communication" [16]. During the acute crisis, they face difficult decisions about ritualizing the baby, autopsies, and final disposition plans. Later, they confront the unfamiliar territory of grief, while often caring for surviving children, restructuring roles, and adjusting back into life. At the individual level, parents and siblings are left to cope "with their own emotional angst" as each member of the family struggles for equilibrium and leaving little energy to devote to the emotional nurturance of others [16]. While relationship stress may intensify after the death of a baby, some research suggests that the divorce rate does not increase. Mekosh-Rosenbaum and Lasker [17] found that less than 6% of marriages ended in divorce after the death of a baby (loss group) versus 4% after a live birth (control group). DeFrain et al. [18] found similar results with less than 2% of mothers and 3% of fathers citing their child's death as the reasons for their divorce. Mental distress and low social support, including by family and friends, were negatively associated with marital satisfaction, and "those who perceive that they were well supported reported having a more positive relationship with their partners."

Surviving children brave a world where they may not recognize the family system as secure. Depending on the age, maturation, and cognitive development of the bereaved sibling, processing the reality of the death and subsequent consequences—as well as its irreversibility—may take many years, perhaps, a lifetime. DeFrain et al. [18] records the stories of Joseph and his younger sister, Mary, both adults recalling the death of their sister to stillbirth

26 years earlier. Joseph says: "I remember picking up on the emotions from people around us . . . we couldn't play, laugh, or run around . . . I remember the feeling." Mothers, often primary providers of surviving children, may be unable to provide the emotional and physical sustenance demanded of them. Both parents may become anxious, fearful, overprotective, and, in particular, mothers are susceptible to symptoms comorbid with trauma such as anxiety and depression. Chronic maternal depression may lead to problems for children, including reactive attachment problems. Children, particularly very young ones, require deliberate effort and energy, and a grieving mother may no longer feel motivated to invest in living children, particularly absent strong social support. This may be one factor involved in the intergenerational transmission of stillbirth's negative, long-term effects.

Peterson [19] found that stillbirth crosses generations and that "women can absorb during childhood the impact" of their mother's loss—the death of a sibling. Thus, they are "particularly vulnerable to fear during their own pregnancy" [20]. Some women report ongoing, intense emotions, such as anxiety, and this influenced their actual and perceived interactions with their own children [19]. Individual responses within the confines of the family are informed by their mental health history and locus of control, sense of cohesion, characterological tendencies, strengths, culture, and history of loss, abuse, or trauma.

The micro system: traumatic loss and existential angst

A mother's existence is so wrapped up in her relationship to her child, her existence merges so much into their being together, that breaking this relationship would be tantamount to destroying her existence.

—Medard Boss

Walsh [2] outlines variables associated with traumatic death and loss within the micro system that require "careful assessment and attention." Those include (1) deliberate, violent death including those in which the survivor narrowly survives, and innocent lives are lost, (2) untimely death, noted as the "hardest to bear," (3) sudden death, (4) prolonged suffering, (5) ambiguous loss, (6) unacknowledged loss, (7) pile-up losses (including multiple life stressors), and (8) past experiences of traumatic loss. Many of these variables are salient in the case of stillbirth, and these traumatic aspects further complicate a mourner's grief process [2].

Women experiencing stillbirth face consanguineous factors associated with the loss, sometimes alone and often awakening substantial existential angst. For example, there are few tangible artifacts to remind her of the baby, and she may desperately cling to anything that recognizes and validates her sense of motherhood [21]. Cognitive functioning may be compromised following a traumatic experience, and her hormones are adjusting to a postpartum world in which no baby exists for her to nurture. While somatization is common after any traumatic loss, the fact that the baby died *within* her body adds a layer of complication: Death came *into* her body and *took away* her baby. Nothing feels so untimely or unjust. She survived, but her baby did not. Her breasts continue to produce milk for the dead baby. Her womb, the once-safe refuge that housed her child, sags but there is no baby to nurse at her breast. Her body yearns for her baby and her arms ache: and there is a powerful, evolutionary impetus behind this drive. The emotional state derived from maternal hormones is incongruent with her reality for she cannot physically bond with her now dead baby. The maternal drive is a potently preoccupying, biological instinct originating in the brain that, when prematurely or traumatically interrupted, sets the stage for anger, jealously, insecurity, "disruptions in social and sexual rhythms," severe stress, and depression. This "emotional instability can have strong biological determinants, even though the process appears psychological or social" [22]. There is a dialect, then, between recognizing and experiencing both birth and death, alternating and existing between two extreme worlds. It is an extraordinary experience eliciting extraordinary reactions that sometimes defy the material or rational. Thus, for some,

spirituality plays a key role in exciting and managing existential angst as grieving families struggle to find meaning in their loss.

Traumatic experiences may ignite an existential crisis from which concerns related to spirituality include finding meaning or purposelessness, disconnectedness or connectedness, misunderstanding or coherence, and the struggle toward transcendence arises. Transcendence addresses that which goes beyond the mundane of the material world. It entails finding hope amidst the hopelessness of grief. For the religious, it may entail an enriched relationship with the Creator, for the spiritual, the connection to the Universe; for the nonreligious, it may extend meaning through a physical legacy that will withstand time such as a work of art or writing a book [23]. Finding meaning, despite a person's individual spiritual orientation, may help a mourner reframe, integrate, and make sense of the loss. This is a core process, as stillbirth often affects a mother's sense of justness, as she ponders: "Why me?" Spiritual affiliation may provide an essential place for deepened relationships with others.

Viktor Frankl [24], in his seminal book *Man's Search for Meaning*, notes that soul-searching, meditation, or prayer may play a role in providing an altered state of consciousness that is necessary for some to discover pathways to heal. Frankl discusses the concept of tragic optimism, that is, the good that can come from tragic experiences by: (1) turning despair into human achievement and accomplishment; (2) deriving from suffering and guilt the motivation to change for the better; and (3) discovering the incentive to take responsible action. However, he goes on to note that this optimism cannot be born of coercion. It cannot be controlled from the periphery, and it cannot be commanded from within the self. Rather, through the gradual actualization of potential meaning inherent in any tragedy, a person may eventually realize tragic optimism [24].

This concept may appeal to many bereaved as a notion having little to do with religiosity and much more to do with posttraumatic growth. According to Frankl, "what is true for hope is also true for . . . faith and love cannot be commanded or ordered." Frankl suggests a maxim for such meaningful growth through: (1) creating something or an act of service, "doing," for others, (2) meeting an extraordinary person or encountering an extraordinary circumstance, and (3) a person's attitude toward human suffering [24].

Insulating factors

In the dual process model of bereavement, the mourner vacillates between a focus on the loss and a focus on living [25], termed loss-oriented versus restoration-oriented. During orientation toward the loss, the bereaved engages in *grief work*, struggles to relocate the deceased, and focuses on emotional ties and attachment, while *avoiding* restoration. While in restoration-oriented mode, the bereaved is actively attending to life, distracted from the innards of grief, and begins to create new relationships, roles, and identities. This model represents a more balanced experience of grief: alternating between facing the loss and being immersed in the grief and existential angst and reconciling the loss. Over time, the bereaved parent can adjust between the two modes and is better able to manage overwhelming emotions. Yet, clearly, this is a more tenuous struggle for most parents in the case of stillbirth.

However, it is important to distinguish normal grief responses, which often persist well beyond the expectations of society, and chronic depressive and trauma-related disorders. Enduring hyperarousal, avoidance, and intrusion as well as dysthymia may certainly indicate psychopathology requiring further attention. Yet, clinicians should use the MISS model as a means to analyze exogenous factors to determine if any psychopathology is one induced by a traumatic event which she is enduring in aloneness. In other words, is her reactive sadness being exacerbated by systemic circumstances? Diagnostic procedures in assessing disorders are tenuous and subjective, and labeling may result in iatrogenic effects. In addition, when a specific diagnosis is made, providers tend to "selectively inattend to aspects of the patient that do not fit into that particular diagnosis and correspondingly over-attend to subtle features that appear to confirm" the

diagnosis [26]. Providers should avoid syndromal thinking and, rather, consider the MISS model in relationship to the patient, contemplating whether mezzo factors such as coadvocacy, increased social support, and validation may assuage current emotional distress and insulate the grieving mother from unnecessary angst in the future. Walsh [2] recommends that providers normalize and contextualize distress, focus on the patient's strengths in coping, follow-up with mental health services for those exhibiting extreme distress, and mobilize family and social support.

Social support is particularly important to women from an array of sources such as in a clinical relationship or faith-based community, or from work colleagues and friends. Research has shown that provider and partner support can alleviate extreme emotional pain and reduce risk for depression and anxiety in mothers following stillbirth [27]. Support groups have also been found to confer benefits including: unsilencing a story a woman wants to tell allowing her to openly discuss in detail her deepest feelings of pain, loss, or guilt; desensitizing the teller to the trauma; connecting bereaved mothers with a common community thus reducing feelings of isolation; providing a place for the story to change form as the teller focuses on different details with each retelling; cultivating nurturing relationships and empowering women through remembrance and ritualization; through the narrative and information sharing processes, helping the teller gain a sense of control during early grief; providing a place for reciprocal compassion, where bereaved women, and even men, can reach out as mentors to other newly bereaved parents; normalizing of emotions and experiences; and providing a place to explore creative ways to cope with the loss through cognitive modeling [12].

While parental grief is often interminable by its very nature, evolving and changing over a lifetime, these restorative effects of social support may promote posttraumatic growth after loss. Social support vis-à-vis highly patient-centered strategies and "care that alleviates vulnerability in all of its forms" [28] may help to buffer the negative effects of stillbirth for both mothers and fathers. Indeed, it may provide the infrastructure for parents toward finding meaning in their very painful loss and encourage as Frankl suggested, at some point, a sense of meaning and purposefulness following suffering. This type of caring requires the psychological and physical attending from one human being to another.

ATTEND: a model of patient- and relationship-centered caring

The exigency for excellence in care

Bereaved mothers, often overwhelmed by the traumatic nature of stillbirth, may take their cues about how to interact with their dead baby from providers. Usually, "women [submit] almost unquestioningly to the expectations of the staff" [9]. For this reason, providers should be careful not to impose their own values and beliefs; rather, gently guide the woman to making the most appropriate choices based on culture, disclosure, options, and her own wishes. (Figure 13.1)

Healthcare professionals and clinicians are obligated to act in their patient's best interest, ensuring a full range of intervention, skills, and a continuum of care, with particular attention to vulnerable populations. Providers are "ultimately responsible for what they say" and how they

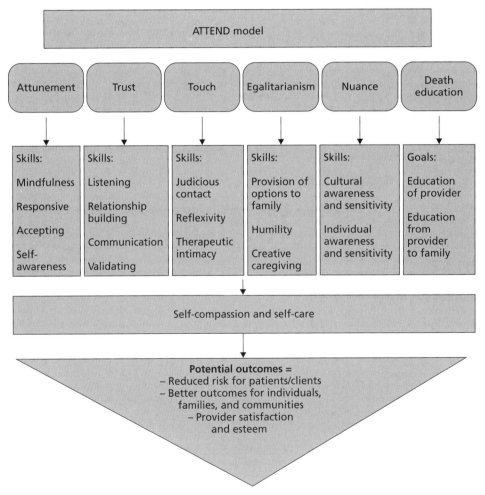

Figure 13.1 ATTEND model of bereavement care.

interact with patients and they should understand the "dimensions of the discourses surrounding" stillbirth [29]. Women, who have experienced the sudden, unexpected death of a baby, should be classified, at least temporarily, as a vulnerable population. Committed to the ethic of caring for others, physicians, midwives, nurses, social workers, psychologists, medical staff, and other professionals are often in the position to advocate for vulnerable populations. Yet, several factors affect a provider's ability to provide this level of care.

At the macro level, economic mandates have obliged both administrators and providers to be "inexpensive and perforce, brief, superficial, and insubstantial" [26]. Psychotherapeutic training has been abbreviated by the crushing will of the "HMO reality," wherein psychiatrists and psychologists are being pressured by the market out of the business of healing, psychotherapeutic relationships and forced, rather, to specialize in psychopharmacologically based, laconic interventions [26]. At the mezzo level, some physicians, particularly obstetricians, may avoid the patient because of their discomfort with death and even sometimes fear of accusatory substandard medical treatment and subsequent legal actions. Thus they tend to avoid honest communication with parents experiencing stillbirth. This tendency increases when the provider is concerned about litigation [30]. Despite this, 75% of physicians surveyed admitted that stillbirth "took a large emotional toll on them personally" and those obstetricians who felt emotionally prepared to cope had significantly fewer negative effects, particularly guilt [31]. Provider guilt may "impair their ability to provide adequate care" following the death of a baby, and this compromised relational interaction may actually lead to an increased risk of patient hostility and litigation [32].

Providers to the families of stillbirth can be found across disciplines, not just in obstetrics: social work, psychology, midwifery, nursing, mortuary sciences, education, and sometimes child welfare. Kastenbaum [33] refers to this as the system of death wherein people, places, times, objects, and symbols affect the grief experience. Community-based providers can include hospice, funeral homes, hospitals, fire and police departments, crisis response teams, and community-based self-help groups.

While providers are often faced with a constellation of familial and individual needs, bereaved parents may be unable to coordinate services, navigate an overwhelming hospital system, or ask the right questions without guidance and support. The onus of responsibility, thus, falls on the providers to develop: (1) a baseline knowledge about the epidemiology of stillbirth and effective trauma and bereavement interventions for grieving families, (2) expertise in verbal and nonverbal communication during a crisis (including a supportive and noncoercive style) which conveys compassion and empathy, (3) a commitment to culturally aware care, and (4) the ability to coordinate appropriate services within the community.

Both medical and mental health providers seem to be returning to a patient-centered model. The Accreditation Council for Graduate Medical Education (ADGME) has established six core competencies which include patient care, medical knowledge, practice-based learning, interpersonal and communication skills, professionalism, and systems-based practice [34]. This is a collaborative model based on family inclusion in psychiatric care. There is also a model for internal medicine that highlights five main areas of concern for the provider–patient relationship to flourish: (1) Who (in the holistic sense) is the patient? (2) What does this patient want from the physician? (3) How is this patient experiencing this event (in this case, stillbirth)? (4) What is the patient's perception and understanding of the cause? (5) What are the patient's feelings about the stillbirth? [35]. There are so many potential responses to each of these five inquiries that it becomes nearly impossible to construct a template within which a provider can fit each patient. Developing rapport—or a relationship—with the grieving family and then responding to their emotions is imperative. Martin Buber's [36] idea of the *I-Thou relationship* recognizes others' experiences as sacred and inimitable. Through authentic exchanges with the patient, empathy flourishes and people can be who they really are, feel what they really feel, and the provider responds accordingly to both. This "narrow ridge" where the I-Thou merges is different for every individual [36]. Here each patient's uniqueness is the centerpiece of care, based on many variables within the micro, mezzo, and macro systems.

The tendency to overgeneralize and hyperstandardize has certainly incited disputes in the literature on best practice following stillbirth. Effective psychosocial care "requires a degree of flexibility, fluidity" and wisdom that is based on clinical research and experience, patient concerns and well-being, and best practice which, together, inform evidence-based practice [37]. There has not yet been a proposed model of psychosocial care specific to infant or child death that illuminates the strengths of evidence-based and patient-centered practice. The ATTEND model offers such a paradigm for providers who wish to incorporate both in their practice.

ATTEND model

The acronym, ATTEND, in this model stands for (A)ttunement, (T)rust, (T)herapeutic touch, (E)galitarianism, (N)uance, and (D)eath education. Attending to another, particularly during a traumatic and emotionally charged experience, can be a challenge for healthcare providers. While much research even in social science focuses on evidence-based practice, more patient-centered approaches suggest that less emphasis should be placed on the rigorous standardization of psychosocial care; rather, with sensitivity, attention should turn toward the undeniably varied aspects of the human experience during and following a traumatic loss. The focus, then, should converge on relationship-based models, such as ATTEND, as these strategies emphasize the uniqueness of each patient and their family. As it relates to the outcomes in MISS model, self-worth was the strongest predictive variable in a bereaved parent's posttraumatic growth, and grief intensity, often exacerbated by provider and societal devaluing of the stillborn baby, can contribute to posttraumatic diminished functioning [15]. The ATTEND model encourages valuing, affirmative, and empathic, rather than traumatizing, provider reactions [21].

Attunement

The American Heritage Dictionary defines attuned as being in accord with or in a harmonious, sympathetic, responsive relationship. Each of these qualities requires a caregiver to engage in mindful practice. Empirically, mindfulness-based approaches in mental health have been effective in more than a dozen recent randomized controlled trials for depressive and anxious disorders. Mindfulness in the provider–patient dyad, and extending into the family system, emphasizes relational ontology. This process facilitates a deep self-awareness of internal processes, such as thoughts, feelings, and biases, as well as the external expression of those states such as linguistics, posturing, communication, and intimate human connections with the other. Within this existential space, two important things often occur: the opportunity for authentic and caring relationships and psychological tolerance that enables a person to be a willing *witness* to the suffering. Emotional pain is exacerbated by the perception "of being separate and alone, thus, suffering may be alleviated by the presence of another who is able to be with and bear the distress" [38]. Much of this tolerance is around the expression of grief and painful emotions, as well as confronting a heightened awareness of death and mortal vulnerability. It is a "being present with" mode rather than a "doing for" mode [39], interweaving aspects of intention, attunement, and attitude. Intention relates to self-regulation, self-awareness, and selfless service that values the other [40]. Attunement with the self helps modulate those internal and external reactions and judgments that so often interfere with the process of full presence with another human being in suffering. Attitude that is mindful includes attributes such as impartial witnessing, acceptance of the moment, patience, trust, openness, gentleness, nonreactivity, and kindness [41].

An example of mindful attunement may include sitting in compassionate silence with couples after the death of a baby or creating a safe space for— and then witnessing—their emotional expression with full acceptance. During these times, it is important for providers to be aware of their own uncomfortableness as it arises, and thus, to refrain from what Freud termed *furor sanandi*, the rage to cure. The opportunities for these types of exchanges may come during the acute crisis, at the postpartum visit, and even months or years later during a subsequent pregnancy or perhaps when a new provider or a referred specialist unfamiliar to the patient discusses their medical history during an unrelated visit. Coordination of care is essential with all providers attending to the needs of an individual patient. Though difficult, at least until a degree of internal tolerance is established, avoidance of these types of critical interactions will most certainly have deleterious effects on the immediate and long-term relationship. Experiential avoidance also diminishes the ability for self-compassion, a protective factor against vicarious traumatization for providers [42]. Conversely, the effects of mindful attunement toward the patient, or even grieving couple and family, can be transformative, particularly given its current state of relative clinical scarcity.

Attunement also includes that of the physical environment. Hospitals which have invested in patient-centered facility remodels have discovered that the "incremental costs were virtually recovered after one year and significant financial benefits" accrued each subsequent year [43]. These changes in the physical milieu included attention toward "peaceful settings" through noise reduction, patient education centers, outdoor views, adequate ventilation (addressing malodorous smells), daylight exposure in each room, and staff support facilities to alleviate stress for providers and ultimately promote healing.

Trust

Compassionate and open communication fosters a mutually trusting relationship. There is evidence to suggest, for example, that patients have expectations of the physician during an adverse event, through empathy, apology, explanation, and acceptance of responsibility, and that such behaviors create trust in the provider–patient relationship. In addition, perception in communication is more important than the actual words spoken [44]. A provider's willingness to listen to the stories of patients is a very important factor in establishing trust.

Sedney et al. [45] identify three main objectives of narrative intervention: (1) enabling the grieving person to better manage grief emotions through verbal articulation; (2) discovering meaning through such articulation; and (3) coalescing with like others. Narrative intervention averts inhibitive responses and can ameliorate the risk of alexithymia [46]. According to Pennebaker [46], inhibition "gradually undermines the body's defenses" and can depress the immune system, heart, and vascular functioning, and even change the biochemical efficacy of the brain and nervous system. This is because inhibitory tendencies increase physical demand on the body by requiring constant constraint and energy to inhibit feelings, thoughts, and behaviors. That may then affect the physical health of the inhibitor and create cumulative stress in the body. Inhibition also influences cognition, disabling the inhibitor from "understanding and assimilating the event, and consequently . . . [they are] likely to surface in the form of ruminations, dreams and associated thought disturbances."

Divulging or disclosing thoughts—in word or in writing—can counter the negative effects of inhibition through the act of opening up and confronting trauma, which may reduce biological stress over time. Storytelling is often therapeutic and the act of telling and retelling the story may provide desensitization to the trauma. Providers in a bereavement role carry the primary responsibility to be a good "listener of stories" [47]. From an evolutionary perspective, the process of habituation is known to cause destimulation. When a stimulus is repeatedly presented, the result is an inhibition of responses [48]. In other words, there may be a desensitization, and thus, a reduction in stress responses, when revisiting grief by telling the story or by reviewing artifacts (photographs, music, and journals) related to the baby's death.

Bird and Cohen-Cole [49] propose a three-function model that includes: (1) gathering data to understand the patient, (2) developing rapport and responding with empathy to the emotions of patients, and (3) patient education. This triad can be highly effective when working with bereaved families. Under this model, communication provides an exchange of useful information, promotes action and interaction, allows the patient to access feelings about an experience, and provides an opportunity for providers to express supportive caring and empathy.

The three-function model addresses the three fields of understanding: the cognitive, emotional, and psychomotor. Gathering data to understand the patient requires that providers take time to become familiar with the unique intricacies of each family and their history. What are their religious or spiritual beliefs? What are the specifics of the loss? How effective is their social support network? What other deaths or traumas may have occurred? What are the current family dynamics? Understanding the grieving family may help the provider better understand complex emotional or psychological responses and potential struggles or conflicts. Thus, it is crucial to pay attention to how communication is delivered, encoded, and perceived to ensure patient comprehension. This can be best achieved through listening that is reflective, acknowledging, supporting, and therapeutic touch.

For example, "What I think I hear you saying is that the last time you felt the baby moving was this morning." In mindful communication, *really* listening to a bereaved couple is paramount in avoiding misinterpretation. It is the most common need of the mourner to have someone available to listen. Pauses between thoughts allow for the organization of successive thoughts. That time may help the mourner articulate feelings into words. Open-ended questions encourage the flow of information and feelings. An example of a closed-ended question would be, "Are you feeling angry at your partner?" This does not allow latitude for an expression of deeper feelings. Several examples of therapeutic, open-ended questions would be, "Tell me more about how you are feeling right now," and "Tell me your story." These encourage the further exploration of feelings and perceptions and allow some control over emotional expressions. Good listeners understand reflective conversation, a technique that encourages mirroring. For clarity and definition, the listener briefly repeats her understanding of the speaker's meaning.

Acknowledgment is active validation of an emotional state. This may reduce self-doubt and questioning for a grieving mother or father. It is helpful when the provider acknowledges that the death of a child is out of the natural order of life. In general, bereaved families do not find platitudes helpful (e.g., "You're young, you can have more children," "Everything happens for a reason," "At least you have other healthy children," or "Your child is in a better place now"). Supportive responses might be, "I cannot imagine what you are going through," or "I'm just so very sorry about Benjamin's death," or "I will be here with you and your family through this terrible time." Of course, the appropriateness of the responses will depend on both the individual patient and her family as well as the nature of her relationship with the provider. In the case of stillbirth, it is extremely vital to disavow use of the term *fetus* when referring to the baby verbally or in the medical records. After all, few physicians would ask their obviously pregnant patient, "How has the *fetus* been this week?" or "Have you decided on a name for your *fetus*?" Words are symbolic and carry with them important meanings.

It is important to be mindful of nonverbal communication modes. Nonverbal communication accounts for more than 90% of the meaning received [50], and techniques such as proxemics, eye contact, tone of voice, facial expression, touch, and posture are the forms of communication that are least under conspicuous control. Yet, the messages that nonverbal communicating convey are often even more significant and meaningful than the spoken word. For example, one randomized, controlled study showed that physicians who sit when delivering bad news are perceived as more compassionate than those who stand [51].

Proxemics is the study of spatial distance—the social space maintained from one person to another. Distancing is often culturally and circumstantially determined [52]. During nonverbal exchanges, a person must be attuned to specific body movements attached to certain meanings. Sometimes the signal from sender to receiver can be distorted and a type of error in communication occurs. When this happens, there is an interruption in the nonverbal space between two (or more) people. The best way to avoid this breach of space is to understand the roles of the individuals in the relationship, the circumstances of the moment, and any cultural prohibitions. There are four boundaries that most people recognize: public, social, personal, and intimate. A general description of these boundaries is as follows:

1. Public space constitutes 12′–25′. This might be a professor to a classroom or a minister at a church service.

2. Social space generally consists of 4′–12′. This might be the acceptable distance at a business transaction, or during a meeting at work or school.

3. Personal space occurs at about 3′ between people. This is the social distance often observed at casual parties or between a physician and a patient during treatment.

4. Intimate space is between 6″ and 18″ and it is commonly recognized as being very personal and is often observed between two people who care for one another.

Physical distance can convey messages of caring and comfort. During an acute crisis, minimizing distance to the patient may be ineffective in building intimacy and trust [53]. Most often, providers will want to be in close proximity, providing comfort and care. For example, rather than engaging in dialogue standing above a grieving mother, eye level and body position should be at or below her level with no more than two feet of unobstructed space between patient and provider. This may require sitting on the floor next to her as she holds and rocks her baby who died, or asking permission to sit on the bed next to her.

Kinesics is the study of body language and includes facial expressions, posture, gestures, or other body movements. Proper use of kinesics will ensure congruency and sincerity in the message from sender to receiver [54]. Behaviors such as looking away from the grieving mother or being distracted easily, lack of facial expression, indifference in voice intonation, or positioning the body facing away from the mother will communicate a lack of concern. Instead, providers should be attentive while working with the grieving mother, convey empathy through facial expressions, use the voice to express sincerity, and face the woman while communicating with her.

Paralanguage, or vocalics, is the production and use of nonverbal sounds: voice qualifiers, vocal segregates, and voice characterizations ("Oh, I see," "Ah!", "I am *so very* sorry"). For example, the way a provider uses her or his voice can communicate either, "I'm feeling *really* uncomfortable with your emotional distress" or "You're *very* important to me right now and I'll be here to ensure your needs are being met." The emphasis on certain words, the tone of voice, and the speed of articulation or the tempo all affect the receiver's perception of the message of caring [54]. Slightly quieter speech, slowed speech, and an emphasis on caring words convey empathy.

Oculesics is the study of the use of eye contact when communicating. Direct eye contact communicates caring and attention toward the other, and it helps the receiver unconsciously accept the truthfulness and sincerity of the sender [54]. Western culture, in particular, values direct eye contact but it is important to be aware of the context when working with grieving families from more traditional cultures. For example, some heritage-consistent American Indians will avoid sustained eye contact. Be sensitive and adapt to the other person's communication style.

Effective nonverbal communication is important in conveying meaning that is congruent with the desired message: Verbal and nonverbal messages need to be congruent, since most of the meaning extracted by the receiver is done so through the nonverbal message. In sum, eye contact (*when culturally appropriate*), a moderated tone and pace of speech, the judicious use of touch (the top of the hand, closest shoulder, or on the back between the shoulders), and strategically applied silence will often convey a supportive presence. However, clinical prudence must be exercised when dealing with certain cultural groups.

Hall [52] suggests that every individual is confronted by daily sensory stimuli that may overwhelm the internalization process. Culture has provided helpful templates, in a sense, by editing and deciphering messages and by providing a template for perception and interpretations. Because "grief is a hardwired feature of human biology . . . biologically determined" the nuance of the experience is often socially and culturally influenced [55]. Families of all cultures need to be able to trust that their providers will be compassionate and respectful. Cultural awareness includes working toward *an aware, but not presumptive* [56], respect-based intervention that includes exploring options with the family, being certain not to impose provider values or beliefs about death. For example, an autopsy is often forbidden in American Indian Nations, according to Sovereign law. Many American Indians forbid postmortem contact and some tribes discourage organ donation. However, providers should not make that decision for the family by ruling out the option of autopsy, organ or tissue donation, or the opportunity to hold the dead baby simply because the family is American Indian. Some American Indians are heritage consistent while others may be more acculturated. Therefore, while knowledge of local ethnography is essential, providers should also allow latitude for individual (and family, when appropriate) decision-making without assumptions about their culture. The culture of a family can also include other social factors such as structure. More and more lesbian couples, for example, are choosing to become birth parents. As the lesbian baby boom gains momentum, more and more mothers and their partners will experience stillbirth. The nontraditional family constitution requires awareness, respect, and flexibility by providers. However, many mothers and their partners report feeling a type of *double-disenfrachisement*. Not only are they grieving the death of their baby, but their experiences are simultaneously decried by the heterosexual and their own lesbian communities [57].

McGoldrick [58] refers to a paradigm she calls the *cultural intersection*. This is the intersection of variables, such as ethnicity, socioeconomic status, cognitive ability, religious beliefs, education, and personality traits, which are likely to influence a mother's beliefs, attitudes, and responses after her baby's death. Additional anecdotal differences may include the experience and perception of pain during pregnancy and birth, communication style, her

beliefs about the cause of the baby's death, and the quality of interaction between the mother and partner, and her providers. The response and duration of grief and mourning expressions depend largely on the variable fusion, the *culture of one*, and the individual's family culture and requires some degree of cultural awareness.

Cultural awareness comes through personalized care that enables the mother to tell and retell the story within her own cultural context. Providers should ask her about her family's rites and rituals, culture, religion, and belief system, while providing an opportunity for her to express her feelings without trying to *fix* her feelings. It is also important to provide nonjudgmental support even when the person's rites and customs feel uncomfortable for the provider. There are five questions clinicians consider particularly important to ask those who are dealing with the emotional aftermath of loss:

1. What are the culturally prescribed rituals for managing the dying process, the deceased's body, the disposal of the body, and commemoration of the death?

2. What are the family's beliefs about what happens after death?

3. What does the family consider an appropriate emotional expression and integration of the loss?

4. What do they consider to be the gender rules for handling the death?

5. Do certain types of death carry a stigma (e.g., suicide), or are certain types of death especially traumatic for that cultural group (e.g., death of a child) [58]?

These open-ended questions build trust and awareness and are appropriate to use with all cultural groups. While outcomes when working with these families are not always predictable, by focusing on their personal perspectives, families may develop a better sense of connectedness that transcends language, nationality, religion, or socioeconomic differences, and a true sense of culturally sensitive care is achieved [56].

Culturally aware communication is the cornerstone of compassionate care. Minority groups and women tend to be high-context communicators. This means they place less meaning on the actual words being spoken, and more emphasis on the nonverbal communication and context [52]. This style of communication is more feeling-centered and intuitive. Conversely, low-context communicators rely heavily on the precise spoken word, and tend to be less perceptive. This results in reduced empathy and awareness, particularly in a crisis situation. In high-context communication, the cultural filters decipher implied meanings arising from the physical milieu, nonverbal communication, relationship interaction, or shared understanding of symbols. In low-context communication, the filters direct attention toward the literal meanings and interpretation of words and less to the subtle cues of nonverbal communication or the context surrounding the words [52]. Providers should pay attention to these listening-centered guidelines for communication: (1) never interrupt the speaker, and allow for a pause between main thoughts; (2) avoid jumping to conclusions; (3) pay attention and engage easily; (4) listen for feelings, beliefs, and ideas and place less emphasis on facts; (5) avoid impulsive reactions; (6) do not allow distractions (turn off cell phones and pagers)—focus on the speaker; (7) maintain respectful nonverbal communication, paying attention to body position and facial expressions; (8) accept the emotional sentiment of the other person; and (9) listen attentively.

Spirituality is one of the most salient themes in studies on culture and plays a very important role for many, though not all, families during times of crisis. Authentic caring for others requires cultural awareness and respect, as well as recognition of the worthiness and value of spirituality. Huls and Kramer-Howe (Table 13.1) [59] identified a need to *encourage* and *empower* providers to use an assessment tool in order to more wholly explore a person's individual sense of spirituality and faith. Previously, the spiritual assessment process typically stopped at the identification of a faith or belief system. However, because spirituality plays a central role in the way people view the world, providers may want to consider whether they should ask permission to venture into this area with grieving families. If using the SHARE assessment paradigm, do so in conversation, not monologue or questioning [59]. The SHARE tool can be used to guide the conversation

(This method can also be modified for use with secularists [the nonreligious] and should not be linear). This method includes five areas for exploration: spirituality, importance, activity, relationship, and empower. Most often, this tool will be used by clinicians and providers who have the time to build a meaningful relationship with the woman and her family.

Doka and Morgan [60] note that "while death is a spiritual event, often the spiritual needs of patients and clients are neglected. . . . An underlying assumption is that while individuals may or may not profess a religion, all have spiritual needs and concerns that must be considered." The SHARE assessment tool is a helpful guide for providers to use.

Patient's values, emotional responses, and communication styles are influenced by many factors including circumstances and culture. Providers should *be aware* of the dominant religious, ethnic, political, and sociocultural norms of local minority groups, but *never assume*.

Therapeutic touch

Therapeutic touch, also known as haptics, has generally been found to reduce tension, improve rapport, and enhance the therapeutic efficacy of providers. Touching is viewed as a rather intimate gesture in most cultures and so it should be used judiciously. However, even some psychotherapists and physicians advocate therapeutic touch when appropriate with clients. "[I]n every branch of the practice of medicine, touching should be considered an indispensable part of the doctor's art" [61]. Neutral touches, instead of noncontactuality, such as the top of the hand or the closest shoulder may be helpful to grieving mothers, especially if an empathic relationship is established and the provider is sensitive to cultural idiosyncrasies. Geib [62] suggests that providers use touch when it is congruent with the degree of trust and intimacy in the relationship and when it is congruent with the patient's circumstances and needs, and patients have reported significantly positive interpretations. Touch communicated caring to patients and enhanced trust, validation, and a feeling of safety, all meaningful outcomes in a provider–patient relationship [63].

Table 13.1 Huls and Kramer-Howe's SHARE model.

1. **Spirituality:** What does spirituality mean to you? How would you describe your belief or faith systems?
   a. Secular view: What meaning, if any, does your loss have for you? How are you able to manage day-to-day life?
   b. Spiritual view: What is God's (or patient's term for their Higher Power) place in what has happened to you? How are you able to manage daily life?
2. **How Important?** What role does your faith/spirituality have in your life?
   a. Secular: What is most important in your life now? Has this changed since your child's death?
   b. Spiritual: What has been most meaningful to you in your faith community? What is most meaningful to you since your child's death?
3. **Activity:** What actions connect you to your beliefs? Do you regularly attend a faith/spiritual group service?
   a. Secular: What calms your grief, anxieties, and sorrow? If anything, what puts you in touch with a sense of strength, peace or hope?
   b. Spiritual: What faith practices (prayer, music, movement, meditation, etc.) do you use to help you manage your emotions/grief?
4. **Relationship:** What is the relationship between your current grief (or present circumstances) and your faith (diagnosis, prognosis, comfort, hope, and so forth)?
   a. Secular: How do you understand this experience to have affected your life? How has this experience changed your relationship with others and with the world?
   b. Spiritual: How has this tragedy changed your relationship with God? How do you feel now in relation to your faith? What spiritual needs do you have?
5. **Empower:** How can we be most effective in supporting your faith/belief?
   a. Secular/Spiritual: If we could do just one thing to help you with this part of your life, what would it be?

Some helpful guidelines when discussing issues related to spirituality include:
- Adopt their language (e.g., use God, Yahweh, Jehovah, Allah, or other client-recognized names).
- If not familiar with practices of that particular faith or belief, ask for a summary or description. Show an authentic, humble interest in understanding that faith/belief.
- Use reflective listening: "So what I hear you saying is that your faith feels really shaky right now?"
- Avoid imposing alternate spiritual beliefs or values on the person.
- Again, accept the individual's emotional state or questioning unconditionally without invoking personal reactions.

Egalitarianism

The principle of egalitarianism in the provider–patient relationship is critical, particularly in obstetrical care, wherein historically, the systemic usurping of women's power in birth was commonplace. The nonpaternalistic and humble provider–patient relationship exists unencumbered by issues of authority. These types of relationships result in more personalized care in the form of home visits, telephone contact after hours, and advocacy on behalf of patients. The outcomes for patients are trust, hope, and valuing [64]. The egalitarian relationship helps the patient feel empowered to make important decisions based on their preferences in a shared decision-making process with a partner and key family members, rather than based on perceived pressure, fears, or anxieties. These decisions should be guided by nonhierarchical communication with providers that includes rationale, anticipated outcomes, and psychoeducation on options and alternatives [65]. Morbidity, intervention fidelity, overall health status, and emotional factors are significantly influenced by the patient–provider relationship, and such "healing relationships seem to work in both directions" [64], benefiting the provider as well as the patient. The humble provider becomes a willing and unpretentious student, overcoming the "arrogance that exaggerates [my own] power at the expense of the power of others" [66].

Nuance

The responsiveness of caregivers to parental grief is increasingly being transformed into a carefully managed stage production . . . It becomes difficult, and ultimately impossible, to listen and respond sensitively to parents' feelings when you are preoccupied with long lists of tasks you are supposed to perform.

—Irving Leon

Philosophers like Fromm, Sartre, and Lacan all believed that "society shapes the individual, and we can only understand individuals if we understand the society, culture, and/or world in which they must continually live and interact" [67]. Rather than focusing on stringent, manualized checklists, providers should focus on the nuances of each patient.

The dissatisfaction with providers that many bereaved families experience is often influenced by nuance, particularly around birth and death; that is, care that is flexible and responsive to subtleties. In the case of stillbirth, for example, there was a fivefold increase in maternal dissatisfaction with the care they received over mothers after a live birth [68]. Provider responses have been found to increase the likelihood of PTSD and depression in women during the postpartum period [69]. And many mothers explained that they were not receiving the care they needed from providers after the death of an older child:

[M]others wanted information on the child's illness, its gravity, causes, prognosis and death. The way in which the information was given was also important. They wanted realistic, honest, and accurate information, but . . . mothers did not always get an answer and professional practitioners kept shifting responsibility for information-giving from one person to another . . . Mothers expected the church to provide help [and] they had both positive and negative experiences of the support provided by the church . . . they wanted communication, advice on practical matters, information on crisis groups, and a genuine interest in their coping with grief [70].

Particularly during the acute crisis of stillbirth, the care she receives from providers can increase psychopathology up to 3 years later [68]. Clinical education is necessary to wholly understand the unique needs of families experiencing the death of a baby or child. Yet, administrators do not always provide necessary training for staff to help them develop these critical interpersonal skills:

[M]ost potential supporters experience intense anxiety about the prospect of interacting with a person who has experienced a life crisis. They may feel confused about how to behave or what to say, and may have little past experience to guide them in these situations. The support provider's anxieties may be heightened by the awareness that the victim is vulnerable, and that inappropriate behaviors might intensify the . . . distress. The potential supporter may be so conscious of what is happening and so worried about responding inappropriately that natural expressions of concern may be unlikely to occur . . . This anxiety may also result in support attempts that are automatic . . . such as "I know how you feel" or "things will get better soon" [71].

Additionally, broader society tolerates the expression of grief for an allowable duration of time, and under specific circumstances of death deemed worthy. Conversely, bereaved mothers simply do not expect that their grief, love, or attachment will ease with time, in direct contradiction with the pressures from others [72].

Listening to the narratives of bereaved mothers may compel providers to reach beyond the obvious interpretation of the actual death event and make them more sensitive to the nuances of loss after stillbirth. Those nuances of loss usually fall into one of two categories: corporeal and symbolic loss. *Corporeal or tangible losses* for women include:
1. The death of the child whom they love (the actual baby who died);
2. The death of their physical presence (the loss of their physical presence in the family);
3. Unrequited expressions of love and affection; and
4. Material immortality (the death of the baby carrying the genetic material of the parent; the death of a biological extension of the self).
Giving birth and death in unison is a paradox. There is often a sense of helplessness, despair, and

fear during the acute crisis when the process of birth ends in death, not life. Kastenbaum [73] talks about the "inconvenient dead," defining them as corpses "in the wrong place, at the wrong time, or in the wrong way." There is no more unwelcome place for death than in the delivery room where all eyes gathered there await the emergence of life.

Symbolic losses may be more difficult to elucidate and may have varying degrees of meaning for each person. These include:

1. The *death* of a familial role (mother or father, sister, brother, grandparent);

2. The *death* of parenthood (the loss of the ability to act as a parent to that specific child);

3. The *death* of a dream (the surrendering of future hope for this child);

4. The *death* of the self (feeling irreversibly transformed, a fraction of one's former self); and

5. The *death* of innocence (the loss of a sense of control and security, and the realization of non-exemption for other loved ones; the loss of peace, serenity, and sometimes faith; and the loss of worry-free future pregnancies).

The death of innocence, or a capitulation of the *assumptive world*, is worthy of further discussion. After stillbirth, there is a subtle sense of vulnerability, the same sense often associated with traumatic losses [74]. Rubin and colleagues [8] go on to summarize these idiosyncratic features:

1. The nature of traumatic bereavement exists on a continuum. "Phenomenologically and psychologically, there are varying degrees and various levels" affecting behavioral, cognitive, and biological, as well as the unconscious mind.

2. Not all who are exposed to traumatic loss will develop long-term dysfunctional reactions.

3. "Traumatogenic" experiences will cause some people to develop persistent symptoms that meet the diagnostic criteria for a myriad of disorders.

4. When symptoms develop, the griever will need to "recreate a network of coherence, safety, security, meaning, and continuity" in order to help her cope with the emotional aftermath.

5. Traumatic responses are subjectively experienced as such.

6. There are multiple variables associated with traumatic bereavement. These authors suggest a more phenomenological approach wherein clinicians "take into account the fundamental notion that individual interpretation of life experiences" is the centerpiece.

A person's assumptive world is often shattered by traumatic losses, as in the case with stillbirth, and all innocence—all faith in the world as just—is lost. These are crucial nuances for the provider to acknowledge.

The probability for adverse psychological and physiological sequelae following stillbirth increases due to the complex effects of pregnancy, childbirth, and then a simultaneous encounter with death, a process that leaves women particularly vulnerable to excessive fear, anxiety, depression, suicidal ideation, mood disorders, and dramatic biochemical changes, often accompanied by enduring separation distress [75]. Contemporary standards of care in the aftermath of stillbirth have incited much debate about the ways in which mothers should be encouraged—or even allowed—to experience their losses and the ritualization of those losses, with very of the dialogue around nuance.

For example, there has been much recent contention around protocol immediately following stillbirth. During the early twentieth century, when both birth and death were institutionalized in the Western world, hospitals took over the management of stillbirth and initiated paternalistic protocols intended to protect women from their own emotional distress. Mothers of stillborn babies never had an opportunity to see or hold the dead baby. Instead, "babies were whisked away and disposed of," in an attempt to minimize the trauma of the experience [76]. Often, by the time mothers were released from the hospital, nurseries had been disassembled and baby items hidden away by well-intentioned family members, and the beloved and long-awaited baby became the dirty family secret about whom no one dared to speak. Not even her.

Sometime during the late 1970s, hospital administrators began to hear the pleas of impassioned physicians such as Emmanuel Lewis. He was highly critical of the "'rugby pass' management of stillbirth . . . the catching of a stillbirth after delivery, the quick accurate back-pass through the labour room door to someone who catches the baby and . . . hides it from the parents and everyone" [77]. In addition, the effects of this paternalism after stillbirth were becoming salient in much of the literature of the early 1980s. Lovell [9] studied 22 mothers of whom 12 never saw or held their stillborn babies. She found that women "usually relied on the judgment of the health professionals . . . and took her cues from the experts," those in authority, as to whether she should or should not see or hold the dead baby [9]. In the absence of contact with her stillborn baby, a mother may worry obsessively over the child's appearance, perhaps exaggerating fears about the baby's features or relentlessly reconstructing the physical appearance. These mothers, according to the author, have difficulty reconciling their losses:

Sandy wonders what happened to her stillborn son: "I have a recurring dream that I'm in the hospital searching for him . . . My name is Sandy, and I'm about stillbirth. I feel it is the most important event in my life. And yet, it is a terrible nothingness..." [The mothers] spoke of their sense of unreality. Most regretted not having seen the baby and letting the hospital deal with the body. This was not necessarily linked to any religious belief.

Mothers who had contact with their baby did not regret their decisions. Rather, they viewed the ritual as very important and believed it helped them to come to terms with their loss.

In reaction to this new shift in attitudes toward stillbirth, standard of care guidelines began to promote ritualization, and mothers were routinely encouraged to see and hold the baby who died. Even in the instance of a congenital anomaly incompatible with life, wherein the newborn suffers severe facial deformation, nurses are advised not to dissuade parents from seeing the baby [78]. Social workers, nurses trained in perinatal death, and pastoral caregivers who often respond to stillbirth confronted the imperative to help mothers "face the reality of the loss" by seeing and holding the baby, "to have a picture . . . to talk about it" [79]. Many hospitals created perinatal bereavement teams of interdisciplinary professionals to manage infant death programs [76]. They may have protocol that includes the collection of mementos, isolette cards, and a lock of hair.

Providers also often facilitate sensitive, postmortem photography, known as *memento mori*, for "some of the same reasons that grieving parents arranged to have photos taken in the nineteenth century" [55]. That is, to capture the visage of a much-loved child, and for many mothers of stillborn babies, to validate their brief existence.

Much of the literature on stillbirth focused on the efficacy of these interventions. Lasker and Toedter [76] noted in their longitudinal research on stillbirth and newborn death that "parents who did experience interventions such as having a photograph or keepsake were significantly more satisfied" than those having not participated in such ritualistic acts. DeFrain et al. [80] studied 350 families experiencing stillbirth, concluding that seeing and remembering the stillborn baby "is essential to the vast majority." A study in the Netherlands found that two factors most significantly affected grief responses and depression in parents: whether parents had an opportunity to say goodbye and home funerals. Parents who were able to bring their child's body home to say goodbye had less intense grief responses than those who engage in institutionalized postmortem ritualization [81]. The researchers attribute this finding to the possibility that "at self chosen moments on which they feel the urge to do so," parents were able to confront the body of their child, thereby "facilitating acceptance of the enormity of the loss" over several days.

However, recent rival research contradicts the benefits of such perinatal death interventions. Theses findings showed that rituals may actually protract grief, and that mothers who held their dead infants experience unresolved mourning. In a study of 53 stillbirth mothers and 53 control mothers, Hughes et al. [82] found that unresolved mourning precipitates a "significant increase in infant disorganized attachment behaviour in children born after a stillbirth." Additionally, "there is a higher risk of disorganization in infants of mothers who have had elective termination of pregnancy or who have seen their dead infant" [82]. In a subsequent study, Hughes et al. [83] examined 65 women who had experienced stillbirth, measuring depressive, anxious, and traumatic symptomatology. The authors concluded "behaviours that promote contact with the stillborn infant were associated with worse outcome" [83]. Thus, rather than facilitating healthy grieving, "seeing and holding the dead infant further traumatizes a woman who is already intensely distressed and physically exhausted." This controversy incited responses from the Western media, academics, and even bereaved mothers themselves, who wrote in to *The Lancet* and other journals, and the outcry on both sides was prolific. One article discouraged pastors from persuading mothers to see their dead babies, purporting that "acts of holding, washing and even dressing a dead infant may actually support denial" [84]. At the same time, bereaved mothers wrote letters to editors of *The Lancet* (2002) about their own experiences:

> I lost my daughter in March, 1998. I was allowed to hold her and dress her, and was given footprints and plaster handprints . . . and was given the option of having some photographs taken with her. I personally feel it was the best thing for me. Angela McCabe, Canada
>
> After reading the paper . . . I felt compelled to write regarding my personal experience. I am the mother of a full term stillborn girl who died 15 years ago. The only regret I have is not spending more time with my daughter. I was encouraged by the staff and my husband to hold her, but was very reluctant . . . today, I thank my husband and the staff for allowing me the few minutes I did spend with my daughter . . . my biggest regret has been my reluctance and the years of silence, not talking about her. The hospital did give us one photograph, a lock of hair, her measuring tape, and her hand and foot print, which I treasure clearly with no regret . . . Even after 15 years, talking about the death of a stillborn child is difficult for everyone, and among African Americans, it seems to be taboo. Deborah Brooks, United States [85].

Nuanced psychosocial care becomes particularly imperative for families when faced with irremediable decisions such as seeing, holding, or photographing a stillborn baby. To assert that *no* mother should see or hold her baby because of an increased risk of adverse symptomatology is as imprudent as the insistence that *every* mother should see and hold her baby after stillbirth to avoid those same risks. Rather than manualizing protocol, these decisions should take place by mothers within the safe confines of a mutually respectful relationship with the provider's guidance and abiding presence, and after the patient has been fully informed about their choices and potential outcomes. Under such circumstances, most mothers will feel empowered to choose to see and hold their stillborn baby and thus will experience fewer symptoms of long-term distress, anxiety, depression, and regret. In fact, a more recent study with a significantly larger cohort of mothers experiencing stillbirth showed that holding and seeing the baby was associated with less anxiety and depression though those results were temporarily reversed during a subsequent pregnancy. The mothers in this study who demonstrated the highest levels of long-term psychopathology where the ones who were offered the choice by providers to see the baby yet they refused that opportunity. This poses the question whether or not assumptive contact might be an option for mothers [86].

Death education

There are two types of death education relevant to psychosocial care: education from provider to patient and continuing provider education. Psychoeducation—communicating with patients about their experiences and offering them options—helps them feel an irreducible sense of control over their very personal tragedies. Providing information about options as well as discussing possible etiological factors would provide improved psychological and emotional outcomes for women [87]. Providers can allow families to make their own decisions about their experiences after they are fully informed. Even offering options about minute details demonstrates a caring and receptive attitude. Providers should look for opportunities to educate patients about their experience during both the actual traumatic experience and the clinical interactions that come later. This will require providers to be well-informed about various aspects related to patient care: for nursing staff and obstetricians, this includes etiology, postmortem evaluations, statistics, and acute individual and familial reactions. For psychotherapists or other providers, it means traumatic bereavement education that includes the effects of loss on the mind and body. Lack of such knowledge may compromise trust and diminish empathy in the provider–patient relationship.

In fact, physicians who experience unfamiliar circumstances or questioning tend to be more uncomfortable with relationship-based models of care and feel less prepared [88]. This could incite avoidance on the part of the provider. Yet, death education targeted toward providers can be helpful in positively affecting self-confidence, making them more comfortable when dealing with bereaved parents [89]. Nurses' comfortable attitudes toward bereavement were directly correlated with their knowledge of the death of a baby. This "highlights the universality of grief" after an infant's death and the need for more education for providers [90]. Nurses wanted more formalized training that emphasizes death studies, "improved communication skills, and greater support from hospital policy and team members relative to bereavement care" [90].

Traumatic bereavement has been shown to correlate with increased healthcare costs [91]. Therefore, to redress this, hospitals should implement a relationship-based patient-centered education program that is family inclusive and that supports, educates, and provides debriefing for all family members on how to help the grieving mother in the months subsequent to the baby's death. The focus must be on the needs of the grieving mother and her family, rather than the provider or facility. Administrative barriers to patient-centered care, such as managed care, economic concerns, and poor organizational management, need to be openly addressed and navigated. This will require a change in the "traditional measures of corporate wealth" in which "financial assets derived from productivity and profits are broadened to include community responsibility, social accountability, and personal fulfillment of employees" [28]. Direct observation

can also be used, and modeling is a powerful aid in teaching effective communication. Senior residents can exemplify empathic communication and help interns become more comfortable in uncertain or distressing situations. Administrators can and should facilitate an environment where these types of active learning experiences can flourish.

The interdisciplinary team and the ATTEND model

Interdisciplinary bereavement teams addressing perinatal death at hospitals ameliorate somatic distress and relieve hostility in grieving mothers. The benefits of these collaborative interactions are particularly discernible in cases where women reported low social support from family and friends [92]. These teams often consist of physicians, nurses, social workers, clergy, midwives, doulas, and sometimes a community member who may also be a bereaved parent. The purpose of the team should be to educate and support staff members, from intake to social work and from maintenance crews to vital recorders, who come into contact with grieving parents, and to monitor patient satisfaction outcomes in the months following stillbirth.

At the micro level, the team should consider issues related to acute interventions such as: (1) ritualization (seeing, holding, and bathing the baby), (2) photography and videography of the birth and bonding time, (3) the development of a grief package for parents that includes books, brochures, and other resources, (4) mementos such as a lock of hair, identification bands, baby blankets or clothing the baby wore, foot and hand molds and prints, (5) symbol of the loss on door of the patient's room, (6) attention to the physical and psychological comfort of the room, including lighting, windows, rocking chair, portable book and music library and cd player, peripheral sounds, and proximity to the newborn nursery, (7) aid in funeral planning, including presenting the option for a home funeral if state law and family culture does not prohibit this, (8) availability of human resources that balances individual and family privacy with the presence of caring staff, (9) opportunities for grandparents, siblings, friends, and others to visit, (10) family photos with the baby, (11) the option to keep the baby in room as long as desired by parents and then the opportunity to request the baby back from the morgue until discharge, (12) presentation of a CBRS in the states with offer this option (27 states currently), (13) a sympathy card signed by patient's providers, and (14) presentation of the postmortem evaluation (autopsy). The team can also meet to address issues related to postvention care. For example, the leader of the team can ensure that remembrance cards are sent at 6 months, 1 year, and 2 years post-loss. They can also coordinate memorial services during holidays, encourage support group participation and therapy, when appropriate, and help connect families to other resources in the community.

In order for an interdisciplinary bereavement team to be successful, administrators need to appropriately balance workload time, necessary to provide essential patient-centered care. While there may be some tension between service provision and resources, valuing patient care should be the primary focus. There are, then, some important implications for providers: **1.** Providers have an ethical responsibility to deconstruct myths about grief after stillbirth and to advocate for greater understanding of the various dimensions of intervention and coping strategies. It is incumbent upon provider communities to ensure that bereaved mothers and fathers have access to information about available local and online support groups.
2. Providers should advocate for changes in administrative policies that would enthusiastically support an integration of modalities for treatment from the moment of loss through the point when the patient no longer feels she needs intervention. In this way, the macro, mezzo, and micro systems synchronize to set the stage for a circle of compassion around bereaved mothers that is based on the MISS model.
3. Hospital providers are in a unique position to advocate for comprehensive continuing education for staff, changing the infrastructure for handling stillbirth, if necessary.
In conclusion, the death of a child is a complex and traumatic experience for families, traversing culture, socioeconomic status, faith/spirituality, and ethnicity. Families need unconditional support from their providers, community organizations, and when appropriate, faith/spiritual-based institutions. Social support—and well-trained providers—can work within community and family systems to provide cohesive and effective interventions to help mothers and fathers cope with the death of a baby to stillbirth.

Vicarious trauma

Working with those who have suffered significant losses has many psychological rewards that are difficult to quantify. However, there are also psychological risks associated with caregiving. The Occupational Safety and Health Administration (OSHA) has declared stress a hazard of the workplace [93]. Unresolved grief and stress can affect a provider's career, self-esteem, family life, and relationships with colleagues. If left untreated, chronic or long-term stress can result in secondary posttraumatic stress symptoms. Flashbacks (mental or visual reexperiencing of a trauma), nightmares, a sudden and painful onslaught of emotions, or an avoidance can potentially affect a provider's ability to relate well with others.

Researchers are now studying topics such as *compassion fatigue, vicarious traumatization*, or *secondary traumatization*, documenting the risk for profound disruptions in the worldview, frame of reference, sense of identity, and spiritualism of all types of providers, from therapists to social workers and physicians to firefighters [94]. Providers themselves, having the responsibility of delivering the tragic news to family members, often experience deep sorrow when a patient's baby dies, and over time, they experience repeated exposure to vicariously traumatic experiences. This ongoing immersion with the grief and trauma of others can take its toll. Facing the deaths of children, in particular, and the accompanying expressions of emotions may prompt providers to revisit their own personal losses and grief. It is very important for providers to recognize manifestations of their own grief and exercise self-compassion.

Unresolved provider stress has been shown to have an adverse effect on patient satisfaction, compliance, and even recovery. Hospital administrators who "take proactive steps to reduce" stress for their providers will realize immense "benefits in terms of patient satisfaction and recovery" [95].

One way to facilitate self-compassion is through mindfulness, that is, attunement and self-awareness around loss. Mindful providers know and understand themselves. They will often recognize (and do not ignore) when they have been affected by a traumatic death. The affects may be emotional and psychological, such as crying, outbursts, sadness, helplessness, or anxiety and in some cases, indifference to avoid emotional pain. There may also be some common physical symptoms of provider grief such as lethargy, tightening in the throat or chest, forgetfulness, intrusive thoughts, nightmares, or the expression of humor at inappropriate times.

Some providers find a degree of resolution to their own grief by following up with the family, reviewing details of the incident, and sharing their feelings with coworkers or other providers. Others may benefit from journaling, psychotherapy, exercising, or learning a new hobby. One of the most empirically validated ways to cope with vicarious trauma is through mindfulness-based stress reduction (MBSR). One 8-week randomized, controlled trial with medical students showed the promising effects of MBSR including a reduction of anxiety and depression and a concomitant increase of empathy when compared to a control group [96]. Other studies have shown that MBSR reduces stress and burnout in high stress careers, overall improved life satisfaction, increases in self-compassion, declinations in ruminative tendencies, and improved patient outcomes [97]. In particular, experiential avoidance exacerbates and prolongs posttraumatic stress in providers, while "self compassion is associated with greater willingness to engage painful thoughts" and memories of trauma [42].

While it is easy to retrospectively identify ways that better care could have been provided, it is also important to identify the good in the care. Providers can reflect on lessons learned from the experience, focusing on the positive, long-term effects that their caring relationship will have on the family. Self-compassion has been shown to reduce self-criticism and ruminative tendencies, and will improve a provider's ability to reflect and learn from an experience [42]. When it is all said and done, providers should strive to be able to say that they have done their best to provide compassionate bereavement care to the grieving mother and her family experiencing stillbirth.

Summary

The death of a child at any age and from any cause is, indeed, a life-changing, traumatic experience. Reconciliation evolves slowly and painfully for many parents as they find their way through, not only the raw grief, but also, the many other elements associated with traumatic events. Parental grief ranks high among the most painful of all other losses, and for many parents, the death of a baby to stillbirth is worthy of the same grief responses as the death of an older child. Exogenous factors affect a woman's experience of mourning after a stillbirth, often exacerbating feelings of disenfranchisement and invalidity. The mother of a stillborn baby needs sensitive guidance so she can meet and say farewell to her baby and engage in rituals that are important to her and her partner. She needs her therapist to sit as a willing patient witness to her pain without attempting to "cure" her of her humanity. Providers should use a patient-centered model, such as ATTEND, to facilitate and normalize responses from grieving parents.

Paradoxically, stillbirth is the coalescence of life and death—the precipice between two opposing forces. It is the ultimate betrayal of the woman by her body: she gave birth to *death* instead of *life*. Until this point in history, all these macro, mezzo, and micro variables have resulted in the pervasive marginalization of bereaved mothers after stillbirth. Now that the time of consciousness has arrived for stillbirth, providers have an opportunity to respond, act with integrity, and change the historical ontology of this tragedy. The time has come to acknowledge the pain of suffering caused by stillbirth and to work toward a sane and compassionate framework of care so that parents can not only return to their pre-loss level of functioning but also have an opportunity to transcend and grow beyond their losses. The time has come to recognize this loss as *the death of a child*. The time has come to give these women—these mothers—back their voices and, in so doing, to end the silence of stillbirth.

References

1. Verhaeghe J. The empowerment of birth. N Life J 2003. Retrieved May 14, 2007, http://www.thefreelibrary.com/New+Life+Journal/2003/December/1-p, 569.

2. Walsh F. Traumatic loss and major disasters: strengthening family and community resilience. Fam Process 2007;46:207–24.

3. Cacciatore J, Bushfield S. Stillbirth: a sociopolitical issue. Affilia 2008;23(4):378–87.

4. Rando TA. Parental loss of a child: differences of grief intensity in bereaved parents. Champaign, IL: Research Press; 1986.

5. Doka K. Disenfranchised grief: recognizing hidden sorrow. Lexington, MA: Lexington Books; 1989.

6. Cacciatore J. The silent birth: a commentary. Soc Work 2009;54(1):91–4.

7. Theut SK, Pederson FA, Zaslow MJ, et al. Perinatal loss and parental bereavement. Am J Psychiatry 1989;146(5):635–9.

8. Rubin SS, Malkinson R, Witztum E. Trauma and bereavement: conceptual and clinical issues revolving around relationships. Death Stud 2003;27(8):667.

9. Lovell A. Some questions of identity: late miscarriage, stillbirth, and perinatal loss. Soc Sci Med 1983;17(11):755–61.

10. Malacrida CA. Complicated mourning: the social economy of perinatal death. Qual Health Res 1999; 9(4):504–19.

11 Layne LL. Motherhood lost: a feminist account of pregnancy loss in America. London: Routledge; 2003.

12. Cacciatore J. Effects of support groups on post traumatic stress responses in women experiencing stillbirth. Omega 2007;55(1):71–91.

13. Layne LL. Transformative motherhood. New York: New York University Press; 1999.

14. Peppers LG, Knapp RJ. Motherhood and mourning. New York, NY: Praeger; 1980.

15. Engelkemeyer SM, Marwit SJ. Posttraumatic growth in bereaved parents. J Trauma Stress 2008;21(3): 344–6.

16. Fletcher P. Experiences in family bereavement. Fam Community Health 2002;25(1):57–71.

17. Mekosh-Rosenbaum V, Lasker J. Effects of pregnancy outcomes on marital satisfaction: a longitudinal study of birth and loss. Infant Ment Health J 1995; 16(2):127–43.

18. DeFrain J, Martens L, Stork J, Stork W. Stillborn: the invisible death. Lexington, MA: Lexington Books; 1986.

19. Peterson G. Chains of grief: the impact of prenatal loss on subsequent pregnancy. Pre Perinat Psychol 1994;9(2):49–58.

20. Verny T. Tomorrow's baby: the art and science of parenting from conception through infancy. New York: Simon and Schuster; 2002.

21. Cacciatore J. Stillbirth: clinical recommendations for care in the era of evidence-based medicine. Clin Obstet Gynecol 2010;53(3):691–99.

22. Williams R. Brain basics: an integrated biological approach to understanding and assessing human behavior. Phoenix, AZ: Biological Psychiatry; 1999.

23. Corr C, Nabe C, Corr D. Death and dying, life and living, Fifth edition. California: Thomson Wadsworth; 2006.

24. Frankl V. Man's search for meaning. New York, NY: Simon and Schuster; 1946/1985.

25. Stroebe W, Stroebe M, Abakoumkin G. Does differential social support cause differences in bereavement outcome? J Community Appl Soc Psychol 1999;9:1–12.

26. Yalom I. The gift of therapy: an open letter to a new generation of therapists and their patients. New York, NY: Harper Collins; 2002.

27. Cacciatore J, Schnebly S, Froen F. The effects of social support on maternal anxiety and depression after the death of a child. Health Soc Care Community 2009;17(2):167–76.

28. Hagenow NR. Why not person-centered care? The challenges of implementation. Nurs Adm Q 2003; 27(3):203.

29. Jutel A. What's in a name? Perspect Biol Med 2006;49(3):425–34.

30. Silver R. Fetal death. Obstet Gynecol 2007;109(1): 153–65.

31. Gold KJ, Kuznia AL, Hayward RA. How physicians cope with stillbirth or neonatal death. Obstet Gynecol 2008;112(1):29–34.

32. Levinson W. Physician-patient communication: a key to malpractice prevention. JAMA 1994;272:1619–21.

33. Kastenbaum R. Reconstructing death in postmodern society. In: DeSpelder L, Strickland A (eds), The path ahead. New York: McGraw Hill; 1977, p. 8.

34. Frierson RL, Campbell NN. Core competencies and training in psychiatric residents in therapeutic risk management. J Am Acad Psychiatry Law 2009;37: 165–7.

35. Platt FW, Gaspar DL, Coulehan JL, et al. "Tell me about yourself": the patient-centered interview. Ann Intern Med 2001;134(11):1079–85.

36. Buber M. Encounter with Martin Buber. London: Allen Lane/Penguin; 1971.

37. Porter-O'Grady TP. A new age for practice: creating the framework for evidence. In: Malloch K, Porter-O'Grady TP (eds), Introduction to evidence based practice. Sudbury, MA: Jones and Bartlett; 2010, pp. 3–29.

38. Dobkin PL. Fostering healing through mindfulness in the context of medical practice. Curr Oncol 2009;16(2):4–7.

39. Segal Z, Teasdale J, Williams J. Mindfulness based CBT: theoretical rationale and empirical status. In: Hayes SC, Follette VM, Linehan M (eds), Mindfulness and acceptance: expanding the cognitive behavioral tradition. New York: Guilford Press; 2004, pp. 31–40.

40. Shapiro SL, Carlson LE. The art and science of mindfulness. Washington, DC: The American Psychological Association Press; 2009.

41. Kabat-Zinn J. Full catastrophe living: using the wisdom of your mind to face stress, pain and illness. New York, NY: Dell Publishing; 1990.

42. Thompson BL, Waltz J. Self-compassion and PTSD symptom severity. J Trauma Stress 2008;21(6): 556–8.

43. Cama R. Linking structure and healing: building architecture for evidence based practice. In: Malloch K, Porter-O'Grady TP (eds), Introduction to evidence based practice. Sudbury, MA: Jones and Bartlett; 2010, pp. 77–98.

44. Wu AW, Huang IC, Stokes S, Pronovost PJ. Disclosing medical errors to patients: it's not what you say, it's what they hear. J Gen Intern Med 2009;24(9):1012–17.

45. Sedney M, Baker J, Gross E. The story of a death: therapeutic considerations with bereaved families. J Marital Fam Ther 1994;20:287–96.

46. Pennebaker J. Opening up: the healing power of confiding in others. New York, NY: Guilford Press; 1990.

47. Rothaupt J, Becker K. A literature review of western bereavement theory: from decathecting to continuing bonds. Fam J 2007;15(1):6–15.

48. Cecil SL, Kraut AG, Smothergil DW. An alert decrement hypothesis of response inhibition to repeatedly presented stimuli. Am J Psychol 1984;97(3):391–8.

49. Bird J, Cohen-Cole SA. The three-function model of the medical interview: an educational device. Adv Psychosom Med 1990;20:65–88.

50. Deep S, Sussman L. Power tools. New York, NY: Basic Books; 1998.

51. Bruera E, Palmer JL, Pace E, et al. A randomized controlled trial of physician postures when breaking bad news to cancer patients. Palliat Med 2007;27:501–5.

52. Hall ET. The hidden dimensions of time and space in today's world: cross-cultural perspectives in nonverbal communication. Germany: Hogrefe & Huber Publishing; 1988.

53. Conlee C, Olvera J. The relationships among physicians' nonverbal immediacy and measures of patient satisfaction with physicians care. Commun Rep 1989;6(1):25–34.

54. Haase RF, Tepper DT. Nonverbal components of empathic communication. J Couns Psychol 1972;19: 417–24.

55. Eberle S. Memory and mourning: an exhibit history. Death Stud 2005;29(6):535–57.

56. Cacciatore J. Appropriate bereavement practice after the death of a Native American child. Fam Soc 2009;90(1):46–50.

57. Cacciatore J, Raffo Z. The experiences of maternally bereaved lesbians. Soc Work (in press).

58. McGoldrick M. Race, culture, and gender in clinical practice. In: McGoldrick M (ed), Re-visioning family therapy: race, culture and gender in clinical practice. New York, NY: Guilford; 1998.

59. Kramer-Howe K, Huls P. S.H.A.R.E: a multidisciplinary tool for accessing spirituality in the stories of mourners. Paper presented at the Association for Death Education and Counseling Conference: Phoenix, Arizona; 2005.

60. Doka K, Morgan J. Death and spirituality. New York, NY: Baywood Publishing Company; 1999.

61. Montagu A. Touching: the human significance of the skin, Third edition. New York, NY: Harper & Row; 1986.

62. Geib P. G. The experience of nonerotic physical contact in traditional psychotherapy. In Smith, E. (Ed.) Touch in Psychotherapy: Theory, research, and practice. Guildford Press: New York, 1998;108–26.

63. Horton J, Clance P, Sterk-Elifson C, Emshoff J. Touch in psychotherapy: a survey of patient experiences. Psychotherapy 1995;32:443–56.

64. Scott JG, Cohen D, DiCicco-Bloom B, et al. Understanding healing relationships in primary care. Ann Fam Med 2008;6(4):315–22.

65. Keirns CC, Goold SD. Patient centered care and preference sensitive decision making. JAMA 2009; 302(16):1805–6.

66. Mayeroff M. On caring: world perspectives. New York, NY: Harper & Row; 1971.

67. Chessick RD. The technique and practice of listening in intensive psychotherapy. New Jersey: Jason Aronson Publishing; 1989.

68. Radestad I, Nordin C, Steineck G, Sjogren B. A comparison of women's memories of care during pregnancy, labour and delivery after stillbirth or live birth. Midwifery 1998;14(2):111–17.

69. Lavender T, Walkinshaw SA. Can midwives reduce postpartum psychological morbidity? A randomized trial. Birth 1998;25(4):215–19.

70. Laakso H, Paunonen-Ilmonen M. Mothers' experience of social support following the death of a child. J Clin Nurs 2002;11(2):176–85.

71. Lehman D, Ellard J, Wortman C. Social support for the bereaved: recipients' and providers' perspectives on what is helpful. J Consult Clin Psychol 1986; 54(4):438–46.

72. Uren T, Wastell CA. Attachment and meaning-making in perinatal bereavement. Death Stud 2002; 26:279–308.

73. Kastenbaum R. On our way: the final passage through life and death. Berkeley, CA: University of California Press; 2004.

74. Janoff-Bulman R. Shattered assumptions: toward a new psychology of trauma. New York: The Free Press; 1992.

75. Slade P. Toward a conceptual framework for understanding post-traumatic stress symptoms following childbirth and implications for further research. J Psychosom Obstet Gynecol 2006;27(2):99–105.

76. Lasker J, Toedter LJ. Satisfaction with hospital care and interventions after pregnancy loss. Death Stud 1994;18(1):41.

77. Lewis E. Mourning by the family after a stillbirth or neonatal death. Arch Dis Child 1979;54:303–6.

78. Sadler ME. When your patient's baby dies before birth. RN 1987;50:28–31.

79. Bright DA. Stillbirth. J Fam Pract 1991;32(3):245–53.

80. DeFrain J, Martens L, Stork J, Stork W. The psychological effects of a stillbirth on surviving family members. Omega 1990;22:2–16.

81. Wijngaards-De Meij L, Stroebe M, Stroebe W, et al. The impact of the circumstances surrounding the death of a child on parents' grief. Death Stud 2008; 32:237–52.

82. Hughes P, Turton P, Hopper E, McCauley GA. Disorganized attachment behavior among infants born subsequent to stillbirth. J Child Psychiatry 2001;42(6):791–801.

83. Hughes P, Turton, P, Hopper E, Evans C. Assessment of guidelines for good practice in psychosocial care of mothers after stillbirth: a cohort study. Lancet 2002;360(9327):114–18.

84. Zengerle FS. The controversy over pastoral care of parents after stillbirth. J Pastoral Care Counsel 2007;61(3):243–6.

85. Psychosocial care of mothers after stillbirth: reader comments. Lancet 2002;360(9345):1601.

86. Cacciatore J, Radestad I, Froen JF. Effects of contact with their stillborn babies on maternal anxiety and depression. Birth: Issues Perinat Care 2008; 35(4):313–20.

87. Radestad I, Steineck G, Nordin C, Sjogren B. Psychological complications after stillbirth—influence of memories and immediate management: population based study. Br Med J 1996;312(7045):1505–8.

88. Muething SE, Kotagal UR, Schoettker PJ, et al. Family centered bedside rounds: a new approach to patient care and teaching. Pediatrics 2009;119: 829–32.

89. Bagatell R, Meyer R, Herron S, et al. When children die: a seminar series for pediatric residents. Pediatrics 2002;110(2):348–53.

90. Chan MF, Wu LH, Day MC, Chan S. Attitudes of nurses toward perinatal bereavement. J Perinat Neonatal Nurs 2005;19(3):240–52.

91. Kissane DW. Neglect of bereavement care in general hospitals. Med J Aust 2000;173:456.

92. Lake M, Johnson T, Murphy J, Knuppel R. Evaluation of a perinatal grief support team. Am J Obstet Gynecol 1987;157(5):1203–6.

93. American Psychological Association (APA). Online etymology. 2007. Retrieved January 26, 2010, http://dictionary.reference.com/browse/psychiatry.

94. Rubel B. Compassion fatigue: nurse grief . . . who cares? J Radiol Nurs 2003;23(2):55.

95. Halbesleben J, Rathert C. Linking physician burnout and patient outcomes. Health Care Manage Rev 2008;33:29–39.

96. Shapiro S, Schwartz G, Bonner G. Effects of mindfulness stress reduction on medical and premedical students. J Behav Med 1988;21:581–98.

97. Gilbert P. Compassion: conceptualization, research, and use in psychotherapy. London: Routledge; 2005.

CHAPTER 14

Medical Management Including Delivery

Donald J. Dudley, MD

Department of Obstetrics and Gynecology, University of Texas Health Science Center at San Antonio, TX, USA

Only recently has the advent of prostaglandin induction of labor markedly changed the management of intrauterine fetal death (IUFD). Prior to this time, fetal death was most often managed expectantly, with the high likelihood of spontaneous labor ensuing in the weeks after the fetal death occurred. However, with ready availability of prostaglandin analogues, women who suffer fetal death often undergo prompt induction of labor soon after the fetal death is diagnosed. In this chapter, I will review the basic clinical management options available to the obstetrician. Unfortunately, there is little strong evidence supportive of most treatment options, and there are few clear standards of care to guide the practitioner as they strive to provide optimal care for women and their families during this tragic obstetric outcome.

Most studies are case reports and case series, with many descriptive studies comparing one technique to another in a nonrandomized manner. Often, interventions to effect vaginal delivery in viable pregnancies are extrapolated to the management of fetal death. While this is a reasonable inference, there are fundamental differences in managing women with fetal death. First, considerations for the fetus no longer are paramount. Safety for the mother becomes the key issue. Second, labor induction techniques must change with earlier gestational ages, as uterine receptivity to some induction agents, such as

oxytocin, change over gestation such that the uterus becomes more sensitive to the uterotonic agents as pregnancy advances. Importantly, managing psychosocial concerns, including appropriate grieving, become much more important. Box 14.1 lists the considerations that should be made when determining a treatment strategy for women experiencing a fetal death.

In this chapter, I will review expectant management, medical induction of labor, surgical induction and delivery, and the role of cesarean delivery in managing fetal death in the second and third trimesters. Additionally, I will address special clinical considerations, including managing a single fetal death in multiple gestation and women with fetal death who have a prior cesarean delivery.

> **Box 14.1 Considerations in the management of fetal death**
>
> Patient wishes
> Gestational age at time of fetal death
> Uterine size
> Prior uterine incision
> Autopsy
> Patient emotional state
> Physical health of the patient
> Cost to health care system
> Side effects of medications
> Availability of medications

Stillbirth: Prediction, Prevention and Management, First Edition. Catherine Y. Spong.
© 2011 Blackwell Publishing Ltd. Published 2011 by Blackwell Publishing Ltd.

Expectant management

One option always available, although infrequently exercised, in the management of IUFD is expectant care. In this instance, the woman suffering the fetal death is followed weekly with clinical evaluation for any potential complications. The overall risk for complications is very small, and in general this risk should not preclude the offer of expectant management.

The natural history of fetus is such that the majority of women will enter spontaneous labor within 2 weeks of the diagnosis of IUFD [1]. While there are few contemporary studies of expectant management for fetal death, older studies have confirmed that expectant management is safe. For example, Dippel in 1934 [2] reported on 306 fetal deaths after 28 weeks and noted no maternal deaths related to expectant management. Similarly, Tricomi and Kohl in 1957 [3] noted that, in 165 women, 90% of women went into spontaneous labor within 14 days and delivery occurred within 21 days in 93% of the women. Only rarely do women retain fetuses for an extended period of time. In the Tricomi and Kohl study, they reported that one woman retained her dead fetus for 120 days, or 49 days past her reported due date.

One reason why practitioners are reluctant to offer expectant management is the perceived risk for a rare condition known as retained dead fetus syndrome (RFDS) [1], or fetal death syndrome [4]. This syndrome is characterized by maternal coagulation defects including hypofibrinogenemia. Originally reported by Weiner et al. in 1950 [5] in women with Rh isoimmunization and fetal death, RDFS was thought to occur because of release of tissue thromboplastin from the dead fetus. Erez et al. [4] reported that women with fetal death have increased in vivo thrombin generation and platelet activation compared to women with normal pregnancies, and that amniotic fluid could be one potential source for tissue factor and thus be one pathway for the pathogenesis of RFDS.

In older studies, the likelihood of RFDS occurring was considered to be due to the length of time the fetus was retained in utero. Pritchard [6] reported the largest case series in 1959. In this case

series of more than 100 women, hypofibrinogenemia occurred only after 5 weeks from the diagnosis of fetal death. In a subsequent study, Phillips et al. in 1964 [7] reported on 69 women who retained a dead fetus for more than 5 weeks. Fibrinogen levels were not noted to decrease until 4 weeks after diagnosis of the IUFD, and then a steady decline was noted until delivery of the fetus occurred. However, hypofibrinogenemia of less than 120 mg/dl was noted only after about 9 weeks after fetal death was diagnosed. Older studies reported that the use of heparin could reverse the hypofibrinogenemia associated with IUFD [8, 9].

The studies regarding the natural history of IUFD were generally performed prior to the widespread use of sonography for fetal diagnosis. Thus, one concern may be that women had likely experienced fetal death well before the clinical diagnosis might occur when diagnosis of the fetal heart beat was with a stethoscope and a skilled practitioner. These studies on expectant management may be skewed such that spontaneous labor may occur later than expected in women who are diagnosed within a day or two of the fetal death. Of course, this also would mean that the risk of RDFS would likely be longer than 4 or 5 weeks as suggested by these older studies.

Should expectant management be considered in contemporary obstetrics, care should be taken to monitor for the possible development of coagulation defects. Weekly fibrinogen concentrations should begin after 3–4 weeks from the time of diagnosis of the fetal death, and prompt delivery entertained if the fibrinogen levels drop into the 100 ng/dl to 150 mg/dl range. However, given the efficacy of current methods for labor induction, RDFS should probably never occur in women unless they have not previously been diagnosed with fetal death or if they have not sought prenatal care or evaluation for potential pregnancy problems.

One recent study compared expectant management to labor induction [10]. In this nonrandomized retrospective study, 108 women underwent spontaneous labor and 100 women were induced by a variety of means, including oxytocin, prostaglandin E_2 (PGE_2), or laminaria placement. About

10% of the cohort had a prior cesarean. None of the patients experienced cesarean delivery, while the time in labor for those undergoing induction was longer as would be expected, 13.7 versus 4.4h. They did note that three women in the expectant group were induced when hypofibrinogenemia was detected. Complications such as retained placenta, postpartum hemorrhage, and blood transfusion were not different between the two groups, although women being followed expectantly developed endometritis more frequently (6% vs. 1%). The authors noted that labor induction minimized psychological stress, maximized autopsy potential, and decreased the risk for endometritis while prolonging the stay in labor and delivery. Conversely, expectant management was associated with the potential for prolonged grieving, minimized autopsy potential, and increased the risk for endometritis, but with a shorter time in the labor and delivery suite. Given these factors, they advocated for routine labor induction over expectant management.

In summary, there are few evidence-based guidelines when deciding upon expectant management or labor induction. Expectant management is relatively inexpensive and safe, but has the disadvantage of having the patient await spontaneous labor. Anecdotally, such waiting may pose significant psychosocial stress for the patient. However, there are few data to support this conclusion. Conversely, labor induction is convenient, yet more costly and may carry higher risks of intervention and the possibility of unsuccessful induction. On balance, either approach can be justified and supported. Therefore, individualized patient care, taking into account all of the above factors and, most importantly, desires of the informed patient, should guide the practitioner in designing an acceptable management plan.

Medical induction of labor

The introduction of prostaglandin agents dramatically changed the management options for fetal death. Prior to this, expectant management, oxytocin, and mechanical dilation were essentially the only options available. However, with the advent of prostaglandins, obstetricians had a reliable medication available with a high level of success and manageable side effects. As a result, medical induction of labor is now commonly offered to women who have suffered IUFD. There are many options available to the obstetrician, and the selection of agents and strategy for the induction of labor in these patients is colored by the available studies as well as the experience and judgment of the obstetrician. One consideration in making the decision of agent and dose is that higher doses can be employed since safety considerations for the fetus are not an issue. Thus, the safety of the mother is singly important. Options for medical labor induction include oxytocin, misoprostol, mifepristone, and PGE_2 analogues.

Oxytocin

Oxytocin has been clinically available since the 1940s and has been commonly employed in the management of IUFD. Notably, there are few studies that guide the practitioner regarding optimal concentrations and means of administration. Currently, intravenous oxytocin titration is the standard method of administration, but oxytocin may be administered buccally, intramuscularly, and intranasally. In general, an optimal situation for oxytocin use would be in women in the third trimester with a favorable cervix (Bishop's score of 6 or greater). At term, when oxytocin receptor expression is high, accepted labor and delivery protocols for intravenous oxytocin induction for a living fetus are recommended. A relatively low dose of oxytocin may be administered, for example, starting at 1–3mU min and increasing by that amount every 15–20 min. Also, higher doses, such as that used in the active management of labor, may be also administered [11]. Oxytocin in this case is started at 6mU min and then increased by 6mU min every 15–20 min. No upper limit for oxytocin use in the management of fetal death has been established, although one would be surprised to see the need for doses higher than 40–50mU min.

Higher-dose protocols, described by Toaff et al. [12], have proven to be successful, but these oxytocin concentrations are higher than described in other protocols and some practitioners may be reticent to apply this protocol. However, for

Table 14.1 Acceptable oxytocin regimens in the management of fetal death.

Starting dose	Increasing dose	Interval
1 mU/min	1 mU/min	Every 30–40 min
3 mU/min	3 mU/min	Every 15–20 min
6 mU/min	6 mU/min	Every 15–30 min
50 U in 500 ml saline at 60 ml/min	10 ml	Every hour

women with fetal death in the second trimester, oxytocin receptor expression is lower and so higher concentrations are needed. If the Toaff protocol is employed, care must be taken to avoid oxytocin toxicity, as this is one scenario where water retention and hyponatremia could occur. However, this complication is rare even with these higher-dose protocols [13]. See Table 14.1 for a summary of the different oxytocin regimens that are acceptable for use in this setting.

For women with an unfavorable cervix, 12-h administration of misoprostol (25–50 µg every 4–6 h) or a prostaglandin insert is an acceptable initiating therapy to attempt to soften and thin the uterine cervix. After the 12-h preparation period, oxytocin is administered at sufficient doses to effect labor. Amniotomy should be performed when feasible, as oxytocin will be more efficacious after membrane rupture.

Prostaglandin E$_2$

Prostin, or dinoprostone, is a PGE$_2$ analogue that has powerful effects on uterine contractility. Discovery of pharmacological preparations of PGE$_2$ has completely changed the management of fetal death, in that these drugs are effective not only at inducing uterine contractions but also overcoming the unfavorable cervix. Prostin should not be used in women beyond 28 weeks of pregnancy, as the risk for uterine rupture increases, and other medications (oxytocin, misoprostol) have equal efficacy with less risk.

One of the first studies regarding the use of PGE$_2$ in managing fetal death employed intravenous infusions of PGE$_2$ in comparison to intravenous oxytocin [14]. This small study of 30 women showed that intravenous PGE$_2$ was more efficacious than oxytocin. Subsequently, the Food and Drug Administration approved the use of vaginal PGE$_2$ suppositories in 1979 for use in women with fetal death up to 28 weeks gestation. In a summary of PGE$_2$, Kochenour in 1987 [1] summarized studies to that time and noted that vaginal PGE$_2$ suppositories were characterized by vaginal delivery within 24 h in 90% of patients. The average induction to delivery interval was approximately 8–9 h, and 5–25% of women required sharp uterine curettage for retained placental fragments. The most common side effects in women with no premedication included vomiting (about 50%), diarrhea (33%), and pyrexia (40% had a temperature elevation of greater than 2°F). Approximately 10% of patients experienced tachycardia, headache, and chills. Some clinicians will often use 10 mg prostin (half of an insert) to determine receptivity of the uterus, but also in an attempt to avoid these common side effects of the drug. Premedication with antiemetics, antispasmodics, and antipyretics is commonly employed to avoid these troublesome side effects. Because PGE$_2$ is such potent smooth muscle contractant, the drug should be avoided in women with asthma, hypertension, hypotension, and cardiac, renal, and hepatic disease.

Prostin vaginal suppositories contain 20 mg of dinoprostone and can be inserted every 4–6 h. Total amount of time for administration is typically over 24–36 h to effect delivery. Treatment for longer than 48 h is discouraged. A common finding is that the cervix will not dilate until just before delivery. Hence, patience in applying the therapy is paramount. Of historical interest is the use of intravenous PGE$_2$ [14]. While efficacious and with minimal gastrointestinal side effects, the use of intravenous PGE$_2$ was largely supplanted by vaginal suppositories because of ease of administration.

Other prostaglandin agents

Intra-amniotic prostaglandin F2α (PGF2α) has been reported to successfully terminate pregnancies complicated by fetal death [15]. In this study, 30 women were given 40 mg PGF2α via intra-amniotic administration, with a mean time to delivery of about 5 h. However, the disadvantages posed by the route of administration and the inability to adjust dosing limits the applicability of the drug. Both extra-amniotic and intravenous administration of PGF2α has been reported [16]. However, in a study comparing extra-amniotic PGF2α with misoprostol, misoprostol was more efficacious, had a shorter induction to delivery time, and fewer side effects [17]. Given this, use of PGF2α has been largely supplanted by misoprostol.

Intramuscular 15-methyl PGF2α, also known as Hemabate, was used fairly extensively in the 1980s [1]. Success rates, as defined by vaginal delivery, exceeded 90% with a mean induction to delivery time of 9 h [18]. However, side effects similar to that seen with PGE_2 were common. Thiery et al. [19] reported on a case series of 255 women who were treated with 15-methyl PGF2α for missed abortion in the second trimester, and they reported 99.6% delivery within 36 h. However, two-third of women had gastrointestinal side effects that could be ameliorated with premedication. Given the extent of side effects, the use of this agent, like the others, has been replaced by misoprostol.

Misoprostol

Oral misoprostol for labor induction for fetal death was first reported in 1987 [20]. Misoprostol is the most thoroughly investigated medication to effect delivery in the women with fetal death and has largely replaced the use of PGE_2 (dinoprostone) and F2α. In fact, the most recent ACOG Technical Bulletin regarding stillbirth does not mention the use of dinoprostone [21]. Misoprostol, a prostaglandin E_1 analogue, has the advantage of having fewer and less severe side effects than PGE_2 and PGF2α with similar or even better efficacy.

The use of misoprostol to terminate pregnancy complicated by fetal death or fetal anomalies has been extensively reviewed in a recent meta-analysis by Dodd and Crowther [22]. This Cochrane review included 38 studies that met criteria with a total of 3,679 women evaluated. For this review, studies had to be randomized controlled trials comparing misoprostol to control or other methods of labor induction. Based upon this review, the authors state that vaginal misoprostol is as effective at effecting delivery within 24 h as other methods described earlier and with a similar induction to delivery interval. Moreover, vaginal misoprostol had a much better side effect profile than other uterotonics, while data regarding the risk of uterine rupture was limited such that no definitive opinion could be offered regarding this complication. Also, Dodd and Crowther conclude that vaginal misoprostol is more effective than oral misoprostol in accomplishing vaginal delivery of a fetal death. They advocate more study to determine the optimal dose and administration frequency, the risk of rare adverse events, and the use of sublingual misoprostol.

In a separate meta-analysis of 14 studies, Gomez Ponce de Leon et al. [23] found that oral misoprostol use was associated with a slightly greater chance of delivering within 24 h, but not 48 h, where vaginal misoprostol was more efficacious. However, oral administration was associated with greater gastrointestinal complications. They found no difference between 600 and 400 μg applications and recommended that the lower dose be used.

In a separate Cochrane review by Nielson et al. [24], of medical treatment for early fetal death (less than 24 weeks), a meta-analysis of 24 studies of 1,888 women was performed to assess the efficacy and safety of different medical treatments for early pregnancy failure less than 24 weeks. These studies included a medical treatment that was compared to another treatment or no treatment (including placebo). They concluded that vaginal misoprostol was both effective and characterized by few side effects and less need for uterine curettage when compared to no treatment of vaginal PGE_2. However, lower-dose regimens of misoprostol were less effective at ending pregnancy. Similar to late pregnancy termination, oral misoprostol was less effective than vaginal misoprostol and the authors noted the need for further study on optimal dosing and frequency of administration.

A major drawback to misoprostol is that there are no specific delivery systems for vaginal application, meaning that tablets have to be split and then

Table 14.2 Vaginal misoprostol dosing and interval schedule [25].

Gestational age	Starting dose	Interval
13–17 weeks	600–800 μg	Every 6 h
18–26 weeks	100 μg	Every 6 h
27–43 weeks	25–50 μg	Every 4 h

inserted (if using less than 100 μg applications). Another significant problem is that there are no studies showing best and most appropriate dosing or route of administration in women with IUFD. A recent review by Gomez et al. [25] provided recommendations for dosing of misoprostol (Table 14.2). In general, higher doses are used earlier in pregnancy with the dosage decreasing with advancing gestation. For example, first-trimester dosing is usually 600–800 μg orally every 6 h, while between 13 and 17 weeks the authors recommend 200 μg every 6 h. From 18 to 26 weeks, 100 μg every 6 h is recommended and then for 27–43 weeks 25–50 μg every 4 h is suggested. The most common side effects are gastrointestinal (about one-third of women given the drug) and pyrexia (in about 7%). Misoprostol administration should be limited to 24 h. After this time period, changing agents to PGE$_2$ should be strongly considered.

Regardless of these unsettled issues regarding misoprostol, it has become a standard method to induce labor in women with fetal death because of its excellent side effect profile, equivalent clinical outcomes to other methods of induction, and substantial cost savings. Misoprostol cost pennies to hospitals as opposed to other medications used for this indication.

Mifepristone

Mifepristone, or RU486, is a competitive progesterone receptor antagonist and has been shown to be an effective abortifacient in the first trimester [26]. However, mifepristone must be used with prostaglandins to effect termination of pregnancy. In 2002, Wagaarachchi et al. [27] reported on almost 100 women with fetal death after 24 weeks who were treated with a single oral dose of mifepristone (200 μg) with combined vaginal and oral misoprostol for 12 h. If the pregnancy was greater than 34 weeks, 100 μg misoprostol was used. They noted that 95 of the 96 delivered within 72 h of administration of mifepristone and the regimen was well tolerated with few side effects. Fairley et al. [28] compared oral mifepristone with oral or vaginal misoprostol at a lower dose (400 vs. 50 μg) in women with fetal death after 24 weeks. They found that the higher dose of misoprostol shortened the induction to delivery time interval by about a third (10 vs. 7 h), but that the lower dose of misoprostol was associated with fewer gastrointestinal complications. The combination of mifepristone with misoprostol has been compared to misoprostol alone in women with fetal death at 21–42 weeks gestation in a study by Vayrynen et al. [29]. Their nonrandomized study of 130 women showed that the induction to delivery interval was not different between the two groups, but that pretreatment with mifepristone at earlier gestational ages improved outcomes.

The usual dose of mifepristone is a single dose of 200 mg orally. The most common side effects include nausea, vomiting, diarrhea, headache, dizziness, and fatigue. While these studies show promise for this combination of medications, more research needs to be done with prospective randomized trials to assess the efficacy, side effect profile, risks, and benefits of these drug regimens.

Surgical induction and evacuation

The primary techniques for surgical induction of labor include amniotomy, the balloon catheter, and dilation and evacuation. Amniotomy has been used as a means of labor induction for decades and was first described over 200 years ago. A recent Cochrane review of amniotomy for induction of labor in women with a live fetus [30] found little objective evidence to recommend this technique for labor induction, but years of clinical experience indicates that amniotomy, in association with oxytocin administration either before or after rupture of membranes, will result in the induction of labor in the majority of cases. One small study from 1980 [31] compared amniotomy alone with amniotomy with oxytocin and hypertonic saline solution injected intra-amniotically. They found that amniotomy, with or without oxytocin, resulted in an average time to delivery of 7–9 h.

Amniotomy

Amniotomy, either after oxytocin administration has commenced or prior to oxytocin administration, is an excellent choice for labor induction. Notably, there are few objective data on the best sequence of interventions or outcomes. Usually, the best candidates for amniotomy are women with a favorable cervical examination, as some cervical dilation or effacement is usually needed for the practitioner to perform amniotomy.

Transcervical catheter placement

A Foley catheter placed transcervically has been used with good success for labor induction with a viable fetus [32]; however, little data is available to support its use in women with IUFD. One small study in 1994 [33] showed that induction of labor with a double-balloon catheter was as efficacious as extra-amniotic prostaglandins in effecting delivery and with few complications. However, this study included only 20 women. A larger study from Africa was reported in 1997 [34], in which 244 women with fetal death, most in the third trimester, were randomized to either extra-amniotic saline via a Foley catheter placed transcervically, or intra-amniotic prostaglandin therapy. They deemed extra-amniotic saline administration as being both safe and effective when compared to intra-amniotic prostaglandins, but that women with saline infused via a Foley catheter required oxytocin administration more frequently.

However, an extrapolation of these studies seems reasonable, and so this technique may be considered. In this case, a 30- or 60-cc Foley bulb is inserted through the cervix into the lower uterine segment and the bulb inflated with saline. The catheter itself is then placed on tension. Some use lower doses of oxytocin concomitantly with the Foley bulb. Usually, after a few hours, the Foley bulb is spontaneously expelled and the

cervix is dilated to about 3 cm. The previously noted Cochrane review [32] showed that extra-amniotic infusion of saline is probably not additive to merely the catheter alone, and so is not recommended. Amniotomy and oxytocin can then be employed to effect uterine contractions.

Surgical evacuation

In many instances, surgical evacuation may be the safest and most expeditious method for ending the pregnancy. Hern et al. [35] reported on their experience of surgical evacuation of the uterus for fetal anomalies and fetal death in 124 women from 15 to 34 weeks gestation. Their routine method for fetal death management at less than 20 weeks gestation included placing laminaria tents prior to dilation and evacuation. At greater than 20 weeks, they induced labor and then performed instrumental extraction or assisted expulsion of the fetus. There was only one complication in this case series, and so the authors concluded that outpatient surgical evacuation was safe and efficacious in women with fetal death. Also, Jacot et al. [36] reported on their experience of second-trimester pregnancy terminations from 15 to 20 weeks gestation. Their technique included placing laminaria tents and then performing D & E. They found that complications were rare and included primarily infectious morbidity. Uterine rupture was rare. For fetal death at less than 24 weeks, surgical evacuation via D & E is recommended if practitioners are available who have expertise in the procedure. However, surgical D & E often precludes the acquisition of an intact fetus for a detailed autopsy. The advantages, and disadvantages, of D & E must be weighed when considering surgical evacuation.

Fetal death in women with prior cesarean delivery

Special considerations must be made for women with a history of a prior cesarean delivery. In women with one prior low transverse cesarean section and a third-trimester fetal death, induction of labor using oxytocin, amniotomy, and the

Foley bulb are all acceptable. The risk of uterine rupture is quite low in these women using these methods. However, prostaglandin analogues should probably be avoided in women with a prior uterine incision at these gestational ages, given a much higher overall risk for uterine rupture [37]. Conversely, prostaglandin analogues may be used in women with a prior cesarean who have fetal death diagnosed in the second trimester. In these cases, the risk of uterine rupture in association with prostaglandins is quite low.

The use of misoprostol in second-trimester pregnancy termination in women with a prior cesarean has recently been reviewed by Berghella et al. [38]. They identified 461 women with prior cesarean who had experienced misoprostol induction in the second trimester, and of those women with one prior low transverse cesarean two (0.4%) experienced uterine rupture. No women of the 46 with two prior low cesareans experienced uterine rupture. However, this work did not specify if any of the indications for ending pregnancy included fetal death. A separate meta-analysis by Goyal [39] identified an overall risk of 0.28% uterine rupture in women undergoing second-trimester misoprostol-induced pregnancy termination, while the risk in women with no prior cesarean for uterine rupture was 0.04%. She noted that 1 in 414 women experiencing this procedure would be expected to experience uterine rupture as a complication.

There are few studies of using misoprostol for managing fetal death in women with prior cesarean delivery. Bhattacharjee et al. [40] reported on 80 women who experienced termination of pregnancy in the second trimester with a history of cesarean delivery. Of these, 16 (20%) had a fetal death. When compared to a control cohort of women experiencing second-trimester pregnancy termination without a prior cesarean, they found no differences in maternal outcomes and there were no instances of uterine rupture. However, uterine rupture has been reported with misoprostol use, both in women with or without uterine scars from prior cesarean delivery [41, 42].

Perhaps the largest experience of delivering women with antepartum fetal death in the setting of prior cesarean delivery was recently reported by the Maternal-Fetal Medicine Units Network [43]. In their analysis of data collected for a cesarean section registry, 209 fetal deaths in 45,988 women were identified. Of these 209, 51 (or about one-fourth of the cohort) experienced repeat cesarean delivery, either electively or in labor. Of the 158 women who experienced a trial of labor, 26 delivered vaginally after spontaneous labor and 116 had labor induced with a wide variety of techniques, including oxytocin alone, prostaglandins, and prostaglandins with oxytocin, among others. Of these women undergoing labor induction, 86% accomplished vaginal delivery. Uterine rupture was detected in five of the women, four of whom were undergoing labor induction (3.4% of women being induced). All four women with rupture while being induced had one prior low transverse incision. Transfusion was required in 7.7% of the patients, 3.3% of women required an intensive care unit stay, and there were no maternal deaths. Notably, none of the women who experienced uterine rupture required transfusion, hysterectomy, or intensive care unit admission.

From these data, the authors concluded that trial of labor was marked by a high rate of vaginal birth after cesarean (VBAC) success, but that there was a higher rate of uterine rupture when compared to women having VBAC with a living fetus. The prior study by the Network had shown a uterine rupture rate of 7/1,000 with a trial of labor and a living fetus [44], while the overall rate in the fetal death cohort was 24/1,000 and then 34/1,000 of those attempting a vaginal birth. The authors note that many of the women were being induced with prostaglandin agents prior to recommendations to avoid these agents in women undergoing VBAC [45]. The authors suggest that labor induction is a valid option for women with fetal death and a prior cesarean section, with the caveat that appropriate resources are available to manage any potential complications.

Women with a prior classical uterine incision should most likely undergo repeat cesarean delivery. Even without the consideration of fetal safety, the risk for uterine rupture is 6–12% [46, 47] and so maternal safety considerations are such that a repeat procedure can avoid the risk of rupture with the potential need for hysterectomy, blood transfusions, and other potential complications that may occur in these women.

Cesarean delivery

Primary cesarean delivery has been reported in women with fetal death [48]. There are clear obstetric indications for cesarean delivery in women with fetal death, for example, fetal macrosomia (estimated fetal weight of greater than 4,500 g), fetal abnormalities leading to obstruction of the birth canal (e.g., solid tumors), and other obstructions to the birth canal (e.g., uterine fibroids). In the report by Mukherj, 121 women (or about 1.4% of all cesareans performed at their site) experienced cesarean delivery with a fetal death. Common indications for cesarean delivery included obstetric hemorrhage, malpresentation, repeat procedures, obstructed labor, a second twin, and eclampsia. Notably, about 10% of cesareans on women with diagnosed fetal deaths were performed for "fetal distress." When there are clear obstetric indications for cesarean delivery, operative therapy should employed with appropriate documentation of reasons for proceeding with cesarean delivery.

Elective primary cesarean delivery for fetal death may occur more often than reported. However, the reasons for this extreme intervention are not clear, while the potential short- and long-term complications from cesarean are well delineated [49]. Choosing expediency over consideration of maternal short- and long-term safety and outcomes seems shortsighted and difficult to support. There are no data to support this intervention as safe or effective. While the delivery may be quickly effected, the long-term effects after fetal death on maternal emotional and physical well-being are not known. Only after carefully weighing these risks should primary cesarean be considered for these women.

Special consideration of destructive operations of the fetus must be made. While rarely performed in the United States today, fetal destructive procedures are employed in low resource areas. Purposeful fetal decapitation, craniotomy, cleidotomy (division of one or both clavicles), and embryotomy (evisceration of abdominal or thoracic contents) have all been suggested as methods to avoid cesarean delivery in settings where cesarean is not readily available or more dangerous than the destructive procedures [50]. In underdeveloped countries, the risk for maternal death is greater from obstructed labor than the risk from fetal destructive procedures [50, 51]. Further, inadvertent fetal decapitation may occur when attempting maneuvers to effect vaginal delivery of a dead fetus, particularly if the time frame from death to delivery is prolonged. While inevitably distressing to the patient, her family, and labor and delivery staff, this circumstance should prompt the practitioner to maintain composure and continue efforts to complete the delivery.

Fetal death in multiple gestation

One special circumstance where expectant management should be strongly considered is when fetal death is diagnosed in one fetus of a multiple gestation. Death of one fetus in a multiple gestation is a rare complication, occurring in up to 5% multiple gestations during the second and third trimesters [52]. This finding is exclusive of the vanishing twin often noted in the first trimester. Notably, death of a single fetus in higher-order multiple gestations (e.g., triplets, quadruplets) may be more common, complicating up to 17% of triplet pregnancies [53]. There are no clear answers to many concerns of fetal death in multiple gestation, such as optimal timing of delivery, role of antenatal testing, and maternal effects of the fetal death [54]. While some studies have reported the risk of RFDS in women with single fetal death in multiple gestation, this risk is likely an overestimation [54].

Managing single fetal death in multiple gestation is hampered by the lack of solid clinical evidence based on studies with sufficient numbers. Management guidelines are based primarily on case series and expert opinion, and ultimately management is made on a case-by-case basis. A key consideration in these women is the chorionicity of the pregnancy. In monochorionic pregnancies, the insult to the surviving fetus may occur at the time of demise [55] and so prompt intervention at the time of diagnosis may not improve outcomes. Moreover, contemporary antenatal surveillance mechanisms (e.g., nonstress testing, biophysical profiles) lack the sensitivity and specificity to provide precise and useful information to guide the decision for delivery. Some practitioners advocate delivery of a multiple gestation with a fetal demise at 37 weeks, assuming fetal surveillance continues to be reassuring [54].

In a systematic review, Ong et al. [56], reported in cases of single twin delivery that the other dies in 12% of monochorionic pregnancies and 4% of dichorionic pregnancies. Further, the risk of adverse neurologic consequences in the surviving twin was 18% in monochorionic pregnancies and only 1% in dichorionic pregnancies. Even with these data, the authors concluded that better prospective data was required before definitive management recommendations could be made.

A recent study by Fichera et al. [57] reported on 23 twin pregnancies with a single demise in which such expectant management was followed. In this report, the authors suggest that fetal ultrasound and magnetic reasonance imaging (MRI) can provide useful prognostic information, although these recommendations are hampered by small sample size.

Given these studies, expectant management is usually the most prudent course of action. After the diagnosis of a single fetal demise in multiple gestation, some form of fetal surveillance is recommended. There are no clear and definitive guidelines on the optimal method of fetal surveillance that should be employed. Many authorities recommend weekly nonstress testing and/or biophysical profiles, with more frequent testing should other comorbidities, such as intrauterine growth restriction, occur. Periodic sonography for fetal growth parameters is recommended. Fetal brain MRI may have value [56], but no prospective trials have proven this to be of benefit. The timing of delivery is individualized based on fetal surveillance and growth. With any evidence of fetal compromise, delivery of the surviving twin should probably be effected. However, even if the surviving fetus, or fetuses, shows no evidence of fetal compromise, elective delivery at 37 weeks has been suggested [54].

Other clinical considerations

Grief management is of particular importance in the labor and delivery setting. Postpartum depression may occur in up to 20% of women after stillbirth [58], and a further 20% may have posttraumatic stress disorder (PTSD) [59]. Nursing staff assigned to these patients should be skilled in helping these women and families cope with their sudden loss. If possible, experienced nursing staff who have completed Resolve Through Sharing (RTS) training in perinatal grief management should be assigned to these patients (http://bereavementservices.org). Women and families who suffer stillbirth experience a rapid sequence of multiple emotions, including grief, guilt, anger, despair, and hopelessness. Skillful intervention at this time by nursing staff, pastoral staff, and medical staff may assist the family cope with loss. In addition, interventions can be planned to attempt to minimize or prevent PTSD. While a common practice in labor and delivery units is to strongly recommend that women and families view the dead infant, other investigators found that behaviors to promote contact with the stillborn infant actually resulted in poorer outcomes, including higher rates of depression, anxiety, and PTSD [60]. These authors recommend that parent's wishes regarding their own psychosocial management be respected. A more detailed psychosocial management approach is described in Chapter 13.

At the time of diagnosis of fetal death, a diagnostic evaluation should commence in the attempt to assign a cause of death. The obstetrician should consider initiating the consent process to obtain a postmortem examination on the fetus. This test continues to be the gold standard to identify a potential cause, or causes, of fetal death [61]. Obtaining such consent is never pleasant nor easy, but this evaluation may be the single most important diagnostic test to offer to the patient. The timing of the initial discussion of the postmortem examination is critical. The best time to offer this test is when the patient asks why the death occurred, almost a uniform experience. In general, the patient and her family should not be asked to decide when the topic is first broached, but be asked again at a latter time after the delivery for their decision. The physician should emphasize to the patient that, in most cases, only after a post-mortem examination can a definitive cause of death be assigned (also see Chapter 12).

After the postmortem examination, the next most important evaluation is pathologic examination of the placenta (also see Chapter 10). The placenta and membranes should be sent for patho-logic evaluation in every case of fetal death. There are few circumstances where this may not be able to occur. In addition, the practitioner should initiate a laboratory evaluation for the causes of fetal death, as is noted in Chapter 12.

Conclusions

Regardless of the methodology employed to effect delivery in women who have suffered fetal death, the obstetrician should create a therapeutic plan before initiating therapy based on the gestational age of the patient, comorbidities that have occurred before and during the pregnancy, and overall condition of the patient. With plan in hand, the practitioner can account for changes in maternal condition in anticipation of vaginal delivery. The patient should be informed early in the process that the entire therapeutic plan may take 24–36 h, so as to set expectations and allow for changes in her overall condition. Unrealistic expectations can compound the grief response and lead to more emotionally charged interactions that may compromise the patient's condition as well as the patient–physician relationship. With compassionate care and sensitive communication from the medical and nursing staff, the patient can receive optimal obstetric care and emotional support to assist them in dealing with their sudden and tragic loss.

References

1. Kochenour N. Management of fetal demise. Clin Obstet Gynecol 1987;30:322–30.
2. Dippel AL. Death of foetus in utero. Johns Hopkins Med J 1934;54:24.
3. Tricomi V, Kohl SG. Fetal death in utero. Am J Obstet Gynecol 1957;74:1092–7.
4. Erez O, Gotsch F, Mazaki-Tovi S, et al. Evidence of maternal platelet activation, excessive thrombin generation, and high amniotic fluid tissue factor immunoreactivity and functional activity in patients with fetal death. J Matern Fetal Neonatal Med 2009;22:672–87.
5. Weiner AE, Reid DE, Roby CC, Diamond LK. Coagulation defects with intrauterine fetal death from Rh isoimmunization. Am J Obstet Gynecol 1950;60:1015–22.
6. Pritchard JA. Fetal death in utero. Obstet Gynecol 1959;14:573–80.
7. Phillips LL, Skrodelis V, King TA. Hypofibrinogenemia and intrauterine death. Am J Obstet Gynecol 1964;89:903–14.
8. Jimenez JM, Pritchard JA. Pathogenesis and treatment of coagulation defects resulting from fetal death. Obstet Gynecol 1968;32:449–59.
9. Lerner R, Margolin M, Slate WG, et al. Heparin in the treatment of hypofibrinogenemia complicating fetal death in utero. Am J Obstet Gynecol 1967;97:373–8.
10. Salamat SM, Landy HJ, O'Sullivan MJ. Labor induction after fetal death: a retrospective analysis. J Reprod Med 2002;47:23–6.
11. O'Driscoll K, Foley M, MacDonald D. Active management of labor as an alternative to cesarean section for dystocia. Obstet Gynecol 1984;63:485–90.
12. Toaff R, Ayalon D, Gogol G. Clinical use of high concentration oxytocin drip. Obstet Gynecol 1971;37:112–20.
13. Turnbull AC, Anderson AB. Induction of labor. 3. Results with amniotomy and oxytocin titration. J Obstet Gynecol Br Commonw 1968;75:32–41.
14. Gordon H, Pipe NGJ. Induction of labor after intrauterine fetal death: a comparison between prostaglandin E_2 and oxytocin. Obstet Gynecol 1974;45:44–6.
15. Antsaklis A, Diakomanolis E, Karayannopoulos C, et al. Induction of abortion by intra-amniotic administration of prostaglandin F2a in patients with intrauterine fetal death and missed abortion. Int Surg 1979;64:41–3.
16. Salamalekis E, Kassanos D, Hassiakos D, et al. Intra/extra-amniotic administration of prostaglandin F2a

in fetal death, missed and therapeutic abortions. Clin Exp Obstet Gynecol 1990;17:17–21.

17. Ghorab MN, El Helw BA. Second trimester termination of pregnancy by extra-amniotic prostaglandin F2a or endocervical misoprostol: a comparative study. Acta Obstet Gynecol Scand 1998;77:429–32.

18. YlikorkalaO, Kirkinen P, Jarvinen PA. Intramuscular administration of 15-methyl prostaglandin F2a for induction of labor in patients with intrauterine fetal death or an anencephalic fetus. Br J Obstet Gynecol 1976;83:502–4.

19. Thiery M, Parewijck W, Decoster JM. Management of second trimester missed abortion with intramuscular 15-methyl prostaglandin F2 alpha. Contracept Deliv Syst 1983;4:153–9.

20. Mariani-Neto C, Leao EJ, Kenj G, De Aquino MM. Use of misoprostol for induction of labor in stillbirths. Rev Paul Med 1987;105:325–8.

21. ACOG Practice Bulletin #102. Management of stillbirth. Obstet Gynecol 2009;113:748–61.

22. Dodd JM, Crowther CA. Misoprostol for induction of labor to terminate pregnancy in the second or third trimester for women with a fetal anomaly or after intrauterine fetal death. Cochrane Database Syst Rev 2010;4:CD004901.

23. Gomez Ponce de Leon R, Wing DA. Misoprostol for termination of pregnancy with intrauterine fetal demise in the second and third trimester of pregnancy: a systematic review. Contraception 2009;79: 259–71.

24. Neilson JP, Hickey M, Vazquez JC. Medical treatment for early fetal death (less than 24 weeks). Cochrane Database Syst Rev 2006;3:CD002253.

25. Gomez Ponce de Leon R, Wing D, Fiala C. Misoprostol for intrauterine fetal death. Int J Gynecol Obstet 2007;99:S190–S193.

26. Tang OS, Ho PC. Clinical applications of mifepristone. Gynecol Endocrinol 2006;22:655–9.

27. Wagaarachchi PT, Ashok PW, Narvekar N, et al. Medical management of late intrauterine death using a combination of mifepristone and misoprostol. Br J Obstet Gynecol 2002;109:443–7.

28. Fairley TE, Mackenzie M, Owen P, Mackenzie F. Management of late intrauterine death using a combination of mifepristone and misoprostol: experience of two regimens. Eur J Obstet Gynecol Reprod Biol 2005;118:28–31.

29. Vayrynen W, Heikinheimo O, Nuutila M. Misoprostol-only versus mifepristone plus misoprostol in induction of labor following intrauterine fetal death. Acta Obstet Gynecol Scand 2007;86:701–5.

30. Bricker L, Luckas M. Amniotomy along for induction of labor. Cochrane Database Syst Rev 2000;4: CD002862.

31. Rozenman D, Kessler I, Lancet M. Third trimester induction of labor with fetal death in utero. Surg Gynecol Obstet 1980;151:497–9.

32. Boulvain M, Kelly A, Lohse C, et al. Mechanical methods for induction of labour. Cochrane Database Syst Rev 2001;4:CD001233.

33. Toppozada MK, Shaala SA, Anwar MY, et al. Termination of pregnancy with fetal death in the second and third trimesters—the double balloon catheter versus extra-amniotic prostaglandin. Int J Obstet Gynecol 1994;45:269–73.

34. Mahomed K, Jayaguru AS. Extra-amniotic saline infusion for induction of labor in antepartum fetal death: a cost effective method worthy of wider use. Br J Obstet Gynecol 1997;104:1058–61.

35. Hern WM, Zen C, Ferguson KA, et al. Outpatient abortion for fetal anomaly and fetal death from 15–34 menstural weeks gestation: techniques and clinical management. Obstet Gynecol 1993;81:301–6.

36. Jacot FR, Poulin C, Bilodeau AP, et al. A five-year experience with second-trimester induced abortions: no increase in complication rate as compared to the first trimester. Am J Obstet Gynecol 1993;168: 633–77.

37. Lydon-Rochelle M, Holt VL, Easterling TR, Martin DP. Risk of uterine rupture during labor among women with a prior cesarean delivery. N Engl J Med 2001;345:3–8.

38. Berghella V, Airoldi J, O'Neill AM, et al. Misoprostol for second trimester pregnancy termination in women with prior cesarean: a systematic review. Br J Obstet Gynecol 2009;116:1151–7.

39. Goyal V. Uterine rupture in second-trimester misoprostol-induced abortion after cesarean delivery: a systematic review. Obstet Gynecol 2009;113:1117–23.

40. Bhattacharjee N, Ganguly RP, Saha SP. Misoprostol for termination of mid-trimester post-cesarean pregnancy. Aust N Z J Obstet Gynecol 2007;47:23–5.

41. Plaut MM, Schwartz ML, Lubarsky SL. Uterine rupture associated with the use of misoprostol in the gravid patient with a prior cesarean section. Am J Obstet Gynecol 1999;180:1535–42.

42. Berghahn L, Christensen D, Droste S. Uterine rupture during second-trimester abortion associated with misoprostol. Obstet Gynecol 2001;98:976–7.

43. Ramirez MM, Gilbert S, Landon MB, et al. Mode of delivery in women with antepartum fetal death and prior cesarean delivery. Am J Perinatol 2010;27:825–30.

44. Landon MB, Hauth JC, Leveno KJ, et al.; National Institute of Child Health and Human Development Maternal-Fetal Medicine Units Network. Maternal and perinatal outcomes associated with a trial of labor after prior cesarean delivery. N Engl J Med 2004;351:2581–9.

45. ACOG Committee Opinion on Obstetric Practice. Committee opinion. Induction of labor for vaginal birth after cesarean delivery. Obstet Gynecol 2002;99:679–80.

46. Halperin ME, Moore DC, Hannah WJ. Classical versus low-segment transverse incision for preterm cesarean section: maternal complications and outcomes of subsequent pregnancies. Br J Obstet Gynecol 1988;95:990–6.

47. McMahon MJ. Vaginal birth after cesarean. Clin Obstet Gynecol 1998;41:369–81.

48. Mukherj J, Kamilya G, Bhattacharyya SK. Caesarean section for the dead baby—an unhappy reality. J Indian Med Assoc 2007;105:318–19.

49. Silver RM, Landon MB, Rouse DJ, et al.; National Institute of Child Health and Human Development Maternal-Fetal Medicine Units Network. Maternal morbidity associated with multiple repeat cesarean deliveries. Obstet Gynecol 2006;107:1226–32.

50. Maharaj D, Moodley J. Symphysiotomy and fetal destructive operations. Best Pract Res Clin Obstet Gynecol 2002;16:117–31.

51. Singhai SR, Chaudhry P, Sangwan K, Singhal SK. Destructive operations in modern obstetrics. Arch Gynecol Obstet 2005;273:107–9.

52. Kilby MD, Govind A, O'Brien PM. Outcome of twin pregnancies complicated by a single intrauterine death: a comparison with viable twin pregnancies. Obstet Gynecol 1994;84:107–9.

53. Johnson CD, Zhang J. Survival of other fetuses after a fetal death in twin and triplet pregnancies. Obstet Gynecol 2002;99:698–703.

54. Cleary-Goldman J, D'Alton M. Management of a single fetal demise in a multiple gestation. Obstet Gynecol Surv 2004;59:285–98.

55. Malone FD, D'Alton ME. Anomalies peculiar to multiple gestations. Clin Perinatol 2000;27:1033–46.

56. Ong S, Zamora J, Khan KS, Kilby MD. Prognosis for the co-twin following single-twin death: a systematic review. Br J Obstet Gynecol 2006;113:992–8.

57. Fichera A, Zambolo C, Accorsi P, et al. Perinatal outcome and neurological follow up of the cotwins in twin pregnancies complicated by single intrauterine death. Eur J Obstet Gynecol Reprod Biol 2009;147:37–40.

58. Forrest GC, Standish E, Baum JD. Support after perinatal death: a study of support and counseling after perinatal bereavement. BMJ 1982;285:1475–9.

59. Turton P, Hughes P, Evans CD, Fainman D. Incidence, correlates and predictors of post-traumatic stress disorder in pregnancy after stillbirth. Br J Psychiatry 2001;178:556–60.

60. Hughes P, Turton P, Hopper E, Evans CD. Assessment of guidelines for good practice in psychosocial care of mothers after stillbirth: a cohort study. Lancet 2002;360:114–18.

61. Gordijn SJ, Erwich JJ, Khong TY. Value of the perinatal autopsy: a critique. Pediatr Dev Pathol 2002;5:480–8.

CHAPTER 15

Management of the Subsequent Pregnancy

George Saade, MD
Division of Maternal Fetal Medicine, Department of Obstetrics and Gynecology,
University of Texas Medical Branch, Galveston, TX, USA

As one of the most common adverse pregnancy outcomes, affecting nearly 1% of all births in the United States, it is not uncommon for a health care provider to encounter a pregnant woman with a previous stillbirth. Such a pregnancy is likely to be managed differently than a pregnancy in a woman who has never been pregnant or a woman who never had a complicated pregnancy. In addition to the heightened anxiety for the pregnant woman, as well as the provider, a number of management decisions are required, such as whether to perform any screening tests or workup. The latter will definitely rely on the causes of the prior stillbirth as well as the maternal medical condition, and these factors are covered in other chapters. However, the most critical decisions involve when and what fetal surveillance to perform, and timing of delivery. The anxiety to the provider is compounded by the lack of clear and high-level evidence to guide such a decision. This chapter will attempt to provide a practical approach based mostly on Level III and some Level II evidence.

Recurrence risk

The complexity and extent of any management plans for a pregnancy following a stillbirth depends on the likelihood of recurrence, which in turn depends on the etiology of the prior stillbirth, which in turn depend on the extent of the workup of the prior stillbirth. Few conditions clearly increase the recurrence risk of stillbirth, specific hereditary disorders and maternal conditions such as diabetes, chronic hypertension, and thrombophilia have a quoted recurrence rate of 0–8% [1–4]. Others have found a recurrence of stillbirth to be 2- to 10-fold increased in a subsequent pregnancy [5, 6]. Using the Missouri maternal linked cohort data from 1978 to 1997, of 400,000 women with first and second pregnancies, the risk of stillbirth was fivefold increased in women with a prior stillbirth (OR 4.7, 95%CI 3.3–6.6; occurring in 22.7/1,000 vs. 4.7/1,000). Furthermore, the recurrence rate was 2.6-fold higher for African-Americans compared to Caucasians (35.9/1,000 vs. 19.1/10,000) [7]. In sum, the recurrence risk is estimated to be 2- to 10-fold increased and depends in part on the etiology of the prior stillbirth, the presence of fetal growth restriction, the gestational age of the stillbirth, and race.

The risk of recurrence in cases of a genetic or structure abnormality is dependent on the specific abnormality, the mode of inheritance, and whether one or both parents are carriers. Workup of the parents and genetic counseling is therefore essential. Prenatal diagnosis, if available, would be useful in determining the presence of the abnormality in the current pregnancy, and in guiding management. In general, if the fetus in the current

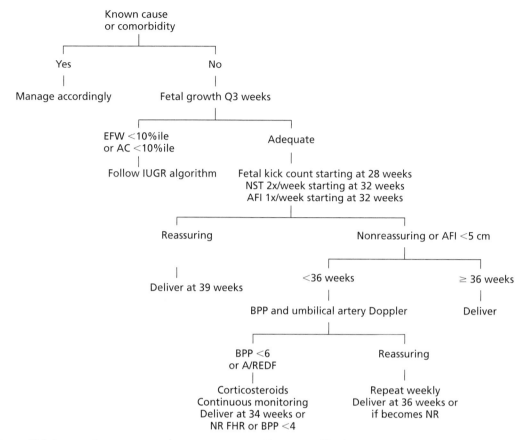

Figure 15.1 Suggested management of pregnant women with a prior stillbirth. Known cause refers to workup of prior stillbirth and include chromosomal and structural anomalies, or other causes such as trauma, infection, and cord accidents. Comorbidity includes maternal diabetes, hypertension, autoimmune diseases, and antiphospholipid syndrome. For management of these patients, refer to the text or other specific chapters. This is a suggested management and may need to be individualized to particular patients. EFW, estimated fetal weight; AC, abdominal circumference; IUGR; algorithm, intrauterine growth restriction algorithm (Figure 15.2); NST, nonstress test; AFI, amniotic fluid index; BPP, biophysical profile; A/REDF, absent/reverse end diastolic flow; NR FHR, nonreassuring fetal heart rate, such as category III or category II with repetitive decelerations; NR, nonreassuring such as BPP < 6 or absent/reverse diastolic flow in the umbilical artery.

pregnancy does not have the abnormality, and there were no other comorbid or contributing factors in the prior pregnancy, then the management of the current pregnancy should be the same as for any other patient.

In a typical practice in the United States, however, women presenting with a prior history of stillbirth are likely to either lack a workup or have an incomplete and uninformative workup. In the others, the workup is most likely to have been negative, and the stillbirth classified as

unexplained. For practical purposes, therefore, the following management is aimed at that category of women with a history of unexplained stillbirth.

Other adverse pregnancy outcomes

Importantly, clinicians caring for a woman who previously experienced a stillbirth should be aware that she is at higher risk for many adverse

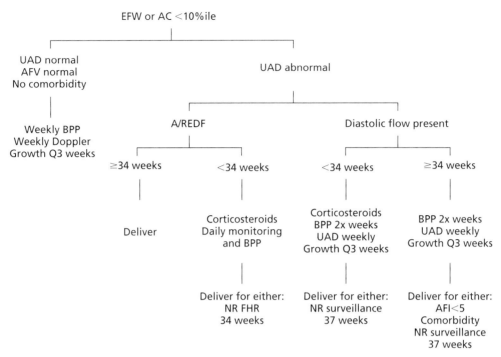

Figure 15.2 Suggested management for pregnant women with a prior stillbirth who are suspected to have fetal growth restriction when following management in Figure 15.1. This is a suggested management and may need to be individualized to particular patients. EFW, estimated fetal weight; AC, abdominal circumference; UAD, uterine artery Doppler; AFV, amniotic fluid volume; BPP, biophysical profile; A/REDF, absent/reverse end diastolic flow; BPP, biophysical profile; NR FHR, nonreassuring fetal heart rate, such as category III or category II with repetitive decelerations; NR surveillance, nonreassuring surveillance such as BPP < 6.

pregnancy outcomes beyond stillbirth alone. The earlier the loss, the higher the risk of an adverse outcome. In 95 women who experienced a fetal death between 13 and 24 weeks, in a subsequent pregnancy, 40% had preterm birth, 5% stillbirth, and 6% neonatal death [8]. Similarly, from a cross-sectional study of the Finnish birth registry, women with a prior stillbirth had increased risks of adverse pregnancy outcomes including placental abruption (5.4% vs. 0.7%), preterm delivery (13% vs. 5.2%), and low birthweight infants (12% vs. 3.6%) [9].

Management of specific conditions associated with stillbirth

For prior stillbirth associated with specific medical disorders, such as hypertension, diabetes, and autoimmune disease, the management includes treatment of these medical conditions. This chapter will not attempt to provide management guidelines for these specific disorders, and the reader should consult other sources. However, it is important to note that for specific medical disorders, such as diabetes and hypertension, aggressive treatment prior to conception and during early pregnancy may help to optimize pregnancy outcome.

The issue of inherited thrombophilia deserves particular mention. The association between thrombophilia and stillbirth remains controversial, with some studies showing an association [10–14] while others do not [15, 16]. Similar to what was noted by Facco et al. [17] for the reported association between thrombophilia and intrauterine growth restriction (IUGR), the association between thrombophilia and stillbirth appears to be mostly in case–control studies and largely because of publication bias, with those showing an association more likely to have been published earlier than those that failed to show an association. One exception to this is a recent longitudinal study which showed an association between factor V Leiden mutation and stillbirth. However, only six stillbirths occurred in that cohort [18]. Whether one believes that there is an association or not is immaterial for management since the more important issue is there is no evidence that screening and treatment of women with thrombophilia prevents stillbirth, or improves outcomes, outside the context of preventing thromboembolism in women with prior history or with major thrombophilia. The most recent ACOG Practice Bulletin does not recommend routine screening of women with history of stillbirth [19]. However, some patients may present already with a diagnosis of thrombophilia made on a prior workup. In these cases, the issue revolves mostly on prevention of thromboembolism. The ACOG recommendation is that in the absence of prior thromboembolism, women with low-risk thrombophilia (factor V Leiden heterozygous; prothrombin *G20210A* heterozygous; protein C or protein S deficiency) do not need any treatment, unless they have additional risk factor (first-degree relative with a history of a thrombotic episode before 50 years of age, or other major thrombotic risk factors such as obesity or prolonged immobility) in which case they may be candidate for postpartum anticoagulation (prophylactic low-molecular-weight heparin [LMWH]/unfractionated heparin [UFH] for 4–6 weeks or vitamin K antagonists for 4–6 weeks with a target international normalized ratio (INR) of 2.0–3.0, with initial UFH or LMWH therapy overlap until the INR is 2.0 or more for 2 days). In contrast, women with high-risk thrombophilia (antithrombin deficiency; double heterozygous for prothrombin *G20210A* mutation and factor V Leiden; factor V Leiden homozygous or prothrombin *G20210A* mutation homozygous) require prophylactic heparin antepartum and postpartum anticoagulation. A history of prior thromboembolism in any of these scenarios changes the management to a more aggressive approach (Table 15.1) [19].

In contrast, unexplained stillbirth is one of the obstetrical clinical criteria for antiphospholipid syndrome. ACOG recommends prophylactic doses of heparin and low-dose aspirin during pregnancy and the postpartum period (6–8 weeks) for women with antiphospholipid syndrome and no thrombotic history (Level C), and consideration should be given to serial ultrasonographic assessment. Antepartum testing should be considered after 32 weeks of gestation, or earlier if there are signs of growth restriction (Level C) [19].

Management of the subsequent pregnancy following an unexplained stillbirth

Management of a pregnancy in a women with a history of stillbirth ideally begins preconceptionally, when a detailed medical and obstetric history can be performed and a thorough evaluation of the prior pregnancy(ies). At this time, discussion should include the importance of smoking, alcohol and illicit drug cessation, and attaining a normal body mass index (BMI), if applicable, given their association with stillbirth. In addition, at this time, a discussion of the options of testing can be provided. In addition, using the information from the prior stillbirth, counseling of the recurrence risk is provided. Commonly women do not present for a preconception visit, and the first encounter is a prenatal care visit where the issues mentioned earlier can be addressed.

At the first prenatal visit, in addition, counseling should be provided regarding the risk of other obstetrical adverse outcomes such as preterm birth and fetal growth restriction. The option of obtaining serum markers in the first and second trimester, monitoring fetal growth closely, the use of fetal kick count monitoring, and antepartum testing may be discussed (Table 15.2).

Certain testing performed for other indications provides some insight of fetal and especially placental development and the potential for adverse pregnancy outcomes including stillbirth. From the first-trimester screening blood work, a low pregnancy-associated plasma protein A (PAPP-A)

Table 15.1 Recommended thromboprophylaxis for pregnancies complicated by inherited thrombophilias.*

Clinical scenario	Antepartum management	Postpartum management
Low-risk thrombophilia[†] without previous VTE	Surveillance without anticoagulation or prophylactic LMWH or UFH	Surveillance without anticoagulation or postpartum anticoagulation if the patient has additional risks factors[‡]
Low-risk thrombophilia[†] with a single previous episode of VTE—not receiving long-term anticoagulation	Prophylactic or intermediate-dose LMWH/UFH or surveillance without anticoagulation	Postpartum anticoagulation or intermediate-dose LMWH/UFH
High-risk thrombophilia[§] without previous VTE	Prophylactic LMWH or UFH	Postpartum anticoagulation
High-risk thrombophilia[§] with a single previous episode of VTE—not receiving long-term anticoagulation	Prophylactic, intermediate-dose, or adjusted-dose LMWH/UFH regimen	Postpartum anticoagulation or intermediate- or adjusted-dose LMWH/UFH for 6 weeks (therapy level should be at least as high as antepartum treatment)
No thrombophilia with previous single episode of VTE associated with transient risk factor that is no longer present—excludes pregnancy- or estrogen-related risk factor	Surveillance without anticoagulation	Postpartum anticoagulation
No thrombophilia with previous single episode of VTE associated with transient risk factor that was pregnancy or estrogen related	Surveillance without anticoagulation or prophylactic or intermediate-dose LMWH/UFH	Postpartum anticoagulation or intermediate-dose LMWH/UFH
No thrombophilia with previous single episode of VTE without an associated risk factor (idiopathic)—not receiving long-term anticoagulation	Prophylactic LMWH/UFH or intermediate-dose LMWH/UFH or surveillance without anticoagulation	Postpartum anticoagulation or intermediate-dose LMWH/UFH
Thrombophilia or no thrombophilia with two or more episodes of VTE—not receiving long-term anticoagulation	Prophylactic, intermediate-dose, or adjusted-dose LMWH or prophylactic, intermediate-close or adjusted-dose UFH	Postpartum anticoagulation or intermediate- or adjusted-dose LMWH/UFH for 6 weeks
Thrombophilia or no thrombophilia with two or more episodes of VTE—receiving long-term anticoagulation	Adjusted-dose LMWH/UFH	Resumption of long-term anticoagulation

LMWH, low-molecular-weight heparin; UFH, unfractionated heparin; VTE, venous thromboembolism.
*Postpartum treatment levels should be greater or equal to antepartum treatment. Treatment of acute VTE and management of antiphospholipid syndrome are addressed in other Practice Bulletins.
[†]Low-risk thrombophilia: factor V Leiden heterozygous; prothrombin *G20210A* heterozygous; protein C or protein S deficiency.
[‡]First-degree relative with a history of a thrombotic episode before 50 years of age, or other major thrombotic risk factors (e.g., obesity, prolonged immobility).
[§]High-risk thrombophilia: antithrombin deficiency; double heterozygous for prothrombin *G20210A* mutation and factor V Leiden; factor V Leiden homozygous or prothrombin *G20210A* mutation homozygous.

Table 15.2 Management of the subsequent pregnancy.

- First-trimester sonogram for accurate dating, given the risk of fetal growth restriction
- First-trimester serum screening, especially PAPP-A
- Early gestational diabetes screen, with rescreen at 24–28 weeks if negative
- Second-trimester maternal serum screening, especially MSAFP
- Fetal anatomic survey at 18–22 weeks
- Close monitoring of fetal growth
  - Clinical
  - Serial ultrasounds
- Maternal assessment of fetal movement (fetal kick counts) ~28 weeks
- Antepartum fetal surveillance

Table 15.3 Strategy for the detection and diagnosis of hyperglycemic disorders in pregnancy.

First prenatal visit
Measure FPG, AIC, or RPG on all or only high-risk women*
    If results indicate overt diabetes, treatment and follow-up as for preexisting diabetes
    If results not diagnostic of overt diabetes and FPG are 92–126 mg/dl (5.1–7.0 mmol/l), diagnose as GDM
    If results not diagnostic of overt diabetes and FPG are <92 mg/dl (5.1 mmol/l), test for GDM from 24 to 28 weeks
      with a 75 g OGTT[†]

24–28 weeks gestation
Two-hour 75 g OGTT, performed after an overnight fast, on all women not previously found to have overt diabetes or
GDM during testing earlier in this pregnancy:
    Overt diabetes if FPG ⩾ 126 mg/dl (7.0 mmol/l)
    GDM if one or more values equals or exceeds thresholds indicated in Table 15.1
    Normal if all values on OGTT less than thresholds indicated in Table 15.1

Postpartum glucose testing
Should be performed for all women diagnosed with overt diabetes during pregnancy or GDM

Note: To be applied to women without known diabetes antedating pregnancy.
*Decision to perform blood testing for evaluation of glycemia on all pregnant women or only on women with
characteristics indicating a high risk for diabetes is to be made on the basis of the background frequency of
abnormal glucose metabolism in the population and on local circumstances.
[†]There have been insufficient studies performed to know whether there is a benefit of generalized testing to
diagnose and treat GDM before the usual window of 24–28 weeks gestation.

defined as less that the fifth centile at 10 weeks significantly increased the risk of stillbirth. From the FASTER trial, in women with this low PAPP-A, the risk of stillbirth after 24 weeks had an odds ratio of 2.15 (1.11–4.15) [20]; other reported a greater than 40-fold risk of stillbirth due to placental dysfunction (abruption, fetal growth restriction) in these women [21]. Using second-trimester screening, an unexplained elevated maternal serum alpha fetoprotein (MSAFP)—a long known marker for placental dysfunction—is associated with an increased risk of stillbirth [22–24]. The combination of low PAPP-A with high MSAFP was synergistic in increasing the risk of stillbirth (OR 36.7, 95% CI 8.0–167) [25].

The odds of being diagnosed with diabetes in the next pregnancy after an unexplained stillbirth are approximately 4 times that for other women [26]. Testing for diabetes should not wait until the third trimester, and consideration should be given to using The International Association of Diabetes and Pregnancy Study Groups (IADPSG) recommendations for diagnosis of hyperglycemic disorders in pregnancy (Table 15.3) [27]. The first step in these recommendations is the detection of overt diabetes in women not previously diagnosed outside pregnancy. While women with prior stillbirth were not specifically addressed, these recommendations seem to be applicable to these patients if diabetes was not excluded in their prior pregnancy. It should be noted that screening after the diagnosis of stillbirth cannot exclude diabetes as an etiology.

Sonograms for accurate dating, anatomic survey, and monitoring of fetal growth are recommended. Accurate establishment of gestational age is one of the most important management steps in women with previous stillbirth since the diagnosis of growth restriction and the timing of initiation of fetal testing and delivery depend on gestational age. Ultrasound to follow up growth is also indicated since uteroplacental insufficiency and fetal growth restriction may be the common pathway for a large proportion of stillbirth [28]. A customized approach to evaluation of fetal growth restriction appears to be better than a population-based approach [29]. Pregnancies complicated with fetal growth restriction should receive more frequent fetal assessment. Assessment of placental and fetal status with Doppler is generally indicated for these pregnancies. While not focusing on women with prior stillbirth, a Cochrane review concluded that Doppler assessment decreases perinatal mortality and results in less obstetric interventions when used in pregnancy at high-risk for adverse outcomes, most of whom were patient with fetal growth restriction [30]. This benefit was not present when the review included studies in low risk or unselected populations [31].

The major issue to consider in a patient who had a prior stillbirth revolves around fetal surveillance, such as which test to use and the frequency of testing. A number of antepartum fetal surveillance tests are available, including fetal movement counting, nonstress testing, and biophysical profile. Which approach to use will depend on the particular practice setup. There are no trials which compared fetal movement counting with no counting overall, let alone in women with prior stillbirth. While there is no evidence that fetal movement counting lowers perinatal mortality, women with prior history of stillbirth are commonly asked to monitor fetal movement daily. The method of fetal movement assessment should be the one that is the most practical for the patient and health care provider. The "count to 10" or "Cardiff" method seems to have the highest acceptance and compliance rates [32]. The patient may choose a specific time during the day, preferably a quiet time at night, and determine how long it takes for the fetus moves 10 times. The time to 10 movements increases progressively after 32 weeks, but should be less than 40 min in more than 90% of patients [33]. If 2 h pass, then further evaluation would be needed.

While not specifically targeting women with prior stillbirth, a Cochrane review concluded that there was no advantage of biophysical profile over conventional fetal monitoring (cardiotocography [CTG] and amniotic fluid assessment) in improving perinatal outcome. However, when the high-quality trials were analyzed, women managed with biophysical profile were more likely to undergo induction of labor and be delivered by cesarean section [34]. Antepartum surveillance is indicated even in the absence of fetal growth restriction. As demonst rated in the study by Weeks et al. [3], 6% of women had abnormal antepartum tests and there was no relationship to the gestational age of the prior stillbirth. The American College of Obstetricians and Gynecologists recommends antepartum testing should begin at 32 weeks or later [35]; other protocols include twice weekly non-stress test (NST)/amniotic fluid index (AFI) (the modified biophysical profile [BPP]) initiated at 32 weeks or 1–2 weeks before the gestational age of the previous stillbirth. Given the concern that the woman may have more anxiety at the gestational age of the prior stillbirth, antepartum testing may be started earlier if needed.

The timing of delivery in these pregnancies remains controversial. In pregnancies with normal fetal growth, reassuring fetal surveillance, and no comorbid conditions, expectant management is acceptable. However, due to maternal anxiety, expectant management after 39 weeks may not be practical. Loosing a baby after 39 weeks when an elective delivery would have resulted in a live neonate with outcome equivalent to one delivered later is untenable [36]. Some advocate for elective induction at 39 weeks of gestation or with pulmonary maturity if earlier delivery is desired. Studies using hazard ratio analysis show that the overall risk of stillbirth per ongoing pregnancy nadirs at 39 weeks [37]. A sizeable number of stillbirths can be prevented if women, regardless of prior pregnancy outcome, are electively delivered by 39 weeks [38, 39]. This would certainly apply to women with prior stillbirth.

The management of the pregnant patient with a prior stillbirth is hampered by our limited ability to predict the outcome in the current pregnancy, or the limited benefit of surveillance and intervention to prevent stillbirth. Ideally, we would provide the patient with a prior history of stillbirth with her individualized risk of stillbirth or adverse pregnancy outcome in a subsequent pregnancy based on all the available information from the stillbirth workup as well as evaluation of risk factors. However, such an approach is not currently possible. Risk scoring systems that have been developed, including those that were not specifically developed for patients with a history of stillbirth, have poor predictive value outside the population in which they were developed. As for the various surveillance methods and interventions, there is limited evidence that they actually prevent stillbirth in the next pregnancy without increasing morbidity from unnecessary interventions. Assigning a risk score, performing a screening test, or assessing the fetus does not prevent stillbirth unless it is coupled with an effective intervention. Currently, the only intervention to prevent stillbirth is delivery. However, unnecessary delivery may increase maternal and neonatal morbidity and mortality. When risk scores with better predictive abilities are developed, maybe then interventions such as delivery at 37–39 weeks can be focused at those women at high risk of adverse outcome.

References

1. Freeman RK, Dorchester W, Anderson G, et al. The significance of a previous stillbirth. Am J Obstet Gynecol 1985;151:7–13.

2. Samueloff A, Xenakis EM, Berkus MD, et al. Recurrent stillbirth. Significance and characteristics. J Reprod Med 1993;38:883–6.

3. Weeks JW, Asrat T, Morgan MA, et al. Antepartum surveillance for a history of stillbirth: when to begin? Am J Obstet Gynecol 1995;172:486–92.

4. Surkan PJ, Stephansson O, Dickman PW, et al. Previous preterm and small-for-gestational-age births and the subsequent risk of stillbirth. N Engl J Med 2004;350:777–85.

5. Greenwood R, Samms-Vaughan M, Golding J, Ashley D. Past obstetric history and risk of perinatal death in Jamaica. Paediatr Perinat Epidemiol 1994;8(Suppl. 1): 40–53.

6. Greenwood R, Golding J, McCaw-Binns A, et al. The epidemiology of perinatal death in Jamaica. Paediatr Perinat Epidemiol 1994;8(Suppl. 1):143–57.

7. Sharma PP, Salihu HM, Oyelese Y, et al. Is race a determinant of stillbirth recurrence? Obstet Gynecol 2006;107:391–7.

8. Goldenberg RL, Mayberry SK, Copper RL, et al. Pregnancy outcome following a second-trimester loss. Obstet Gynecol 1993;81:444–6.

9. Heinonen S, Kirkinen P. Pregnancy outcome after previous stillbirth resulting from causes other than maternal conditions and fetal abnormalities. Birth 2000;27:33–7.

10. Rey E, Kahn SR, David M, Shrier I. Thrombophilic disorders and fetal loss: a meta-analysis. Lancet 2003; 361:901–8.

11. Dudding TE, Attia J. The association between adverse pregnancy outcomes and maternal factor V Leiden genotype: a meta-analysis. Thromb Haemost 2004;91:700–11.

12. Nelen WL, Blom HJ, Steegers EA, et al. Hyperhomocysteinemia and recurrent early pregnancy loss: a meta-analysis. Fertil Steril 2000;74: 1196–9.

13. Lissalde-Lavigne G, Fabbro-Peray P, Cochery-Nouvellon E, et al. Factor V Leiden and prothrombin G20210A polymorphisms as risk factors for miscarriage during a first intended pregnancy: the matched case-control 'NOHA first' study. J Thromb Haemost 2005;3:2178–84.

14. Preston FE, Rosendaal FR, Walker ID, et al. Increased fetal loss in women with heritable thrombophilia. Lancet 1996;348:913–16.

15. Dizon-Townson D, Miller C, Sibai B, et al. The relationship of the factor V Leiden mutation and pregnancy outcomes for mother and fetus. National Institute of Child Health and Human Development

Maternal-Fetal Medicine Units Network. Obstet Gynecol 2005;106:517–24.

16. Silver RM, Zhao Y, Spong CY, et al. Prothrombin gene G20210A mutation and obstetric complications. Eunice Kennedy Shriver National Institute of Child Health and Human Development Maternal-Fetal Medicine Units (NICHD MFMU) Network. Obstet Gynecol 2010;115:14–20.

17. Facco F, You W, Grobman W. Genetic thrombophilias and intrauterine growth restriction—a meta-analysis. Obstet Gynecol 2009;113:1206–16.

18. Said JM, Higgins JR, Moses EK, et al. Inherited thrombophilia polymorphisms and pregnancy outcomes in nulliparous women. Obstet Gynecol 2010;115:5–13.

19. Antiphospholipid syndrome. ACOG Practice Bulletin No. 68. Washington, DC: ACOG; 2005.

20. Dugoff L, Hobbins JC, Malone FD, et al. First-trimester maternal serum PAPP-A and free-beta subunit human chorionic gonadotropin concentrations and nuchal translucency are associated with obstetric complications: a population-based screening study (the FASTER Trial). Am J Obstet Gynecol 2004; 191:1446–51.

21. Smith GC, Crossley JA, Aitken DA, et al. First-trimester placentation and the risk of antepartum stillbirth. JAMA 2004;292:2249–54.

22. Waller DK, Lustig LS, Smith AH, et al. Alpha-fetoprotein: a biomarker for pregnancy outcome. Epidemiology 1993;4:471–6.

23. Wenstrom KD, Owen J, Davis RO, Brumfield CG. Prognostic significance of unexplained elevated amniotic fluid alpha-fetoprotein. Obstet Gynecol 1996;87:213–16.

24. Spencer K. Second-trimester prenatal screening for Down syndrome and the relationship of maternal serum biochemical markers to pregnancy complications with adverse outcome. Prenat Diagn 2000;20: 652–6.

25. Smith GC, Shah I, Crossley JA, et al. Pregnancy-associated plasma protein A and alpha-fetoprotein and prediction of adverse perinatal outcome. Obstet Gynecol 2006;107:161–6.

26. Robson S, Chan A, Keane RJ, Luke CG. Subsequent birth outcomes after an unexplained stillbirth: preliminary population-based retrospective cohort study. Aust N Z J Obstet Gynaecol 2001;41:29–34.

27. International Association of Diabetes and Pregnancy Study Groups. International association of diabetes and pregnancy study groups recommendations on the diagnosis and classification of hyperglycemia in pregnancy. Diabetes Care 2010;33:676–82.

28. Gardosi J, Mul T, Mongelli M, Fagan D. Analysis of birthweight and gestational age in antepartum stillbirths. Br J Obstet Gynaecol 1998;105:524–30.

29. Gardosi J, Francis A. Adverse pregnancy outcome and association with small for gestational age birthweight by customized and population-based percentiles. Am J Obstet Gynecol 2009;201:28.e1–8.

30. Alfirevic Z, Stampalija T, Gyte GML. Fetal and umbilical Doppler ultrasound in high-risk pregnancies. Cochrane Database Syst Rev 2010;1:CD007529; DOI: 10.1002/14651858.CD007529.pub2.

31. Alfirevic Z, Stampalija T, Gyte GML. Fetal and umbilical Doppler ultrasound in normal pregnancy. Cochrane Database Syst Rev 2010;8:CD001450; DOI: 10.1002/14651858.CD001450.pub3.

32. Mangesi L, Hofmeyr GJ. Fetal movement counting for assessment of fetal wellbeing. Cochrane Database Syst Rev 2007;1:CD004909; DOI: 10.1002/14651858. CD004909.pub2.

33. Kuwata T, Matsubara S, Ohkusa T, et al. Establishing a reference value for the frequency of fetal movements using modified 'count to 10' method. J Obstet Gynaecol Res 2008;34(3):318–23.

34. Lalor JG, Fawole B, Alfirevic Z, Devane D. Biophysical profile for fetal assessment in high risk pregnancies. Cochrane Database Syst Rev 2008;1:CD000038; DOI: 10.1002/14651858.CD000038.pub2.

35. ACOG practice bulletin. Antepartum fetal surveillance No. 9. Washington, DC: ACOG; 1999.

36. Tita AT, Landon MB, Spong CY, et al.; Eunice Kennedy Shriver NICHD Maternal-Fetal Medicine Units Network. Timing of elective repeat cesarean delivery at term and neonatal outcomes. N Engl J Med 2009;360:111–20.

37. Smith GC. Life-table analysis of the risk of perinatal death at term and post term in singleton pregnancies. Am J Obstet Gynecol 2001;184:489–96.

38. Hankins GD, Clark SM, Munn MB. Cesarean section on request at 39 weeks: impact on shoulder dystocia, fetal trauma, neonatal encephalopathy, and intrauterine fetal demise. Semin Perinatol 2006;30:276–87.

39. Landon MB, Hauth JC, Leveno KJ, et al.; National Institute of Child Health and Human Development Maternal-Fetal Medicine Units Network. Maternal and perinatal outcomes associated with a trial of labor after prior cesarean delivery. N Engl J Med 2004;351:2581–9.

Multidimensional Integrative Stillbirth Systems Model

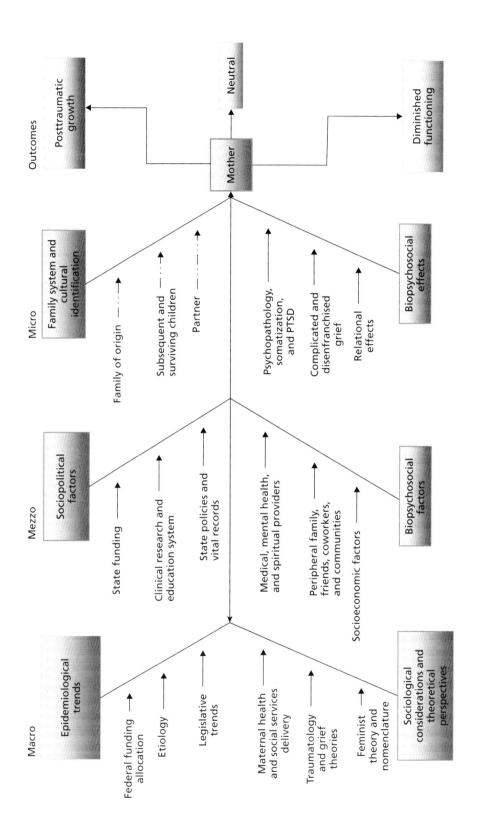

Index

Note: Page numbers followed by "*f*," "*t*," and "*b*" refer to figures, tables, and boxes, respectively.